The
GENEALOGY
of PLANT
FOODS

"A veritable who's who of the plants we eat, this book shares the backstories of foods I thought I knew well. Turns out we were only marginally acquainted. Everything I didn't know is here: the history, evolution, culinary landscape, and nutritional bounty of the amazing seeds, roots, flowers, and fruits that have nourished life on Earth from its beginnings."

VICTORIA MORAN, AUTHOR OF
MAIN STREET VEGAN AND *AGE LIKE A YOGI*

"A deeply fascinating book that explores the origins of our food and serves as a valuable reference on the medicinal properties and preparation methods of each food it describes. It beautifully illustrates how people across the world are interconnected through the foods we share as a global humanity. A delightful enrichment of my library."

WOUTER BIJDENDIJK, AUTHOR OF *PLANT POWER*

The
GENEALOGY
of PLANT
FOODS

The Spiritual, Nutritional,
and Medicinal Power
of the Foods That Sustain Us

NATHANIEL ALTMAN

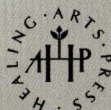

Healing Arts Press
Rochester, Vermont

Healing Arts Press
One Park Street
Rochester, Vermont 05767
www.HealingArtsPress.com

Healing Arts Press is a division of Inner Traditions International

Note to the reader: *This book is intended to be an informational guide. The remedies, approaches, and techniques described herein are meant to supplement, and not to be a substitute for, professional medical care or treatment. They should not be used to treat a serious ailment without prior consultation with a qualified health care professional.*

Cataloging-in-Publication Data for this title is available from the Library of Congress

ISBN 979-8-88850-309-6 (print)
ISBN 979-8-88850-310-2 (ebook)

Printed and bound in India at Replika Press Pvt. Ltd.

10 9 8 7 6 5 4 3 2 1

Text design and layout by Kenleigh Manseau
This book was typeset in Garamond Premier Pro with Krete and Hoefler Text used as display typefaces.
Photographs by Nathaniel Altman. Where not otherwise stated, photographs are in the public domain or creative commons via Wikimedia.

To send correspondence to the author of this book, mail a first-class letter to the author c/o Inner Traditions, One Park Street, Rochester, VT 05767, and we will forward the communication, or contact the author directly at **nathanielaltman.com**.

Scan the QR code and save 25% at InnerTraditions.com. Browse over 2,000 titles on spirituality, the occult, ancient mysteries, new science, holistic health, and natural medicine.

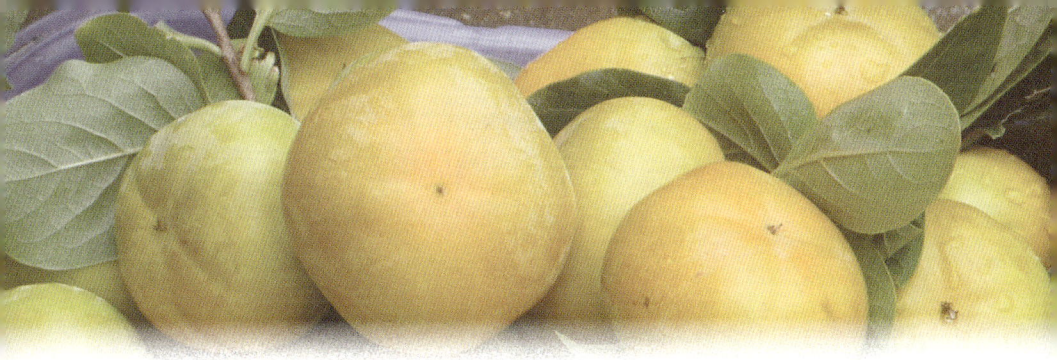

Contents

Fruits

Vegetables

Herbs and Spices

Grains

Pulses

Nuts and Seeds

Other Foods

⇥⇤

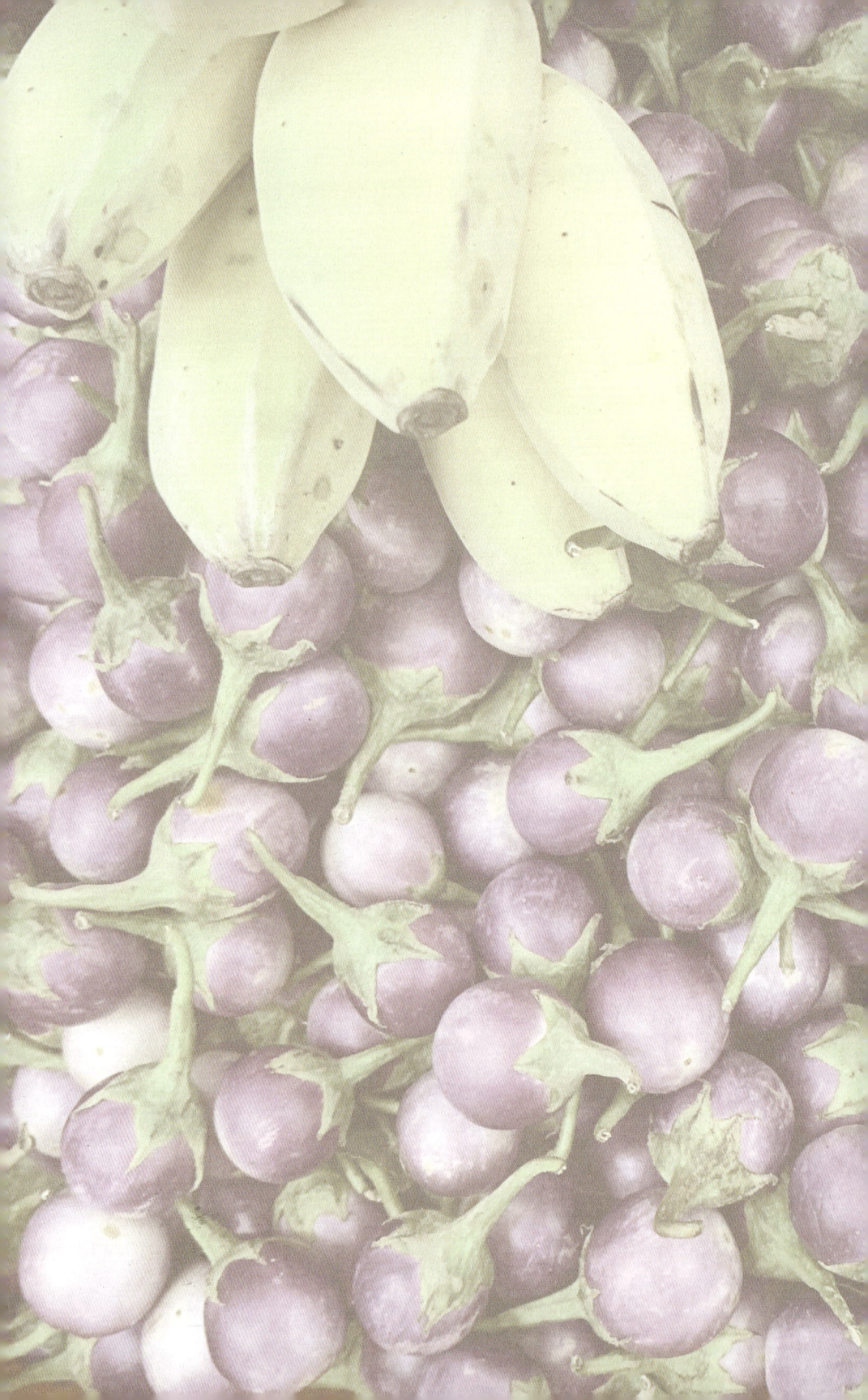

Introduction

Tracing a New Genealogy

People are fascinated by food. In addition to nourishing our bodies, food has played a major role in our cultural traditions, spiritual practices, literature, poetry, and art for thousands of years. Literally hundreds of cookbooks are published every year in the United States alone, and magazines, newspapers, TV programs, and internet blogs and vlogs focus on how to prepare and enjoy the vast variety of foods available to us from supermarkets, farmers markets, and backyard gardens. There has even been an increase in "food tourism," where people travel primarily to experience both new and familiar types of cuisine. We are currently experiencing a resurgence in healthy eating, with more and more consumers demanding foods that are both delicious and good for their health.

Despite the central role food plays in our lives, most people take the food we eat for granted. Many do not realize that every food we eat becomes part of the cells of our bodies. When we eat an apple, for example, the vitamins, minerals, fiber, and a wealth of *phytochemicals*—chemical compounds found in plant foods—are digested by our bodies, eventually becoming part of our body's cells and playing a vital role not only in our survival but our good health as well. In fact, every plant food has been recognized throughout history as having medicinal value; recent science has not only validated many traditional beliefs, but is also exploring ways food can be used to both prevent and even treat a wide range of diseases including diabetes, heart problems, Alzheimer's disease, and cancer. It should come as no surprise that many Indigenous communities around the world have recognized the vital connection between humans and food for millennia, and consider sitting down for a meal as a sacred act, a time for gratitude and respect.

Few understand the complex processes involved with bringing our food to the dining room table, from preparing the soil, planting and caring for the seeds, growing healthy plants, harvesting, packing, transportation, and finally the mechanics involved in selling foods at supermarkets, greengrocers, farm stands, and farmers markets. Unlike people living in parts of the world where nutritious food is often scarce, many who live in rich countries like the United States take food for granted. One result of this is that approximately 40 percent of the food we buy winds up in the garbage, uneaten.

Why This Book?

Like many others who are interested in genealogy, I devoted several years to investigating my family's history. Although early family records have been impossible to locate, the information I was able to find about my ancestors was both fascinating and life-changing. By knowing about my family's roots, I gained new insights into my own life's path and gained tremendous respect for my ancestors, the difficulties they faced in Eastern Europe, and the sacrifices they made to establish new lives here in the United States. I owe my life to them, and am grateful.

As an author of several books about food and nutrition, I have always been interested in the origins of food, and during an extended period of self-isolation during the recent COVID-19 pandemic, I decided to learn more. To my surprise, I soon discovered that the vast majority of foods consumed in North America originally came from other parts of the world, just like most of our human ancestors. And

I found that many of these "new immigrants" faced problems similar to those of our immigrant ancestors. For example, foods like tomatoes, eggplants, and potatoes were initially shunned due to the belief that they were poisonous, as they belong to a family of plants called nightshade, which includes the plant belladonna, also known as "deadly nightshade." Eggplant was only accepted after Thomas Jefferson—who played a key role in American agriculture—served it to guests at the White House.

Like most people, I had no idea where most of our foods originally came from, and how they arrived to our shores. For example, most people assume chili peppers originated in Mexico, India, or Thailand, where they are an essential part of these national cuisines. Yet, recent anthropological and genomic research shows that chili peppers are actually indigenous to the Amazon Basin, and that their seeds spread north to Mexico—primarily by birds. The birds' taste buds did not register the heat of the peppers, so they had no trouble eating them. And because their digestive systems could not digest the seeds, they were excreted as the birds migrated north, eventually taking root and growing into plants.

Human migration also helped to spread chili peppers. Cultivation of chili peppers began in Mexico, and Spanish explorers introduced them to Spain in the sixteenth century. From there, they were introduced to Africa, Europe, and Asia by traders along the famous Silk Road, and became staple crops in India, Thailand, and China.

While writing this book, I gained new and profound insight into the early beginnings of the foods we eat and about the long, complex, and often difficult journeys they made to new lands. When I eat a simple carrot, for example, I am now aware that its roots began in Türkiye and the Middle East, and that it was introduced to Europe—probably by Arab traders—over ten centuries ago. Carrots eventually made their way to the New World during the 1600s, when immigrants brought carrot seeds with them from Europe and planted them in their gardens.

Over the next several hundred years, carrots became a major commercial crop in North America. I can now buy carrots at any greengrocer or supermarket; I can eat them raw, drink them as juice, or prepare them in a wide variety of soups, casseroles, and stir-fries. I now appreciate even more this food that nourishes and protects me (especially my eyesight). I will never take a carrot for granted again!

By getting to know the origins, history, and benefits we obtain from the foods we eat, I believe we will appreciate them more and not take them for granted. In addition, a deeper knowledge of foods and their culinary, nutritional, and health–related benefits can lead to making better choices for ourselves and our loved ones.

Although there is a lot of diverse information available about individual foods on blogs, food industry websites, and magazine articles, clear and simple information about the origins and histories of the plant foods we eat cannot been found in a single, easy to read, documented volume. Surprisingly, the last major work on the subject was *The Origin of Cultivated Plants* by French–Swiss botanist Alphonse de Candolle, originally published in 1883 and first translated to English in 1886.

In addition to anecdotal information about various foods, much new information about the history, nutritional value, and medicinal value of many of the foods we eat has only recently become available in often-obscure, peer-reviewed scientific, medical, and agricultural journals. This information is based on "new science," including genomic research, DNA studies, and laboratory and clinical evidence. So, I decided to put all this information together in one comprehensive, documented, and reader-friendly volume.

The Need

At a time when life expectancy in the United States has declined and diet-related disease has become a leading cause of premature death, Americans need to make more conscious food choices, and eat more of the hundreds of healthy, nutritious, and delicious foods that are available to us. Yet, rather than tell people what they should eat, I aim to present information in a lively, historical, and anecdotal context to appeal to my readers' innate curiosity. As a result, each section of this book is designed to offer clear and concise information about our favorite plant foods—more than one hundred of them. Each section will briefly describe each food, explore its origin(s) and how it arrived in different countries (with particular focus on the United States), how it is used, its nutritional and medicinal highlights, and where is it primarily grown today.

Each section is based on documented scientific and nutritional sources including medical journals and peer-reviewed scientific studies. This information will reacquaint readers with foods they may have known and loved since childhood, and also introduce them to new foods they may have never tasted before.

One of the major objectives of this book is to highlight the medicinal value of each food at a time when diet-related diseases compete with smoking as a leading cause of death. Although the idea of food as medicine dates back thousands of years to Hippocrates, the results of a new study published in the September 2023 issue of the medical journal *Circulation*, involving research on nearly four thousand people, showed conclusively that a diet rich in plant foods helps improve health by reducing glucose levels, blood pressure, "bad" cholesterol, and body weight.

There is another current that underlies the importance of this book. During a time when people are dividing themselves from others along religious, racial, political, and national lines, food can be a great unifier. On one hand, many of the foods humans eat and love came from other countries: potatoes from Peru; avocados, corn, and beans from Mexico; peaches and oranges from China; apples from Kazakhstan–Kyrgyzstan; and blueberries, squash, and strawberries from the United States.

Despite our many differences and disagreements, the love of certain foods is something we deeply share—both Muslims and Jews are crazy about hummus, which is made with chickpeas and olive oil native to the Middle East, where both religions were born. Coffee—indigenous to Saudi Arabia and Ethiopia—is prized by coffee lovers of every political and religious persuasion throughout the world. Borsht—a delicious soup made from beets (which originated by the Mediterranean Sea)—is loved by Ukrainians and Russians alike. If we want to learn about people from other countries and their traditions, we need to just sit down and enjoy their food!

Humans partake in one of nature's most powerful and intimate acts—that of ingesting foods that not only nourish us and keep us alive and healthy, but actually become part of our bodies. This shared experience transcends our differences, and certifies that—above all—we share common needs, hopes, and actions as members of one big human family.

The focus of *The Genealogy of Foods* is on foods of plant origin. Although the origins of the wide variety of meat, fish, dairy products, and eggs are both fascinating and of historical importance, they deserve a separate book (or books) of their own. In addition, most of the animals we eat—as well as those that provide dairy products and eggs—obtain their sustenance from some of the grains (along with soybeans) that we will cover in the text.

How to Use this Book

The Genealogy of Food has been designed to be as user-friendly and enjoyable to read as possible. The foods in each chapter are arranged according to how each plant is normally consumed, whether we harvest its fruit, vegetable, grain, or seed or nut, and so on. Individual sections begin with a brief description of a food, along with its botanical name. A brief "genealogy" of the food then follows, often revealing little-known historical facts and anecdotes that will inspire and surprise.

Each section goes on to explore the traditional culinary uses of each food, with tips on how it can be used in the kitchen today. You will also find essential nutritional information, along with a brief review of health and medicinal benefits each food provides, as revealed by the latest scientific and clinical studies. Many of these benefits are due to the chemicals found in these plant foods, known as phytochemicals. Although the therapeutic values of many foods have been known for centuries, the discovery of phytochemicals—thanks to recent advances in biological and chemical research—reveals how and why this occurs. Most sections conclude with information about where the food is primarily grown, both domestically and abroad.

References located at the end of each plant section feature information about the websites, books, and scientific journals that provided the information about the plant. Many of these resources can be accessed online. If you wish to learn more about the foods described in this book, as well as about specific phytochemicals and how they can improve health, you are encouraged to study further.

Nathaniel Altman
Brooklyn, New York

Botany 101
Taxonomy and Cultivation

Botanical Names

Most of the plant names included in this book have been classified by a two-tiered naming system known in scientific circles as binomial nomenclature. This system, which was developed by the Swedish biologist Carl Linnaeus in 1735 includes all living things, using Latin names to classify them. In botany, the first name identifies the *genus* of the plant, and is always capitalized. In the plant world, the genus ranks below "family" and above "species." The second part of the name, which is also known as the *specific name* or *specific epithet*, refers to the species of the plant within the genus. For example, the botanical name for the pear is *Pyrus communis*. "*Pyrus*" is the name of the genus, while "*communis*" is the individual species.

The botanical name of the tomato is *Solanum lycopersicum*. *Solanum* is a genus within the nightshade family, known in Latin as Solanaceae. This genus contains many species of flowering plants, including potatoes and eggplants. The potato is identified as *Solanum tuberosum*, while the botanical name of the eggplant is *Solanum melongen*. Other well-known members of the Solanaceae family of plants are bell peppers and some species of chili peppers—but they belong to the *Capsicum* genus, and are identified as *Capsicum annuum*.

Hybrids

The vast majority of the plant foods included in this book are the result of hybridization, a process that involves the breeding of two "parent plants" with different types of genes. Hybridization can occur naturally among some species, or can take place through human engineering.

In simple terms, a hybrid is the offspring of a cross between parents from two different species or subspecies. As we'll explore later on, a hybrid cross between a pomelo tree and a sweet orange tree produced the grapefruit tree. Hybridization can also increase the genetic variability within a single plant species, which is seen by botanists as vital for the survival of the fittest and a boon to natural selection. The goal of agricultural hybridization is to develop offspring that are superior to the parental types, selecting for desirable traits such as more flavor, longer storage life, or better appearance, and getting rid of traits that are deemed undesirable, such as an abundance of seeds or susceptibility to certain insect pests. Sweet orange varieties, for example, are said to be the result of a cross between a non-pure mandarin orange and a hybrid pomelo that had a substantial mandarin component.

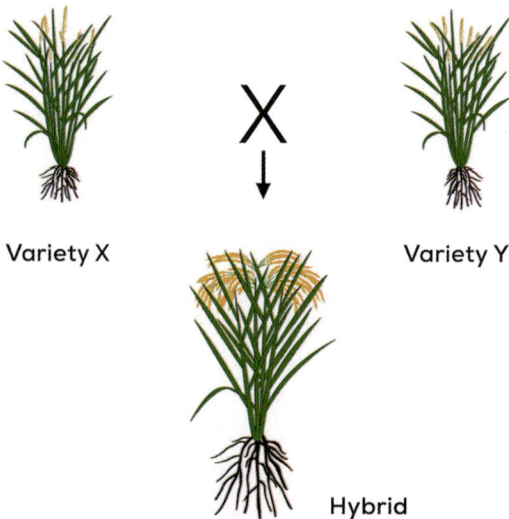

Variety X X↓ Variety Y

Hybrid

The hybridization of rice.
After a diagram from the International Rice Research Institute, 2006.

Hybridization can occur naturally (as in the case of grapefruit) due to cross-pollination by insects or animals. It can also be purposely engineered by farmers or plant scientists. The famous Bing cherry is a cross between maternal parent cultivar Black Republican and paternal cultivar Royal Ann (also known as Napoleon) cherries by Oregon farmers in 1875, while some of the latest apple, orange, and tomato hybrids have been carefully engineered in laboratories by plant scientists, to produce new varieties of each plant. The celebrated Fuji apple is one such hybrid. It was developed at the Tōhoku Research Station of the Ministry of Agriculture and Forestry in Japan, from the Red Delicious and the Virginia Ralls Janet apple cultivars in the late 1930s.

The hybridization of plants has taken place over thousands, even millions, of years, and is responsible for the amazing variety of the plant foods we consume today. For example, there are now more than ten thousand tomato varieties available that came about due to hybridization.

Some plant varieties came into being as a natural result of mutation. The popular navel orange, for example, is believed to be a mutation that took place between 1810 and 1820 in a Selecta orange tree that was planted on the grounds of a monastery in Bahia, Brazil.

A Note about Grafting

Grafting is another way to propagate plants. Grafting occurs when tissues of plants are joined so as to continue their growth together, as one plant. The two major parts of a graft are the *stock*, or *rootstock*, which is selected for its roots, and the *scion*, a part of another plant that is selected perhaps for its stems, leaves, flowers, or fruits. The scion contains the genes desired to be duplicated by the grafted plant. For successful grafting to occur, what is called the "vascular cambium tissues" of the stock and scion plants must be placed in contact with each other until the living graft has "taken," a process that usually involves a period several weeks.

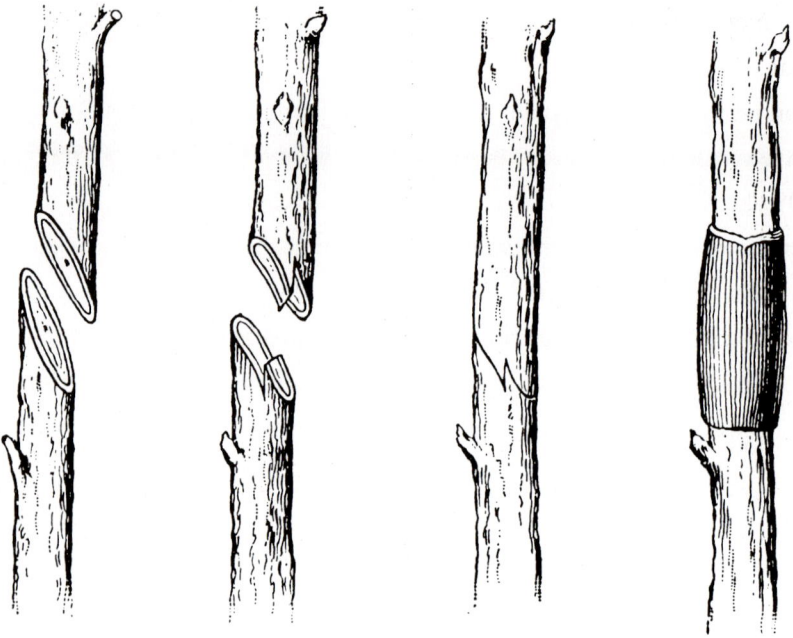

The "splice" grafting of plants.
Horace H. Cummings, Nature Study by Grades
(New York: America Book Company, 1909).

Grafting is an ancient horticultural practice that goes back thousands of years to both Mesopotamia and China. It has been used in the propagation of many fruit-producing plants, such as grape vines and trees like apple, avocado, orange, grape, peach, pear, and various nuts.

The development of new plant hybrids, whether created intentionally or by chance and exploited commercially in agriculture or horticulture, is ongoing, and will be important for both farmers and food consumers in the future. Environmentalists, farmers, and food scientists alike are concerned about the effects of climate change on the world's food supply, and are focusing on how flooding, drought, increasing soil salinity, extreme temperatures, and herbicide resistance by insects will affect crop variety and yields in the future. There is also an interest in developing foods that require less commercial fertilizers and pesticides, many of which pose dangers to human health.

New plant hybridizations will be needed to develop plant varieties that will thrive despite these challenges, which will require communication and cooperation among food technologists, farmers, and consumers. An article published in the journal *Nature* (Bailey-Serres et al. 2019, 109–118) addressed the challenges for the future: "The integration of genetic resources and transformative technologies, from genome editing to synthetic biology, are necessary to capture traits that increase global food security and reduce the effects of agriculture on the environment."

Resources

1. J. Bailey-Serres, J. E. Parker, E. A. Ainsworth et al., "Genetic strategies for improving crop yields," *Nature* 575 (2019), 109–118.

Nutrition 101
Key Dietary Components

Dietary considerations have often played a minor role in traditional medical therapy. Despite many clinical and laboratory findings showing that certain types of diets (especially those high in saturated fat, cholesterol, sugar, and salt) may contribute to a variety of degenerative diseases—such as cancer, atherosclerosis, hypertension, and diabetes—the mainstream medical community has always emphasized medications, radiation, and surgery to treat these health problems rather than looking to correct their underlying causes. It isn't that physicians don't care, but that many simply do not have an adequate understanding of diet and nutrition to begin with. They receive minimal instruction about nutrition in medical school, which often totals six hours of class time. Unless they decide to educate themselves about diet and nutrition, physicians may know less about the subject than their patients.

Although this is not a book about nutrition, per se, this chapter lists important components of a healthy diet—for information only. The following terms will be used throughout the book to describe important attributes of each food. Consult a qualified dietitian or nutritionist for specific advice regarding your personal dietary needs.

Proteins

Proteins are a large category of molecules that support the body's cell structure, immune system, movement, chemical reactions, hormone synthesis, and more. Protein is important for growth, as it builds muscle and regulates the body's water balance.

Proteins are made up of tiny building blocks called amino acids. Nine of the twenty amino acids found in the human body are "essential"—which means your body needs them but can't make them on its own, so you need to get them from your diet. Meat and dairy foods contain all nine. While most plant foods do not contain all nine essential amino acids, eating a variety of protein-rich foods throughout the day, such as peanut butter on whole grain bread or rice and beans, will help assure you are consuming all nine.

Carbohydrates

Carbohydrates provide energy. Sugars and starches are carbohydrates, and are found in many plant foods. During digestion, sugars and starches are broken down into simple sugars. They are then absorbed into the bloodstream, where they're known as blood sugar, or *blood glucose*. Nutritionists recommend that we limit foods with added sugars and refined grains, such as sugary drinks, desserts, and candy, which are high in calories but low in nutrition. They suggest instead that carbohydrates are better when obtained from fruits, vegetables, and whole grains.

The glycemic index (GI) measures how quickly carbohydrates from foods enter the bloodstream and increase blood sugar levels. Foods with a "low" GI—like green vegetables, barley, strawberries, and legumes—are rated at fifty-five or less, "medium" GI foods—like brown rice, sweet potatoes, and blueberries—have a rating of fifty-six to sixty-nine, while "high" GI foods—like white bread, white rice, white potatoes, and most cakes, cookies, and candy—are in the seventy or above range. The purpose of consuming low-GI foods is that they are less likely to raise blood sugar levels.

Dietary Fiber

Fiber is found in most plant foods, and is essential for digestive health and eliminating toxins from the body. Carbohydrates that are also rich in fiber are known as *complex carbohydrates*, which have been found to regulate glucose levels in the blood. Eating foods rich in fiber may help maintain healthy weight, and prevent colon and rectal cancers and type 2 diabetes. Fiber-rich foods include vegetables, whole grains, and legumes.

Minerals

Minerals are essential to our survival; each mineral plays a vital role in good health. In addition, minerals often work together with other compounds found in food which increases their overall nutritional and health benefits. They are divided into two main groups: *major minerals*, which we need to consume in larger amounts, and *trace minerals*, which are needed by the body in smaller amounts. Major minerals include calcium, chloride, magnesium, phosphorus, potassium, and sodium. Trace minerals include chromium, cobalt, copper, iodine, iron, manganese, molybdenum, selenium, and zinc. In the sections that follow, the minerals found in each food will be identified.

Here is a brief list of some of the most important minerals found in plant foods, and their functions:

- Calcium is vital for maintaining healthy bones and teeth, and also supports blood clotting, muscle contraction, and nerve impulses.
- Iron produces hemoglobin, a compound that carries oxygen within the blood. Iron deficiencies can lead to anemia.

- Magnesium aids in the formation and maintenance of healthy bone tissue, and helps support cardiovascular health.
- Manganese plays a crucial role in the body's antioxidant defense system, and has been found to play a role in glucose and fatty acid metabolism.
- Potassium, along with sodium (and chloride), helps maintain fluid balance inside and outside of cells, and plays a primary role in regulating blood pressure.
- Selenium helps support thyroid hormone metabolism, and forms an integral part of several antioxidant enzymes and proteins, thus reducing oxidative stress in the body.
- Zinc plays a major role in maintaining a healthy immune system, along with supporting normal growth and repair of body cells and tissues.

Phytochemicals

In addition to presenting little known and, often, newly discovered facts about the history of foods, this book also addresses the importance of certain molecular compounds in foods, called phytochemicals. For many readers, this may be the first time you have heard of them.

Phytochemicals are simply chemicals produced by plants. They include indoles, retinoids, tocopherols, polyphenols, glucosinolates, carotenoids, and phytosterols. Thanks to recent advances in food research, scientists are not only discovering chemicals in plants that they hadn't found before, but also how these phytochemicals are beneficial for human health. Ongoing research at leading universities and medical centers around the world has led nutritionists and medical professionals to recommend plant foods high in phytochemicals, not only to prevent many diseases but also because some may even help reverse a variety of chronic health problems including type 2 diabetes, cardiovascular disease, neurological disease, and even cancer.

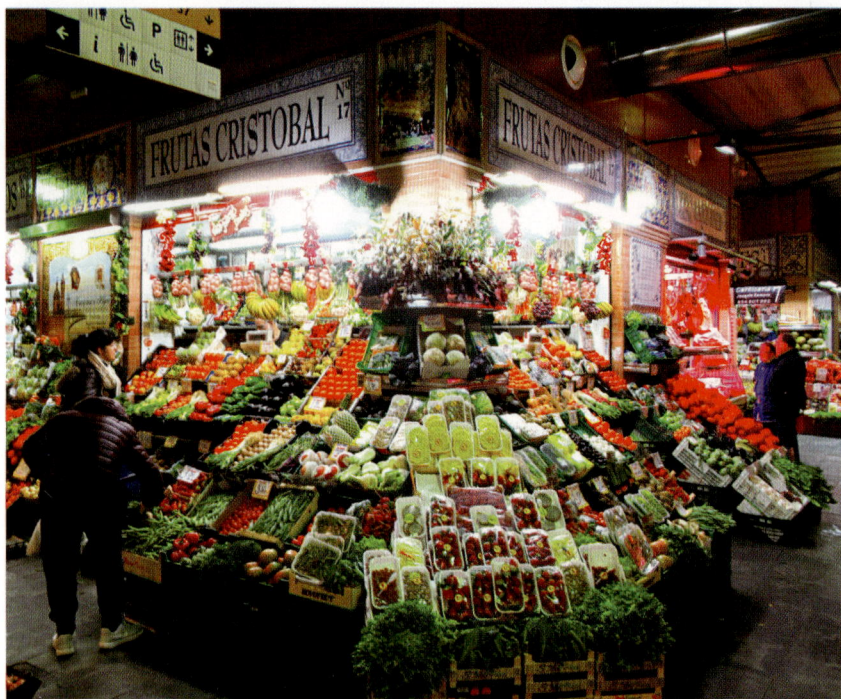

Huge selection of plant foods at a greengrocer.

Thanks to recent developments involving chemometric applications in conjunction with various analytical methods, such as chromatographic and spectroscopic analysis, more than four thousand phytochemicals have been identified. Yet only a fraction have been studied in depth, and many more are still undiscovered.

Phytochemicals in foods can help lower blood pressure, reduce cholesterol, regulate blood sugar, improve sleep, calm the nerves, and even help prevent cancer. Recent scientific discoveries have found that antioxidants, anti-inflammatories, antimicrobials, and other phytochemicals in plants provide significant benefits that promote human health and longevity due to their disease-preventing properties. They are typically found in an array of plant-based foods, which are described in detail in the following sections. The best way to increase the amount of phytochemicals in your body is to consume a varied plant-based diet rich in fresh fruits, vegetables, legumes, nuts, seeds, and whole grains. Nutritional supplements should be used carefully, following consultation with a qualified health professional.

Most phytochemicals belong to the following groups:

Polyphenols

These include phytochemicals such as flavonoids, ellagitannins, lignans, resveratrol, quercetin, and isoflavone. They exhibit antioxidant properties in laboratory studies, but how they affect human health is only partially understood. They are found mostly in grape skins, wine, olive pulp, oranges, tea, soy, and chocolate—but are found in dozens of other plant-based foods as well.

Glucosinolates and Isothiocyanates

These phytochemicals are found primarily in cruciferous plants such as broccoli, cabbage, kale, and brussels sprouts. Their primary task is to protect plants from pests and disease. A growing body of research has shown that these phytochemicals can also help fight different forms of cancer, as well as a variety of other chronic degenerative diseases like heart disease and diabetes in humans who consume them.

Carotenoids

Carotenoids are chemicals that produce color in plants, such as carrots, sweet potatoes, and pomegranates. They include alpha- and beta-carotene, lycopene, lutein, zeaxanthin, and anthocyanins. Carotenoids are found in spinach, kale, and other green leafy vegetables, as well as carrots and sweet potatoes. Those found in carrots, for example, have been shown to improve night vision and support eye health. Others, like anthocyanidin, as in strawberries and red raspberries, have been found to protect the cardiovascular system.

Phytosterols

The chemical structure and function of phytosterols are similar to those of human cholesterol. They are primarily found in legumes such as beans, peas, and chickpeas. They are believed to reduce "bad" cholesterol in the blood, and thus help prevent hypertension (high blood pressure) and other cardiovascular problems.

Although the following sections of this book will highlight the often-fascinating histories of the foods we eat and their uses, you will also learn about the latest information of how phytochemicals in these foods are essential to health and well-being. Many of the phytochemicals will be as unfamiliar to readers as they were for me when I first began to write this book. However, every effort has been made to discuss each phytochemical briefly and in simple, nontechnical language.

Antioxidants

Many phytochemicals are antioxidants, which prevent oxidative chemical reactions in the human body. Oxidative chemical reactions produce molecules called "free radicals," which can be damaging to cells and lead to a variety of health problems such as heart disease, diabetes, and other chronic health conditions. Free radicals are also being studied for how they promote the aging process.

Yet, free radicals are not necessarily "bad." In fact, many are essential to life. Physiological amounts of some free radicals (including superoxide and hydroxyl radicals) are produced by the body to deliver energy to the body's cells. In addition, free radicals have a crucial role in killing bacteria, fungi, and viruses—without those free radicals, we could not survive on Earth. For example, when exposed to a flu virus the body creates free radicals to destroy it. Free radicals also play an important role in regulating chemicals the body needs for its survival, such as hormones.

Free radicals are manufactured by the body—they are produced in extra-high amounts during vigorous exercise, but people who are in good physical shape are easily able to detoxify them—and are formed by certain medications. Free radicals can also be absorbed from the environment. Air pollution (including ozone-laden smog, motor vehicle exhaust, and cigarette smoke), toxic waste, certain food additives, pesticide residues, and radiation (such as from X-rays and airplane travel) all produce free radicals that can affect us in different ways.

When we have too many free radicals in our bodies, cell damage can occur. In his book *Free Radicals and Disease Prevention*, David J. Lin lists how excess free radicals can cause harmful effects to cells. They can:

- Break off the membrane proteins, destroying a cell's identity.
- Fuse together membrane lipids (fats) and membrane proteins, hardening the cell membrane and making it brittle.
- Puncture the cell membrane, allowing bacteria and viruses easy entry.
- Disrupt the nuclear membrane, opening up the nucleus and exposing genetic material.
- Mutate and destroy genetic material, rewriting and destroying genetic information.
- Burden the immune system with the above havoc and threaten the immune system itself by undermining immune cells with similar damage (Lin 1993, 19-21).

As a result, free-radical damage has been linked to a number of degenerative diseases including atherosclerosis, cancer, cataracts, diabetes, allergies, mental disorders, and arthritis. Excess free radicals also play a role in the aging process and decreased immune response, opening the door to a variety of health disorders.

Although our bodies maintain their own antioxidant defenses to keep free radicals in check, antioxidants are also found in plant foods including fruits (especially those rich in red, blue and purple hues, like cherries, blueberries, and blackberries), vegetables, legumes, and grains. Many plant foods contain beta-carotene (vitamin A) and vitamins C and E, which are all effective antioxidants, as are minerals such as selenium and zinc. Many other chemicals in plants have antioxidant properties as well.

Because excess free-radical activity can seriously deplete our body's antioxidant reserves, nutritionists recommend that we augment those supplies with foods rich in antioxidants. Natural antioxidants can help inhibit or control excessive oxidation, and are found in a multitude of plant foods. They help protect proteins, fats, and other substances in the body from oxidative damage, and can help stabilize cell membranes. Antioxidants have also been found to influence chemical "messengers" both within and between body cells.

Basically speaking, a healthy diet consists of fresh, whole, and oxygen-rich foods that also provide an abundant amount of antioxidants such as beta-carotene, vitamin C, and vitamin E. Depending on their nature, these antioxidants will either protect cells from free-radical damage or serve as scavengers to "mop up" excess free radicals in the body.

A team of researchers at the Department of Nutrition at the Institute of Basic Medical Sciences, University of Oslo in Norway, analyzed over 3,100 different foods, evaluating their antioxidant content—expressed as "mmol/100 g," or millimole (1/1,000th of a gram) of antioxidant per 100 grams of food. Their findings were published in *Nutrition Journal* in 2010 (Carlsen et al. 2010).[2] The researchers divided foods into different categories. Among the beverages, espresso coffee scored 12.6 mmol/100 g, followed by hibiscus tea (6.99), Lipton green tea (6.8), red wine (2.5), filter-brewed coffee (2.13), and pomegranate juice (2.1).

Among nuts and seeds, walnuts with *pellicule*—the thin skin or membrane surrounding the nutmeat—scored 21.9, pecans with pellicle 8.5, sunflower seeds 6.4, and chestnuts with pellicle 4.7. Dark chocolate (70–99 percent cacao) samples averaged 10.9, while one popular 85-percent cacao bar from Switzerland scored 13.6.

Certain vegetables and fruits also scored high in antioxidant content, including dried apples (3.8), dried apricots (3.1), blue cauliflower (3.3), dried plums (3.2), curly kale (2.8), red and green chili peppers (2.4), red raspberries (2.3), and strawberries (2.16). Herbs and spices generally scored very high in antioxidant content, but most of us use them in small quantities. Those with the highest content included mint leaves, oregano, rosemary, sage, and thyme.

Vitamins

Beta-carotene

Beta-carotene is a provitamin, which means the body can convert it to another vitamin, in this case vitamin A. The best sources of beta-carotene include fresh carrots, leafy greens, squash (especially yellow squashes, like pumpkin), yams, sweet potatoes, and broccoli. The best fruit sources for beta-carotene include cantaloupes, apricots, and peaches.

Vitamin C

The best sources of vitamin C include citrus fruits (like oranges, tangerines, grapefruits, mandarin oranges, and lemons), tomatoes, strawberries, leafy green vegetables, broccoli, brussels sprouts, and green peppers. Three or more daily servings are recommended from this group, although many oxidative practitioners recommend additional supplementation.

Vitamin E

Cold pressed and unrefined vegetable oils (such as canola, olive, safflower, and soy) are very high in vitamin E. Whole grains (including oatmeal and brown rice), dried beans and other legumes, and leafy green vegetables are good sources as well.

B Vitamins

A number of vitamins make up the B vitamin family: B_1 (thiamin), B_2 (riboflavin), B_3 (niacin), B_6 (pyridoxine), B_9 (folate or its synthetic variety, folic acid), and B_{12} (cyanocobalamin). Together, they are known as "vitamin B complex." The B vitamins are a necessary aid for proper digestion and the efficient utilization of carbohydrates, as well as helping to break down proteins so they, too, can be efficiently used by the body. They also aid cell growth and help keep the nervous system in optimal condition, which is important in immune regulation. Vitamin B complex has also been found to be an antioxidant cofactor, which means the B vitamins play a supportive role in enabling the antioxidants listed above to work more effectively.

B vitamins are found primarily in whole grains, dried beans and peas, and seeds and nuts—especially oats, wheat germ, and peanuts. A varied diet including these foods will help to preserve good health, and can complement most oxidative treatment programs.

Vitamin K

Vitamin K is found in many of the plant foods discussed in this book. This vitamin (also known as K_1, to distinguish it from K_2, which is found in animal based foods) is required for blood coagulation. It also controls the binding of calcium in bones and other tissues.

Resources

1. David J. Lin, *Free Radicals and Disease Prevention.* New Canaan, CT: Keats Publishing, 1993, 19-21.
2. Monica H. Carlsen et al, "The Total Antioxidant Content of More Than 3100 Foods, Beverages, Spices, Herbs and Supplements Used Worldwide," *Nutrition Journal* 9, no. 3 (2010).

Altman, Nathaniel. *The New Oxygen Prescription.* Rochester, VT: Healing Arts Press, 2017, 14–17, 347–352.

"Carbohydrates: How carbs fit into a healthy diet." *Nutrition and Healthy Eating.* Mayo Clinic. Accessed March 6, 2024.

Carlsen, Monica H. et al. "The Total Antioxidant Content of More Than 3100 Foods, Beverages, Spices, Herbs and Supplements Used Worldwide." *Nutrition Journal* 9, no. 3 (2010).

Joseph, Michael. "15 Essential Minerals (and the Best Sources)." Nutrition Advance website. August 25, 2023.

Lin, David J. *Free Radicals and Disease Prevention.* New Canaan, CT: Keats Publishing, 1993, 19-21.

Rautio, Sarah. "Food Micronutrients Explained—Antioxidants, anti-inflammatories and phytochemicals." Michigan State University Extension. October 2, 2017.

Fruits

Fruit as a category normally refers to the fleshy structures (or produce) of plants that contain seeds. They are typically sweet or sour, and are edible in their raw state, such as apples, bananas, grapes, peaches, oranges, and berries. A fruit results from the fertilizing and maturing of one or more flowers.

The term "fruit" comes from the Latin word *fructus*, whose root is *frui* (to enjoy). The fruit of a plant, like an apple or a banana, is the part of a plant which we enjoy eating. The bark or leaves of an apple tree, for example, would be less than enjoyable to eat!

Some plants that are botanically classified as fruits are normally eaten as vegetables, such as eggplants, tomatoes, squash, cucumbers, and peppers. Although they may be classified as fruits, they are included in this book as they correspond with their everyday culinary use—as vegetables.

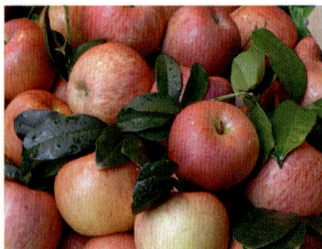

Apple

When most Americans think of apples, they think "Washington state." Although Washington is the biggest producer of apples in the country (followed by New York and California), few people know that apples did not originate in Washington—or even in the United States.

Apples (*Malus domestica*) are believed to have originated over nine million years ago in Central Asia, specifically in what are now Kazakhstan, Uzbekistan, and Kyrgyzstan. The trees originally bore small fruits, like today's crabapple. Historians believe the tiny fruits were eaten by birds and other small mammals who would then disperse the seeds, thereby allowing propagation. Over millennia, the fruits became bigger in order to appeal to a classification of animals called *megafauna*, which includes prehistoric horses, deer, and bears.

It is believed that, like many other ancient foods, the apple eventually spread to China and western Asia—and also to Europe—over the Silk Road. The Silk Road was a network of Eurasian trade routes that existed between the second century BCE until the mid-fifteenth century. Some historians prefer to use the term "Silk Routes" because it better describes the intricate web of both land and sea routes connecting Europe and Asia to the Middle East, the Indian subcontinent, eastern Africa, and northern Africa. Spanning some four thousand miles (6,400 kilometers), these trade routes played a major role in facilitating economic, cultural, philosophical, and religious exchanges between East and West, and all points in between.

The apple arrived in Europe in early Greek and Roman times. The Roman naturalist Pliny the Elder (23/24–79 CE) wrote extensively about apples, including their propagation through seeding and grafting.

Among early Christians the apple became a symbol of knowledge, immortality, temptation, and sin. Yet, according to the Bible, there is nothing to show that the forbidden fruit of the tree of knowledge was necessarily an apple—it was more likely a pomegranate, a fruit whose growth originated in the Holy Land. Apples also played a role in Greek, Roman, and Norse mythology, which regarded apples as providing eternal youth to those who ate them. Apples are said to have existed in what is now Britain before the Romans arrived, and apple trees were grown extensively by the sixteenth century, from both planting seeds and grafting. In his *Gerard's Herball: Or, Generall Historie of Plantes*, published in 1597, English herbalist John Gerard urged the British gentry to propagate only the best grafted apple trees on their estates.

Apples were first brought to the Jamestown Colony in Virginia in 1607, and the plants thrived. The first apple orchard in the American colonies was planted around 1625 by a clergyman who had a farm on Boston's Beacon Hill.

From there and other places in what are now the northeastern United States and southern Canada, many different varieties of apple were propagated thanks in part to John Chapman (1774–1845), better known as Johnny Appleseed. He was an American nurseryman and conservationist who became a folk legend by introducing apple growing to farmers in Pennsylvania, Ohio, Indiana, Illinois, West Virginia, and Ontario. He also planted apple seeds at random as he wandered through the countryside.

Thomas Jefferson was an enthusiastic apple grower, and wrote, "They have no apples here to compare with our Newtown Pippin." Henry David Thoreau wrote about his preference for apples that were "sour enough to set a squirrel's teeth on edge and make a [blue] jay scream." The 1872 edition of A. J. Downing's *The Fruits and Fruit Trees of America* listed more than a thousand apple varieties.

In the 1920s, inexpensive railway shipping and the advent of refrigeration led to orchards distributing apples year round. This in turn led to marketing decisions that reduced commercial apple varieties to fewer than ten, including the ubiquitous Red Delicious, Golden Delicious, and Granny Smith—the three most popular varieties of apple grown in the United States today.

However, a resurgence of interest in heirloom apples has taken root in North America, and seeks to expand the market for both vintage and lesser-known apple varieties such as Baldwin, Cortland, Empire, Gala, Golden Russet, Honeycrisp, Jonathan, McIntosh, Mutsu, Fuji, Rome, and Macoun—a personal favorite of mine that was introduced by the New York Agricultural Experiment Station (now Cornell AgriTech) in 1923. Many heirloom apple seeds have been preserved at Cornell University's germplasm repository in Geneva, New York. New apple varieties are constantly being developed at Cornell's AgriTech campus in Geneva, including the Cordera, Pink Luster, and Firecracker varieties, introduced in 2020.

The apple is among the most beloved and popular fruits in the world, and can be enjoyed as fruit (either whole or cut up), juice, cider, apple cider vinegar, applesauce, apple butter, roasted apples, dried apples, apple smoothies, and as a major ingredient in pies, cakes, and breads. Apples can also be included in main dishes such as meat and vegetable pies, stuffing, egg dishes, and fritters.

Apples are highly nutritious. In addition to dietary fiber, apples provide a range of vitamins and minerals including vitamin A and potassium. Research shows that the antioxidants in apples can reduce inflammation caused by oxidative stress, a cause of accelerated aging, cardiovascular diseases, cancer, and type 2 diabetes. In addition to the apple's antioxidant activity, the pectin found in apples has been linked to stimulating the growth of "friendly bacteria" in the colon, which prevents inflammation, aids digestion, and strengthens the immune system. Apples also contain a variety of micronutrients. A recent article in the *Journal of Food Science* (Oyenihi 2022, 2291–2309) stated that: "Apples are rich sources of selected micronutrients (e.g., iron, zinc, vitamins C and E) and polyphenols (e.g., procyanidins, phloridzin, 5-O-caffeoylquinic acid) that can help in mitigating micronutrient deficiencies (MNDs) and chronic diseases (Oyenihi 2022, 2291–2309)." While it may not be literally true that "An apple a day keeps the doctor away," the apple is one of the healthiest foods one can eat.

China is presently the world's largest grower of apples, followed by the United States, Poland, Italy, and France. The top five apple producing states in the U.S. are Washington, New York, California, Michigan, and Pennsylvania. More than eleven billion pounds of apples are grown in the United States during a typical year.

Resources

Browning, Frank. *Apples*. New York: North Point Press, 1998.

"Exploring the origins of the apple." *Science Daily*. May 27, 2019.

Hanson, Beth, ed. *The Best Apples to Grow and Buy*. Brooklyn, NY: Brooklyn Botanic Garden, 2005.

Iowa State University. "Apples." Agricultural Marketing Research Center website. April 2024.

Khoury, C. K., H. Achicanoy, and A. Bjorkman et al. "Origins of food crops connect countries worldwide." *Proceedings of the Royal Society B: Biological Sciences* 283 (2016): 20160792.

Oyenihi, A. B., Z. A. Belay, A. Mditshwa, and O. J. Caleb. "'An apple a day keeps the doctor away': The potentials of apple bioactive constituents for chronic disease prevention." *Journal of Food Science* 87, 6 (2022): 2291–2309.

Rodger, Erin. "Crunchy, complex: Cornell releases three new apples." *Cornell Chronicle.* September 2, 2020.

Roth, Claire. "The curious early history of apples." Science. Deutsche Welle. Accessed October 4, 2023.

Sawe, Benjamin Elisha. "Where do Apples Come from Originally?" *WorldAtlas.* Accessed October 4, 2023.

Wynne, Peter. *Apples: History, Folklore, Horticulture, and Gastronomy.* New York: Hawthorne Books, 1974.

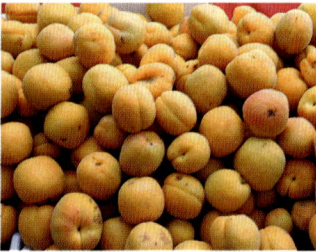

Apricot

Photo by Daderot

In the United States, the vast majority of apricots (*Prunus armeniaca*) are grown in California, where Spanish missionaries introduced the fruit from Europe. The first apricot tree is believed to have arrived in Virginia from Europe in 1720. Considered among the world's most delicious yet delicate fruits, the apricot was cultivated in China and Central Asia as early as 2000 BCE. It was spread to the west along the Silk Road, and found lasting favor with the Persians, who called it "yellow plum" (*zardaloo*). The name itself is derived from the Arabic *al-barqūq* (the plums). The apricot was further spread throughout the Middle East and Europe, and eventually to every region of the world except Antarctica. The "common apricot" is the most cultivated type, though there are more than a dozen species of apricots grown today.

Almost all of the apricots destined for the fresh market must be picked by hand while they are still firm. This adds to higher cost, and is one reason why the annual per capita consumption of fresh apricots in the United States is only 0.11 pounds. Apricots are best eaten raw, although fresh apricots have become a favorite ingredient in Middle Eastern dishes, especially those containing lamb. Dried apricots have been prized as both a snack food and an ingredient in cooked dishes. Apricot paste—known as *amardine*—is considered a delicacy in the Middle East, and involves using crushed apricots with the pits removed; the apricots are then spread into sheets and dried in the sun.

In the Middle East, the apricot is nicknamed "The Golden Fruit" for its nutritional value and medicinal properties. Like peaches and plums, apricots are packed with nutrients—including vitamin A, vitamin C, dietary fiber, and potassium—which are good for heart health, eye health, and to help protect the digestive system. They also contain high concentrations of bioactive phytochemicals like carotenoids, phenolics, and flavonoids. Foods high in carotenoids have been found to reduce the risk of head, neck, and prostate cancers, while phenolics possess powerful antioxidant properties that help protect us from cardiovascular disease, cancer, and type 2 diabetes. Flavonoids have been linked to a reduced risk of cardiovascular diseases and cancer, and improved cognitive function, especially in older adults. In particular, apricots contain the flavonoid *quercetin*, a component of which may help prevent neurodegenerative diseases like Alzheimer's and Parkinson's.

Ground apricot kernels have been used in Chinese Traditional Medicine for thousands of years to support both respiratory and digestive health; they remain an essential ingredient in commercial

Chinese cough lozenges. The term "Expert of the Apricot Grove" (杏林高手) is still used by the Chinese as a poetic reference to traditional physicians.

Türkiye is the world's largest producer of apricots, followed by Uzbekistan and Iran. Much of Türkiye's apricot crop is dried and exported. Although not a major producer, an estimated 75 percent of apricots grown in the United States come from California, with an additional 24 percent grown in Washington.

Resources

Alajil, O., V. R. Sagar, C. Kuar et al. "Nutritional and Phytochemical Traits of Apricots (*Prunus Armeniaca L.*) for Application in Nutraceutical and Health Industry." *Foods* 10, 6 (2021): 1344.

Denker, Joel. "Moon of the Faith: A History of the Apricot and its Many Pleasures." *The Salt.* NPR. June 14, 2016.

Iowa State University. "Apricots." Agricultural Marketing Research Center website. January 2023."*Prunus armeniaca*." Wikipedia. Accessed March 6, 2023.

Jillian. "The History of Apricots." Jillian's Blog. Kingsburg Orchards. April 18, 2013.

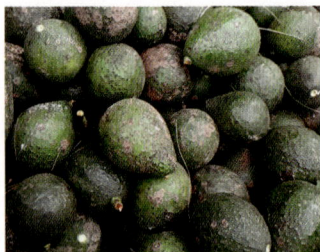

Photo by Eddy A. Saban Sequén

Avocado

Historians believe that the avocado (*Persea americana*) originated in Coxcatlán, in what is now the state of Puebla, located in southern central Mexico. The indigenous, undomesticated variety known as

Criollo is small, with dark black skin, and contains a large seed. It can still be found in local markets in and around Puebla today.

The Indigenous peoples of ancient Mesoamerica began consuming this delicious and nutritious fruit some ten thousand years ago. Prior to its domestication, it is believed that the survival of the avocado may have been dependent on the ability of now-extinct large mammals that were able to ingest the fruit's mildly toxic pit after swallowing the large berry whole. They later deposited the seed in their feces, which allowed the plant to propagate throughout central Mexico.

The avocado (known as *aguacate* in Spanish, derived from the Nahuatl word *āhuacatl*) was an extremely important fruit among the Indigenous people of what is today called Mexico. In addition to providing physical sustenance, it was also believed to possess mythological powers. The ancient Aztecs believed the avocado provided strength (especially sexual prowess) to whomever consumed it; among the Maya, the avocado was so important that the fourteenth month of their calendar (K'ank'in) is represented by the glyph for the avocado. The ancient Maya also believed that important people reincarnated as trees after death, including as an avocado tree. It was also believed that Mesoamerican peoples first domesticated the avocado five thousand years ago, making the cultivation of avocados as old as the invention of the wheel.

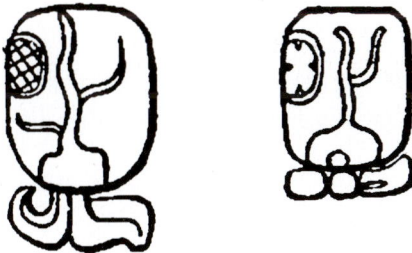

Drawing of K'ankk'in by the American archeologist Sylvanus Griswold Morley, in *An Introduction to the Study of Maya Hieroglyphs* (1915).

The avocado eventually made its way across the Atlantic when Spanish explorers returned to Europe from the New World in the sixteenth century. By 1521, cultivation of the avocado had spread through Central America and into parts of South America before being exported back to Europe by the Spanish.

As with many other fruits and vegetables, more than a dozen different avocado cultivars (a cultivar is a plant that has been grown from stem cutting, grafting, or tissue cultures to ensure it retains the characteristics of the plant parent) have been developed over the centuries. Several avocado varieties were developed in San Diego by members of the Theosophical Society at Point Loma, a Utopian spiritual community that flourished between 1897 and 1942. Point Loma's experimentation began in 1915 with four avocado trees, and by 1925, Point Loma's avocado grove included more than 250 trees of some thirty varieties. These early efforts are believed to have inspired the commercial cultivation of avocados in California.

If you have the opportunity to visit a traditional market in Mexico, you'll find several avocado varieties on sale that you can choose from. In addition to the Criollo, popular varieties include Bacon, Patrón, Pinkerton, Fuerte, and Hass. The Hass is by far the most cultivated avocado worldwide, and is grown in about 80 percent of avocado farms in California, most of which are located in San Diego County. All Hass avocado trees have been grown from grafted seedlings propagated from a single tree that was grown from a seed introduced by the amateur American horticulturist Rudolph Hass in 1926. It is believed that the Hass avocado came about by taking the branches of the Patrón avocado plant and grafting them to the roots of the Criollo.

Over the years, the avocado tree has been introduced in places where the climate is appropriate for its cultivation. In addition to Mexico and California, avocados are grown in more than sixty countries around the world including Colombia, Peru, Indonesia, Kenya, and Brazil. In addition to guacamole, avocados are eaten directly with a spoon, and are popular additions to salads and sandwiches. The avocado is now the fourth most important tropical fruit in the world, and Mexico is the main supplier, with more than 2.4 million tons produced by 2020.

Avocados contain a variety of nutrients including carotenoids (especially lutein and zeaxanthin) which act as a type of antioxidant in humans and are believed to improve eye health. Avocados also contain monounsaturated fats, potassium, and fiber, along with vitamins B, E, and K. Its minerals include potassium and magnesium. According to the Harvard University School of Public Health (The Nutrition Source), "The nutritional profile of avocados fits well with healthful dietary patterns such as the Mediterranean and DASH (Dietary Approaches to Stop Hypertension) diets."

Resources

"A History of Avocados." Avocados from Mexico website. Accessed March 6, 2023.

"Avocado." Wikipedia. Accessed March 6, 2023.

"Avocados." The Nutritional Source. Harvard T.H. Chan School of Public Health. Accessed March 6, 2023.

"Avocados and the Ancient Maya." *Ancient Maya Life*. Accessed March 6, 2023. https://ancientmayalife.blogspot.com/2018/01/avocados-and-ancient-maya.html

Galindo-Tovar, María Elena, Amaury M. Arzate-Fernandez, Niso Ogata-Aguilar et al. "The Avocado (*Persea Americana, Lauraceae*) Crop in Mesoamerica: 10,000 years of History." *Harvard Papers in Botany* 12, no. 2 (2007), 325–334.

Greenwalt, Emmett A. *California Utopia: Point Loma: 1897-1942*. San Diego: Point Loma Publications, 1978, 139-40; 143-44.

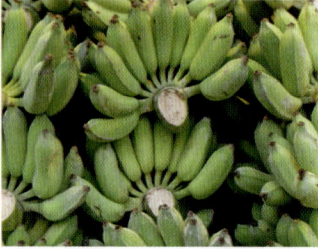

Banana and Plantain

Cultivated bananas and plantains are giant herbaceous plants within the genus *Musa*. Today's bananas and their relatives, plantains, descended from a wild banana herb that grew in the tropics about ten thousand years ago. It appears that a plant dropped its inedible, seedy fruit on the rainforest floor, which caused a change in its DNA. The plant's offspring grew tall and seedless, which made the fruit easy to eat.

Bananas originated in Southeast Asia, from India to Polynesia; scientists have placed their actual center of diversity between Malaysia and Indonesia. There are well over a thousand domesticated Musa cultivars (cultivated varieties), and their genetic diversity is high. This indicates multiple origins from different wild hybrids between two principle ancestral species.

Our Stone Age ancestors discovered this delicious fruit and began to grow it. Bananas and plantains are the fourth most popular fruits in the world today, with a yearly production of over 100 million tons. While, in the West, bananas are considered an ideal "dessert" food, many who live in the tropics consider bananas and plantains essential to their survival. Per capita banana and plantain consumption in Papua New Guinea is 112 kilograms a year; per capita consumption in Laos is 110 kg. By contrast, Canadians eat just 15.1 kilograms of bananas per capita each year, while Americans consume only 11.8 kilograms. Nevertheless, bananas are the most popular fruit in the United States, followed by apples and grapes.

What are the differences between bananas and plantains? Plantains are larger than bananas, with a thicker skin and a higher starch content. Bananas are eaten raw when ripe (yellow skin), while plantains can be eaten when ripe (yellow or brown skin) or unripe (green skin). Plantains are frequently cooked like vegetables in Asian, Latin American, African, and Caribbean dishes. When I visited Colombia for the first time, as an exchange student at age sixteen, my hosts served fried plantains at lunch, which I found unfamiliar yet very tasty. I originally thought they were a type of fried potato.

Eventually, traders brought edible banana varieties from Southeast Asia to Africa by boat. The cultivated fruit began to spread across Africa, Europe, and the Americas; it is believed that bananas were first introduced to the New World by Tomás de Berlanga, a Catholic friar who brought banana plants to Santo Domingo (now the Dominican Republic) from the Canary Islands in 1516. Bananas were soon introduced to other European colonies in the Caribbean and Latin America. The banana's development into a major worldwide trade commodity has its roots in the nineteenth century. Individual merchants began shipping plantains from the Caribbean to American and European markets in the early 1800s.

Of the bananas grown for export, almost all are "dessert" bananas destined for markets in the United States and Europe. The Gros Michel variety was the most popular banana up to the 1950s, but was replaced by the Cavendish cultivar which is hardier and slightly less sweet. In general, the United States consumes bananas grown in Central and South America (primarily Ecuador and Colombia), whereas consumers in the European Union import most of their bananas from the Caribbean. Other major banana producers include India, China, Indonesia, and Brazil. The biggest exporters are in Latin America (especially Ecuador, Costa Rica, and Colombia), followed by tropical countries in Asia, led by the Philippines. Major banana importers are the European Union, the United States, China, Russia, and Japan.

Bananas are a healthy food. They are a good source of dietary fiber, potassium, vitamin B_6, and vitamin C. Bananas also supply various antioxidants and phytonutrients including dopamine (a neurotransmitter) and catechins, which are important for heart health and digestion. Bananas have a relatively low glycemic index (GI) of 42–58, depending on their ripeness. The glycemic index measures how quickly carbohydrates in food enter the bloodstream and thereby increase blood sugar. Ripe bananas have a higher GI; people with type 2 diabetes should avoid eating large quantities of very ripe bananas.

Throughout history, cultivated bananas have been threatened by various types of pathogens. Since the vast majority of bananas are grown as a monoculture, an entire species can be wiped out by the same disease. This has led plant scientists to develop new cultivars that are more resistant to pathogens. Eventually the Cavendish, which is under threat, will be replaced by one or more recently developed cultivars. In addition, growers are evaluating the value of cultivating many different banana varieties rather than relying on a single one.

Resources

Arnarson, Atli. "Bananas 101: Nutrition Facts and Health Benefits." Healthline.com. February 23, 2023.

"Banana Consumption per Capita." Helgi Library. Accessed August 6, 2023.

Banana Market Review 2022. Rome: Food and Agriculture Organization of the United Nations, 2023.

de Candolle, Alphonse. Origin of Cultivated Plants. New York: D. Appleton and Company, 1908, 304.

Heslop-Harrison, J. S., and T. Schwarzacher. "Domestication, genomics and the future for banana." Annals of Botany 100, 5 (2007): 1073–84.

"Plantains vs Bananas: What's the Difference?" The Food Network, August 7, 2023.

"What Is a Banana, Really?" Bayer Global website. Accessed August 6, 2023.

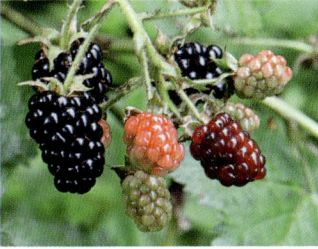

Blackberry

Photo by Ragesoss

Blackberries (*Rubus fruticosus*) are believed to have originated thousands of years ago in various regions of the northern latitudes, including North America, Europe, and Asia. With more than 375 varieties—both cultivated and wild—blackberries are said to have more geographic origins than any other fruit.

Blackberries were valued as medicinal in ancient Greece, where the physician Galen prescribed a decoction of blackberries to treat gout. Blackberries were also used medicinally in ancient Rome to treat bowel problems and fever, and were prescribed by European folk healers to treat whooping cough and colitis. Tea made from its roots has been used to reduce labor pain, while the leaves of the blackberry have been chewed for toothache.

Early Anglo-Saxons baked the fruit in pies to celebrate the first fruit feast of Lughnasadh, at the end of summer. Blackberry brambles were often planted around European villages to thwart entry by human marauders and large animals. Medieval Europeans also believed that blackberries could protect against incantations and curses when gathered at a certain phase of the moon.

Native Americans utilized blackberries not only as a food source but also medicinally, as well as for dying animal skins. They also used the canes of the blackberry plant to make twine. Blackberries have long been enjoyed as human food, and have generally been available free for the picking by roadsides and in fields. I remember picking wild blackberries with my grandfather during the summer months in a field behind our home in upstate New York, wearing heavy clothing to avoid being stuck by brambles.

Blackberries are generally eaten raw and added to cereals, salads, fruit shakes, and smoothies. They are also used to make jams, jellies, and pie fillings. Blackberry leaves are brewed as herbal tea, especially in Europe.

Like other berries, blackberries are both healthy and nutritious. They are especially high in vitamin C, vitamin K, and manganese—a trace mineral that protects body cells from free-radical damage, supports the immune system, and promotes brain function and bone growth. Blackberries are also rich in healthy phytochemicals like polyphenols (antioxidants that have been found to reduce inflammation), and help prevent heart disease, diabetes, and certain types of cancer. A recent scientific article appearing in *Pharmacognosy Reviews* (Verma et al. 2014, 101–104) stated that "Various blackberry plants are useful in the treatment of cancer, dysentery, diarrhea, whooping cough, colitis, toothache, anemia, psoriasis, sore throat, mouth ulcer, mouthwash, hemorrhoids, and minor bleeding."

Although blackberries have been growing wild in North America for thousands of years, blackberry cultivation in the United States didn't begin until the 1850s. Oregon is the major producer of cultivated blackberries in the United States today. Fresh blackberries are also imported from Mexico—the world's largest producer—while frozen blackberries are mostly imported from Chile.

Resources

"Blackberries," Agricultural Marketing Resource Center website. September 2021.

Cleveland Clinic. "The Small Yet Powerful Blackberry: Why You Should Eat Some Today." healthessentials. August 31, 2022.

Grant, Amy. "The History of Blackberries in Cultivation." Gardening Know-How. July 12, 2018.

Harding, Deborah. "The History of the Blackberry Fruit." Garden Guides website. September 21, 2017.

Verma, Rameshwar et al. *"Rubus fruticosus* (blackberry) use as an herbal medicine." *Pharmacognosy Reviews*8, no. 16 (2014): 101–104.

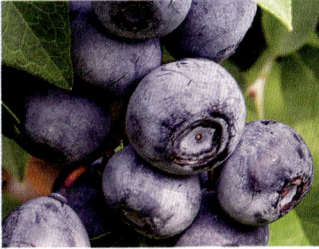

Blueberry

Photo by Jim Clark

Blueberries (*Vaccinium*) are indigenous to the northeastern United States and southeastern Canada; wild blueberries have been an important food for Native Americans for thousands of years. Since blueberries tend to keep longer than other types of berries, Indigenous peoples, such as the Algonquin, often dried wild blueberries to enjoy them during the winter. One of their favorite dishes was called *sautauthig*, which included dried blueberries and dried, cracked corn mixed with water. Some historians believe that sautauthig was served at the first Thanksgiving.

I have fond childhood memories of picking wild blueberries in the woods near my grandparents' summer cottage in Lake Peekskill, New York. My brother and I would bring back a small basket filled with fresh blueberries and enjoy them with ice cream while seated at our grandmother's kitchen table. The berries were small but incredibly tasty.

There was little interest in cultivating blueberries in the United States until the 1890s, when Elizabeth White, the daughter of a New Jersey cranberry farmer, became interested in the blueberry's potential as a commercial crop. In the early 1900s, Frank Coville, a botanist at the United States Department of Agriculture, began research on North American blueberries with the intention of developing improved varieties for commercial cultivation. His studies led to the publication of his book *Blueberry Cultivation* in 1911, and Ms. White bought one of the first copies. She soon contacted Coville and offered him the use of a plot of land on her farm to cultivate the fruit. Coville and others gradually developed several types of blueberries suitable for commercial use, although blueberries could not be classified as a highly successful crop.

Yet, when modern nutritional researchers began to discover that blueberries (along with other berries) contained a wealth of antioxidants and essential micronutrients during the 1990s, blueberries were catapulted into the world of "superfood." They found that blueberries are rich in vitamin C and vitamin K—which is involved in blood clotting and may support bone health—along with the mineral manganese, which supports protein, carbohydrate, and lipid metabolism. Blueberries also contain antioxidants such as flavonoids, that are believed to improve memory and delay age-related cognitive decline. Phytochemicals like *anthocyanin*, also found in blueberries, are believed to protect against heart disease, cancer, and diabetes and help maintain bone strength, blood pressure, and healthy skin. Wild blueberries—like the kind I used to enjoy as a child—are said to provide twice the antioxidants of cultivated berries, and contain more phytochemicals such as anthocyanin. An article in the peer-reviewed journal *Advances in Nutrition* addresses the therapeutic value of anthocyanins:

> Of their various phytochemicals, anthocyanins probably make the greatest impact on blueberry health functionality. Epidemiological studies associate regular, moderate intake of blueberries and/or anthocyanins with reduced risk of cardiovascular disease, death, and type 2 diabetes, and with improved weight maintenance and neuroprotection. (Kalt et al. 2020, 224)

The authors of the article concluded that, "[. . .] it is widely agreed that the regular consumption of tasty, ripe blueberries can be unconditionally recommended."

Fresh blueberries can be enjoyed either alone or as an ingredient in fruit salad; they can also be added to hot or cold cereal, yogurt, or smoothies. They can be added to muffins, pies, and other baked goods. You can easily substitute frozen berries for fresh in most recipes. Many people buy fresh blueberries when they are in season and freeze them to enjoy on winter days.

The elevation of blueberries to superfood status has increased domestic blueberry production fivefold in recent years, to an estimated 500 million pounds. The United States is the world's largest producer of blueberries, where they are grown commercially in thirty-eight out of fifty states. Michigan is the leading producer of cultivated blueberries in the country, followed by New York, New Jersey, North Carolina, Georgia, and Florida. In Canada, British Columbia is the major producer of cultivated blueberries, while Québec, Nova Scotia, and New Brunswick are the nation's leading producers of wild blueberries. Blueberries are also grown in Chile, Argentina, Mexico, and Colombia, and are exported to the United States and Canada during the winter months in North America.

Resources

Blakely, Julia. "Native Fruit: The Wild Blueberry." *Smithsonian Unbound.* November 13, 2018.

"*Blueberries.*" University of California, Davis. Accessed June 4, 2023.

"Canadian Blueberries, from farm to fork." Statistics Canada. Accessed June 4, 2023.

"The history of blueberries: From Native American staple to domesticated superfood." University of Illinois Extension. January 19, 2019.

Kalt, W., A. Cassidy, L. R. Howard et al. "Recent Research on the Health Benefits of Blueberries and Their Anthocyanins." *Advances in Nutrition* 11, 2 (2020): 224–236.

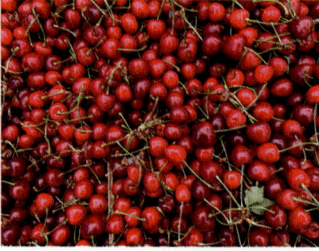

Cherry

Cherries are undoubtedly one of the most delicious of fruits. They are cultivated in both sweet (*Prunus avium*) and sour (*Prunus cerasus*) varieties, encompassing more than twenty different cultivars. Most of the cherries North Americans enjoy are grown in Washington and California.

Sweet cherries originated in Asia Minor, in the fertile regions between the Black Sea and the Caspian Sea. They were believed to have spread to Europe by birds, which ate them and defecated the seeds. Early writers reported that cherry trees grew wild in what is now Armenia, as well as in Greece (especially on Mount Olympus) and Macedonia.

The Greeks were the first to cultivate cherries. The philosopher Theophrastus was the first Greek writer to mention cherries, in about 300 BCE. Pliny the Elder (23–79 CE), the Roman naturalist and author of *Naturalis Historia* (Natural History), suggested that the Roman general Lucullus brought cherries back to Italy when he returned from the Pontus region in Anatolia, part of today's Türkiye.

Cherries are believed to have been introduced to North America in 1852 by Peter Dougherty, a Presbyterian missionary who lived in northern Michigan. The plantings were so successful, neighbors started to grow their own trees, which were of the sour cherry variety. At about the same time, French settlers from Normandy brought cherry pits to plant along the St. Lawrence region, near the Great Lakes of eastern Canada.

One of the most important developments in cherry history was the introduction of the Bing cherry, which is the most widely planted cherry variety in the United States. It was developed at the farm of horticulturist Seth Lewelling in Milwaukie, Oregon, in 1875. Named in honor of his Chinese foreman, Ah Bing (who played an essential role in this cultivar's development), the Bing cherry was a cross between Black Republican and Napoleon cultivars from France, also known as Royal Ann in Oregon.

Sweet cherries are chiefly produced for the fresh market, whereas sour (or tart) cherries are largely processed. Michigan grows about 75 percent of the tart cherry crop, while Oregon and Washington produce about 60 percent of the sweet cherry crop in the U.S. Other states with commercial cherry crops are Utah, Wisconsin, New York, Pennsylvania, and California.

The fruit of the sweet cherry is flavorful and rich in dietary fiber, minerals, organic acids, riboflavin, niacin, and antioxidants. Tart cherries are considered nutrition powerhouses, brimming with antioxidants and essential nutrients like beta-carotene, vitamin C, potassium, magnesium, and iron. The antioxidants in cherries protect against inflammation and fight free radicals that can cause cell damage and contribute to chronic health problems like heart disease, cancer, and diabetes. Several recent medical studies found that eating cherries on a regular basis can relieve muscle pain and ease the swelling and pain of arthritis. Finally, the serotonin and melatonin found in cherries contribute to restful sleep.

Resources

de Candolle, Alphonse. *Origin of Cultivated Plants*. New York: D. Appleton and Company, 1908, 205–6.

Cleveland Clinic. "The Cherry On Top: 8 Health Benefits of Cherries." healthessentials. March 27, 2023.

Eubank, Ann. "The Tragic Roots of America's Favorite Cherry." *Atlas Obscura*. June 19, 2018.

"History of Cherries." National Cherry Festival. Cherry Festival website. Accessed June 5, 2023.

Kappel, Frank. "Cherry." *The Canadian Encyclopedia*. March 16, 2015. https://www.thecanadianencyclopedia.ca/en/article/cherry

Long, Lynn. "Bing Cherry." *The Oregon Encyclopedia*. Accessed June 5, 2023.

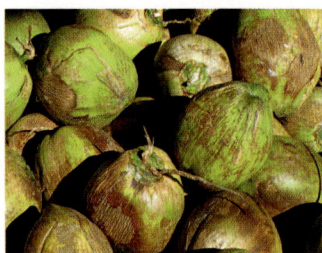

Coconut

Writing in Washington University's blog *The Source*, author Diana Lutz remarked:

> The coconut (the fruit of the palm *Cocos nucifera*) is the Swiss Army knife of the plant kingdom; in one neat package it provides a high-calorie food, potable water, fiber that can be spun into rope, and a hard shell that can be turned into charcoal.

She also mentions that coconuts can float, which helps explain how they were originally spread around the world by ocean currents.

Coconut is an ancient food that is found in many tropical areas of the world; nineteenth-century researchers believed that the coconut originated somewhere in Asia due to the immense varieties of coconut trees that were found there. More recently, the coconut was studied using DNA analysis of more than 1,300 examples gathered from around the world by Dr. Kenneth M. Olsen, a plant evolutionary biologist at Washington University in St. Louis. He pinpointed two distinct origins of the coconut: one in the Pacific basin (Southeast Asia) and the other in the Indian Ocean basin, which includes modern-day Sri Lanka, India, and Bangladesh. Other studies tend to support these findings.

Fossils discovered in what is now New Zealand show that the coconut palm thrived there some 15 million years ago. Other research shows that fossils unearthed in Kerala—the "Land of Coconuts"—in India, and in Khulna (an administrative division in today's Bangladesh) are even older. The coconut palm's multiplicity of uses has earned it nicknames in India such as the "Tree of Life," "Tree of Heaven," "Tree of Abundance," and "Kalpavriksha"—a tree that provides all necessities of life. In India, coconuts have played a major role in Hindu pujas, festivals, marriage ceremonies, and other spiritual and religious events for thousands of years.

Coconuts are believed to have first been introduced to other parts of the world by ocean currents, and later carried by explorers and traders to Europe and the New World. For example, the Spaniards brought coconuts to the Pacific coast of colonial Mexico from the Philippines, which was also governed by Spain.

The versatile coconut provides five kinds of food products: coconut water, coconut "meat," coconut milk, sugar, and coconut oil. Coconut water (mostly imported from the Philippines), widely sold for drinking in North America, contains high amounts of vitamin C, as well as electrolytes (required for proper nerve and muscle function, maintaining acid-base balance, and keeping us hydrated), potassium, and magnesium. Coconut meat is a popular addition to cakes, pies, candy bars, trail mixes, and other snacks. Coconut milk, derived from grated coconut meat, is a popular ingredient in Indian, Indonesian, Panamanian, and Philippine cuisines.

In the tropics, one can enjoy refreshing coconut water by slicing open the top of the outer, green husk with a machete and drinking it directly. When you are done, what remains of the coconut may be split open, providing a delicious soft white flesh that can be enjoyed with a spoon.

The coconut also has a long history of use in Ayurvedic medicine, an ancient Indian system of natural healing that goes back five thousand years. Coconut water, milk, meat, and oil have been used by Ayurvedic practitioners to treat dozens of health problems, including digestive disorders, skin problems, cold and cough, venereal diseases, and gingivitis.

Resources

Ahuja, S. C. et al. "Coconut - History, Uses and Folklore." *Asian Agri-History* 18, no. 3 (2014): 221–248.

de Candolle, Alphonse. *Origin of Cultivated Plants*. New York: D. Appleton and Company, 1908, 433.

"History of the Coconut Tree." Gardenerdy website. Accessed July 10, 2023.

Lutz, Diana. "Deep History of Coconuts Decoded." *The Source*. Washington University in St. Louis website. June 24, 2011.

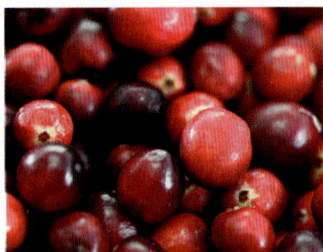

Cranberry

Photo by Cjboffoli

Cranberries (*Vaccinium macrocarpon*) are one of the few fruits that are indigenous to the United States. They are native to the swamps and bogs of northeastern United States and parts of Canada, and are now grown commercially in human-made wetlands and bogs. Americans consume nearly 400 million pounds (181 million kilograms) of cranberries a year—some twenty percent over Thanksgiving alone.

According to *Cranberry Agriculture in Maine: Grower's Guide* (1996 version):

The American cranberry [. . .] grows wild from the mountains of Georgia to the Canadian Maritimes, and as far west as Minnesota. It has been cultivated in the Cape Cod area since the early 1800s and was an active industry in Maine during much of the last century. The cultivated cranberry industry then spread to New Jersey by the 1830s, Wisconsin by the 1850s, and the Pacific Northwest by the 1880s. (The University of Maine Extension website)

Cranberries are bright red in color and are very tart—they are rarely eaten raw. Although mostly prepared as a side dish to serve with Thanksgiving dinner, cranberries are a great addition to everything from savory casseroles and rice dishes to cakes, muffins, and cookies. Commercially made cranberry juice (diluted in water and with added sugar) is a popular beverage, and dried cranberries (again, with added sugar) are a popular snack food. Dried berries can be mixed with nuts and seeds and eaten as a tasty and nutritious trail mix. And, like raisins, dried cranberries are often added to cereal and yogurt.

Cranberries are a very healthy food. In addition to providing high amounts of vitamin C, manganese, and dietary fiber, cranberries are rich in beneficial phytochemicals, especially *proanthrocyanidin* antioxidants, which are essential for maintaining good health and have also been found to specifically prevent urinary tract infections. These phytochemicals also support heart health, improve digestion, and potentially even prevent cancer ("Cranberry" 2021). They also cleanse the mouth of harmful bacteria, thus reducing the development of tooth decay.

In a 2007 review of healthful properties of the cranberry in the peer-reviewed *Journal of Nutrition* (Neto 2007, 186S), the author wrote that phytochemicals found in cranberries "inhibit the growth and proliferation of breast, colon, prostate, lung, and other tumors, as do flavonols, proanthocyanidin oligomers, and triterpenoids isolated from the fruit." She added that "the unique combination of phytochemicals found in cranberry fruit may produce synergistic health benefits," suggesting that the phytochemicals in cranberries work together in different ways to help protect the body from cancer and other serious health problems. She concluded that such findings "suggest a potential role for cranberry as a dietary chemopreventive [i.e., the use of a food or other substance to prevent the development of cancer]."

A more recent article in the journal *Molecules* highlighted the beneficial impact on human health and disease prevention from cranberry consumption, and in particular "its effect against urinary tract inflammation with both adults and children, cardiovascular, oncology diseases, type 2 diabetes, metabolic syndrome, obesity, tooth decay and periodontitis, Helicobacter pylori bacteria in the stomach, and other diseases" (Nemzer et al. 2022, 1502).

Cranberries are grown primarily in Massachusetts, Wisconsin, New Jersey, Oregon, and Washington in the United States; British Columbia and Québec in Canada; and Chile.

Resources

Cleveland Clinic. "Are Cranberries Healthy? 6 Surprising Benefits." healthessentials. January 26, 2022.

"Cranberry: Purported Benefits, Side Effects & More,"
Memorial Sloan Kettering Cancer Center website, February 25, 2021.

"Cooperative Extension: Cranberries." The University of Maine Extension website. June 8, 2025.

Iowa State University. "Cranberries." Agricultural Marketing Resource Center website. January, 2023.

Nemzer, B. V., F. Al-Taher, A. Yashin et al. "Cranberry: Chemical Composition, Antioxidant Activity and Impact on Human Health: Overview." *Molecules* 27, no. 5 (2022):1503.

Neto, Catherine C. "Cranberry and its Phytochemicals: A review of In Vitro Cancer Studies." *The Journal of Nutrition* 137, no. 1 (2007): 186S–193S.

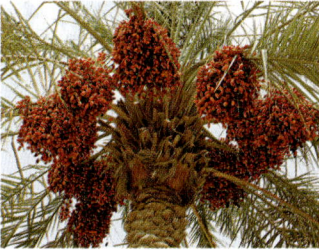

Date

Photo by Nepenthese

Dates, the delicious and healthy fruit of the date palm (*Phoenix dactylifera*), are among the oldest known fruits in the world. While its exact place of origin is open to debate, the date palm most likely originated in either Mesopotamia (including present-day Iraq, Iran, Syria, Kuwait, and Türkiye) or in western India, at least five thousand years ago. Date cultivation then gradually spread through the Arabian Peninsula, the Middle East, and North Africa. Date culture is believed to have arrived in Egypt by 200 BCE, and later spread—east to the Indian subcontinent and west to Spain—by traders. The date palm is believed to have arrived in China from Persia (present-day Iran) during the third century CE.

Dates were essential to the survival of ancient civilizations, both as food and as a source of income. As a result, they held great spiritual and cultural significance, and became a sacred symbol of fecundity and fertility. Date palms and evidence of date culture can be found in ancient Assyrian and Babylonian tablets, including the famous *Code of Hammurabi*. Egyptian, Syrian, Libyan, and Palestinian writings contain references to date palms and their fruit. Dates continue to play an important role during the Muslim holiday of Ramadan, when they are enjoyed after long days of fasting. They are also an important part of the feast at the end of Ramadan, the Eid al-Fitr.

The Spanish were the first to introduce date palms to California and Arizona in the seventeenth and eighteenth centuries, when Jesuit

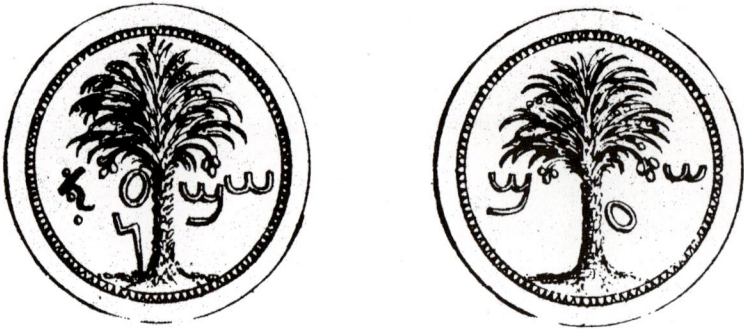

The Date Palm on Ancient Hebrew Coins.
From Calmet, Dictionary of the Holy Bible, *London, 1724.*

and Franciscan monks planted the trees at their missions. Date palms were also planted by farmers in various parts of California, including the Coachella Valley, whose climate is similar to those of date-growing regions in the Middle East.

During the early 1900s, thousands of offshoots representing more than a dozen date palm varieties were imported to California from North Africa and the Middle East. Many farm stands opened along major highways in the Coachella Valley, marketing dates as an exotic food from the faraway and mysterious Middle East, with advertising featuring camels, women in traditional dress, Arabian-style buildings, and, of course, date palm trees. The Coachella Valley remains the center of date cultivation in the United States, with additional groves in Arizona. Dates are also grown in northern Mexico, including in the states of Baja California (Norte and Sur), Sonora, and Coahuila.

There are more than 250 cultivated varieties of dates. The best known are Medjool, Deglet Noor, and Zahidi, with the first two varieties being grown widely in California. They are found in most grocery stores, with the lesser-known varieties found in many Middle Eastern, specialty grocery, or natural foods stores throughout North America and Europe.

Dates are eaten fresh or dried, though dried dates have more flavor and greater mineral content. Dates can be purchased whole (with or without pits) or dehydrated in pieces or diced. They can be enjoyed in cereal, puddings, bread, cakes, cookies, candy bars, ice cream, trail mix, and smoothies. Fresh dates can be made into juice, vinegar, wine, beer, sugar, syrup, honey, chutney, pickle, paste, dips, and as food flavoring.

Dates are a good source of dietary fiber and are rich in calcium, iron, magnesium, and potassium. They also contain a variety of antioxidants that support good digestion, prevent diabetes, and help protect the body from certain types of cancer. However, nutritionists advise that eating large amounts of dried dates can increase blood glucose levels, and advise those with high blood sugar to eat fresh dates instead.

Dates also have medicinal uses. They have long been used as an astringent for treating intestinal problems. Dates have also been used to treat sore throat and colds, relief of fever, cystitis, edema, and liver problems. In India, the gum or exudate of dates is used for treating diarrhea. Dried dates have also been used by pregnant women in the Middle East to help induce labor.

Resources

Chao, C.T., and R.R. Krueger. "The Date Palm (Phoenix dactylifera); Overview of Biology, Uses and Cultivation." *HortScience* 42(5): 1077–1082.

"Dates," Agricultural Marketing Resource Center website, January 2023.

de Candolle, Alphonse. *Origin of Cultivated Plants*. New York: D. Appleton and Company, 1908, 302.

"Dried Dates: Are They Good for You?" WebMD. September 23, 2022.

Wright, G. C. "The Commercial Date Industry in the United States and Mexico." *HortScience* 51,11 (2016): 1333–38.

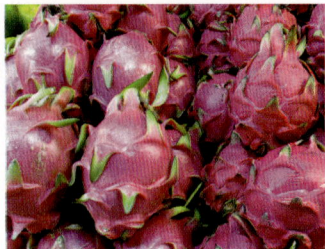

Dragon Fruit

I first encountered dragon fruit (*Hylocereus undatus)* during a visit to Taiwan in 1995. I found the fruit, bright pink in color and featuring a variety of graceful petals, both exotic and delicious, with soft, tiny, black, sesame-like seeds embedded in a subtly sweet, white pulp.

I always believed that dragon fruit was indigenous to Taiwan or at least to other parts of Southeast Asia, but I was wrong. It is actually native to southern Mexico, the Pacific side of Guatemala, Costa Rica, and El Salvador, as well as Venezuela, Colombia, Ecuador, Curaçao, Panamá, Brazil, and Uruguay. Although a relatively new arrival to Europe and North America, it has been enjoyed by discriminating Latin-Americans since pre-Columbian times.

Known as *pitaya* in Spanish and "strawberry pear" in English, dragon fruit is actually a fast-growing, perennial, terrestrial, epiphytic (i.e., a plant that grows on another plant but does not feed from it), vine-like cactus that requires trellises to grow. Described as "the most beautiful fruit in the cactus family," there are at least 250 varieties of pitaya in various colors such as pink, red, purple, yellow, and orange, with white, grey, red, or bright purple pulp, depending on the variety. It is grown mostly in its homeland (Latin America) as well as south Florida, the Caribbean, Hawai'i, Australia, Taiwan, Vietnam, Malaysia, and Israel.

You probably won't find pitaya in the produce section of every supermarket; it is mostly sold fresh in Asian, Latino, and specialty food markets. Pitaya is often enjoyed on its own or added to salads, shakes, and smoothies. Some people slice it and throw it on the grill. Dragon fruit is also commercially processed and added to energy and fruit bars, ice cream, jellies and jams, pastries, and yogurt. Recent research suggests that the dietary fiber from dragon fruit peels can be used to partially replace fat in ice cream. Most of the dragon fruit sold in North America and Europe is imported from Vietnam (pitaya was introduced to what was Indo-China by the French over one hundred years ago; Vietnam is now the world's largest producer) and Central America.

Pitaya has been called a superfruit due to its high nutritional content and proven medicinal value. A recent article in the journal *Pharmaceutics* (Nishikito et al. 2023, 159) by researchers in Brazil, Portugal, and the Philippines explained why dragon fruit enjoys this exalted status:

> Studies have shown that pitaya can exert several benefits in conditions such as diabetes, dyslipidemia [a metabolic disease characterized by high or low levels of fat—including cholesterol and triglycerides—in the blood], metabolic syndrome, cardiovascular diseases, and cancer due to the presence of bioactive compounds that may include vitamins, potassium, betacyanin, p-coumaric acid, vanillic acid, and gallic acid.

In addition to dietary fiber, dragon fruit contains vitamin C, riboflavin, niacin, calcium, phosphorus, magnesium, and iron. Dragon fruit is rich in antioxidants, which help prevent inflammation and cell damage—a major cause of cancer, heart disease, and diabetes. One major antioxidant in dragon fruit is *lycopene*, which occurs naturally in pink fruits and vegetables. While research is ongoing, lycopene may also promote good oral health, bone health, and blood pressure.

Pitaya is also a *prebiotic*, which boosts the production of *probiotics* lactobacilli and bifidobacteria that promote the growth of healthy gut bacteria. And, as it is over 80 percent water, eating dragon fruit is a good way to hydrate the body on a hot summer day.

Resources

Crane, Jonathan H., and Carlos F. Balerdi. "Pitaya (Dragonfruit) Growing in the South Florida Home Landscape." University of Florida IFAS Extension website. January 7, 2020.

"Dragon Fruit: What It Is and Why It's Healthy." healthessentials. Cleveland Clinic website. February 22, 2023.

Iowa State University. "Dragon Fruit." Agricultural Marketing Resource Center website. March 2023.

Nishikito, D. F., A. Borges, L.F. Laurindo et al. "Anti-Inflammatory, Antioxidant, and Other Health Effects of Dragon Fruit and Potential Delivery Systems for Its Bioactive Compounds." *Pharmaceutics* 15, no. 1 (2023): 159.

"Pitaya (Dragon Fruit) History and Homeland." Ejdersim website. Accessed July 13, 2023.

Rebecca, O. P. S., A. N. Boyce, and S. Chandran. "Pigment identification and antioxidant properties of red dragon fruit (*Hylocereus polyrhizus*)." *African Journal of Biotechnology* 9, 10(2010): 1450–1454.

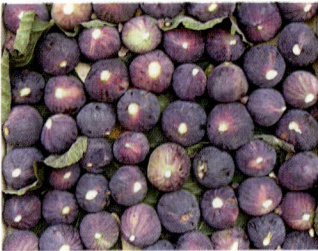

Fig

Figs (*Ficus carica*) are a member of the mulberry family. They are indigenous to an area extending from Asiatic Türkiye to northern India, although natural fig tree seedlings can be found in most Mediterranean countries.

The fig is one of humanity's oldest and most cherished foods. Fig trees were among the earliest fruit trees to be cultivated by *homo sapiens*, beginning around 4000 BCE. Domestication of the wild fig led to the development of bigger and sweeter fruits. Figs were grown primarily around the Aegean Sea and throughout the Levant, which included northern Africa from Morocco east, to Iran in Asia, and northwest from Iran through Europe to what are now Croatia and Romania. The ancient Greeks are said to have received figs from Caria in western Anatolia (now Türkiye). The cultivation of figs by Greek farmers in Paros was first mentioned by the poet Archilochus in 700 BCE. The fig became an important staple food in Greece, and the Spartans were said to have eaten them at their public tables. The Greeks are credited with introducing the fruit to Palestine and Asia Minor.

Figs were well-known in Egypt, where they were called *teb*, and references to these fruits have also been found on tablets in the pyramids of Giza. In France and Italy, fossilized figs have been found in tertiary and quaternary deposits. In ancient Rome, the fig was held sacred by Bacchus, the nature god of fruitfulness and vegetation. A fig tree is associated with the legend of Romulus and Remus—the founders of Rome—standing where their cradle came to rest on the banks of the Tiber after their abandonment near the wolf's cave. It is probable that the Phoenicians spread the culture of the fig tree to Cyprus, Sicily, Malta, Corsica, the Balearic Islands, the Iberian Peninsula, and France.

The first figs were believed to have arrived in China from Persia by traders on the Silk Road. The best-known Western fig, the *Ficus carica*, arrived in China during the early Tang dynasty (618–907 CE). By the sixteenth century, this fig and many others were planted, probably by missionaries, around the lower Yangtze River Basin, joining other varieties already there.

Figs can be enjoyed fresh or dried. They make an excellent and healthy snack food, and can also be served roasted or grilled, or added to salads. Dried figs are a popular ingredient in baking (cakes, cookies, and breads) and also in traditional savory dishes. They can also be used in preserves, jams, and jellies. Figs have been classified as red, white, and black, and more than twenty cultivars have been developed over the years. Popular varieties include the Kadota, Celeste, Mission, Conadria, Green Ischia, and Kari Lob.

Figs have been recognized since ancient times as being good for health. They are rich in vitamins A, B_1 (thiamin), and B_2 (riboflavin), and minerals including calcium, iron, phosphorus, magnesium, sodium, and potassium. Figs contain a type of antioxidant called *phenols*, which studies have shown may lower the risk of heart disease and cancer by preventing cell damage due to free radicals.

Over the centuries, figs have been found to help regulate blood pressure, aid in elimination, support weight control, protect menopausal women from breast cancer, relieve sore throats, and have even been shown to have aphrodisiac properties. In Western folk medicine, poultices made from fresh or dried figs and fig leaves have been used to treat skin problems; latex from stems and leaves have been taken internally as an expectorant and diuretic. Fig leaves have also been valued for their antidiabetic effects and their ability to expel intestinal worms.

The fig has long been important in Traditional Chinese Medicine as slightly cooling, which helps regulate activity of the stomach, lungs, and large intestines. The fruit is considered a gentle detoxifier and a good remedy for chronic dry cough and digestive problems.

Figs continue to be grown extensively in the Mediterranean region, with Türkiye, Egypt, and Morocco being the world's largest producers. Many of the dried figs consumed in the United States are imported from these countries. Fig trees were first introduced to Florida in 1575 by Spanish explorers, and Franciscan missionaries introduced the aforementioned Mission fig to Mission San Diego, California's first Franciscan mission, in 1769. Additional fig cultivars were also imported to the California area from Mediterranean countries, including Türkiye. Although fig production in the United States has declined in recent years, most of the fresh and dried figs produced in the United States are grown in California.

Resources

Chrysopoulos, Philip. "The Fig - An Iconic Greek Fruit Since Ancient Times." GreekReporter.com. March 6, 2021.

de Candolle, Alphonse. *Origin of Cultivated Plants*. New York: D. Appleton and Company, 1908, 296.

"Fig / Ficus carica / Moraceae." Fruits and Vegetables. Frutas-Hortalizas website. Accessed July 12, 2023.

"Fig: Plant and Fruit." *Encyclopedia Britannica*. June 29, 2023.

Keng, Lee Jok. "Figs in Traditional Chinese Medicine." Figara11. September 2021.

Peters, Mike. "Tasty Figs Get New Attention in China's Plates, Farms." ChinaDaily.com. May 15, 2016.

Sarkhosh, Ali and Peter C. Anderson. "The Fig." IFAS Extension. University of Florida website. 2021.

"The Fig Tree: A History of the Fruit and its Cultivation." The Market at DelVal. December 23, 2022.

Veberic, Robert, and Maja Mikulic-Petkovsek. "Phytochemical Composition of Common Fig (*Ficus carica L.*) Cultivars" in *Nutritional Composition of Fruit Cultivars*. New York: Academic Press, 2016.

"Which Country Produces the Most Figs?" Helgi Library. Accessed July 12, 2023.

"Why California?" California Figs website. Accessed July 12, 2023.

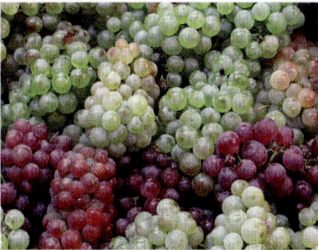

Grape

The art and science of growing grapes (viticulture) is probably as old as human civilization itself. Archeological evidence suggests that our ancestors began growing grapes (*Vitis vinifera*) as early as 6500 BCE. By 4000 BCE, the cultivation of grapes extended from Transcaucasia (comprising present-day Georgia, Azerbaijan, and Armenia) to Asia Minor (the western peninsula of Asia that includes much of modern-day Türkiye) and through the Nile Delta of Egypt. King Hammurabi of Babylon (the author of the famous *Code of Hammurabi*, comprising 282 laws) established rules for the wine trade in 1755 BCE.

The Hittites, an ancient Anatolian people who lived primarily in what is now Türkiye, are credited with spreading grape culture westward as they migrated from Anatolia to Crete, Bosporus and Thrace, as early as 3000 BCE. Later, the Greeks and Phoenicians extended grape growing to Carthage, Sicily and the rest of southern Italy, Spain, and France. The Romans are credited with spreading the cultivation of grapes throughout Europe. According to a history of grape growing published by the University of Missouri:

> At the time of the fall of the Roman Empire, grape culture and wine making primarily were associated with monasteries. Later, the use of wine extended beyond religious rites and became entrenched in culture as a social custom. This increased demand for grapes, and grape culture grew steadily from the sixteenth to the twentieth century. (Trinklein 2013)

Grapes were also found growing in North America, but both their flavor and quality were considered poor for both winemaking and eating. As a result, most of the grapes that are grown in the United States are of European varieties believed to be first introduced to the Americas by Christopher Columbus. As with most of the fruits and vegetables we consume today, today's grapes are the result of centuries of experimentation and hybridization.

Most of the grapes that are grown in the world are devoted to winemaking, totaling some 7.2 trillion gallons (27 trillion liters) in a recent year. Spain, Italy, France, and Türkiye account for some 80 percent of the world's wine production. California is by far the largest wine producer in the United States, followed by Washington state and New York.

Raisins make up the second largest segment of grape production, totaling some eight hundred thousand tons a year. They were first introduced to California and Mexico by Spanish missionaries during the eighteenth century. In the United States, the main region that grows grapes destined to be raisins is the San Joaquin Valley in California. The United States and Türkiye are the world's largest producers of raisins, with California producing nearly all of the raisins grown in the U.S.

Most of the raisins eaten today are of the seedless Thompson variety, developed in the 1880s by William Thompson, an English immigrant to California. In addition to being a stand-alone snack food, raisins are often added to cereal, and are a popular ingredient in granola, muesli, cookies, muffins, breads, curries, and sauces.

Fresh grapes (also known as table grapes) make up approximately 12 percent of world grape production. Since fresh grapes tend to be perishable, they are usually consumed in their countries of origin, although, as a resident of New York City I have often bought grapes imported from Europe and northern Africa. Europe and North America lead the world in both fresh grape production (particularly California and New York, in North America) and consumption. The average American consumes about eight pounds of fresh grapes each year. Grapes are also made into juice, jellies and jams, and grapeseed oil.

As a fruit, grapes are packed with nutrition. They are a good source of vitamins C and K, and also contain protein, carbohydrates, dietary fiber, and minerals including potassium and iron. Grapes are also a source of important micronutrients such as polyphenols, catechins, and anthocyanins, which have protective antioxidant properties that prevent cell damage and help protect the heart, eyes, and brain. Grapes also contain *resveratrol*, a powerful antioxidant found in their skins. In addition to anti-aging properties, resveratrol has been linked to promoting heart and eye health, and reducing the growth of colon cancer. Red grapes (and red wine) contain ten times more resveratrol than green or yellow grape varieties.

Resources

Iowa State University. "Raisins." Agricultural Marketing Resource Center website. March 2023.

Shubrook, Nicola. "Top 5 Health Benefits of Grapes," BBC Goodfood. Accessed August 10, 2023.

"The Laws of Wine Drinking According to the Hammurabi Code," This Day in Wine History website. Accessed August 10, 2023.

"Top 5 Benefits of Grapes," BBC Goodfood. Accessed August 10, 2023.

Trinklein, David. "Grapes: A Brief History." Integrated Pest Management. University of Missouri website. August 7, 2013.

Wikipedia. "Grape," Accessed August 10, 2023.

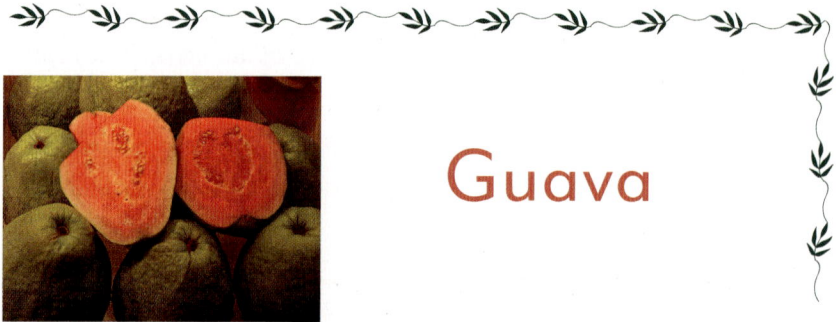

Guava

More than 2.3 million tons of guava (*Psidium guajava*) are grown every year, making it one of the world's most popular tropical fruits. The origin of the guava baffled many early researchers because, by the nineteenth century, guavas were growing throughout the tropical regions of the world. The French-Swiss botanist Alphonse Pyramus de Candolle, author of *Origin of Cultivated Plants* (1908, 143), wrote: "The study and origin of the guava presents in the highest degree of difficulty," yet added: "In order to simplify the search after the origin of the species, I may begin by eliminating the Old World, for it is sufficiently evident that the guava came from the Americas."

Dr. de Candolle was correct: recent archeological evidence shows that sweet and crunchy guavas were first grown (and presumably enjoyed) in what is now coastal Peru as early as 800 BCE. Since that time, guava cultivation gradually spread through South and Central America, having reached Mexico by 200 BCE. From Mexico, cultivation continued on to the Caribbean islands. Guavas were believed to have been "discovered" in Haiti during the seventeenth century by Spanish and Portuguese traders, who introduced the fruit to India, Southeast Asia, and the Pacific Islands.

The guava plant is not a tree, but a small shrub. Over the centuries, many varieties of guavas have been developed that include many different shapes, sizes, colors, textures, and flavors. The most popular varieties are large and pear-shaped with a white inner flesh, although varieties with deep pink flesh are also very popular.

People have traditionally enjoyed guavas raw and cut up with the seeds removed. They are also popular in salads or prepared as juice. Stewed guava shells are made into a popular dessert in Latin America, and guava jelly is a much-loved sweet. Guavas are also added to ice cream, cakes, pies, and chutney—especially in India.

Guavas are an excellent source of vitamin C, and contain significant amounts of vitamin A, iron, calcium, phosphorus, and potassium. They have also been used as a natural medicine to treat diarrhea, infections, heart problems, and allergies. Guavas play a role in modern medicine as well. According to a recent article in the journal *Clinical Phytoscience* (Naseer et al. 2018, 1), "This plant finds applications for the treatment of diarrhea, dysentery, gastroenteritis, hypertension, diabetes, caries and pain relief and for improvement in locomotors coordination."

Contemporary laboratory studies have found that the flavonoids, tannins, gallic acid, and botulin acid found in guava leaves possess both antibacterial and antifungal properties. The phenolic compounds in guava have been found to destroy cancerous cells and help keep the skin looking younger. Guava leaf extract is being used in treating cough, diarrhea, oral ulcers, and swollen gums. There is even some evidence that ethanolic extract of guava can increase both sperm quality and quantity, and can be used for treatment by infertile males.

India is presently the world's largest producer of guavas, followed by China, Mexico, Egypt, and Brazil.

Resources

de Candolle, Alphonse. *Origin of Cultivated Plants*. New York: D. Appleton and Company, 1908, 243.

Arevalo-Marin, Edna, et al. "The Taming of *Psidium guajava*: Natural and Cultural History of a Neotropical Fruit." *Frontiers in Plant Science*. 28 September 2021.

"Guava." University of Kansas American Indian Health and Diet Project website. Accessed August 12, 2023.

"Health Benefits of Guava." Web MD. Accessed August 12, 2023.

Naseer, S., S. Hussain, N. Naeem, et al. "The phytochemistry and medicinal value of *Psidium guajava* (guava)." *Clinical Phytoscience* 4, 32 (2018).

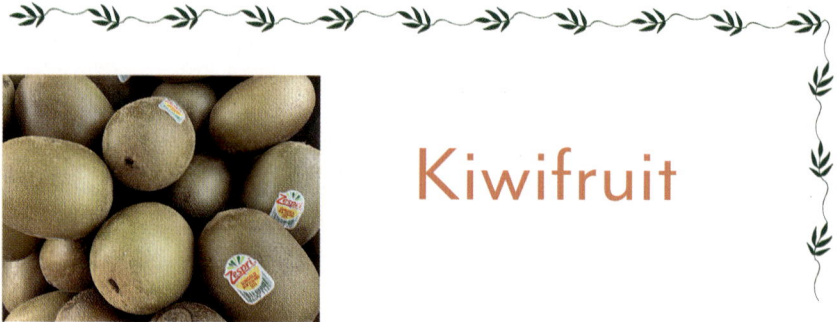

Kiwifruit

Despite its name, the kiwifruit (*Actinidia deliciosa*) is not native to New Zealand, but to China. It is a cultivar of the *Actinidia chinensis*, which was believed to have originated in Hubei and Sichuan provinces, and was first written about during the Song dynasty during the twelfth century. The original variety grew wild, and was mostly used in Traditional Chinese Medicine as a medicinal fruit. The fruit and roots were boiled as tea to treat excessive sweating, arthritis pain, and obesity. Called *xiao yang tao*, kiwifruit is the national fruit of China today.

Seeds were first brought from China to New Zealand in 1904, by Mary Isabel Fraser, the principal of Wanganui Girls' College. They were planted in 1906 by a local nurseryman, and the vines first bore fruit in 1910. People thought the fruit had a gooseberry-like flavor and began to call it "Chinese gooseberry," even though it's technically *not* a gooseberry.

The kiwifruit, considered a true berry, has fuzzy, brown skin (there is also a yellowish variety). The firm, translucent, green flesh has numerous edible, small, purple-black seeds embedded around a white center. The fruit has a delicious, slightly acid flavor, and is usually eaten raw, either as a stand-alone food or added to salads or breakfast cereals.

New Zealand farmers began exporting the fruit to the United States in the 1950s. As this was during the height of the Cold War, the term "Chinese gooseberry" was not well received, and sales were minimal. (In Taiwan, which was called "Free China" at the time, the fruit was known as "monkey head"—also a poor choice for a marketable name.) A resourceful New Zealander named Jack Turner suggested the name "kiwifruit" in 1959. Like the kiwi—New Zealand's national bird—the kiwifruit is small, brown, and furry.

Kiwifruit is highly nutritious. It is a potent source of essential vitamins A, B, C, E, and K, provides appreciable levels of dietary fiber, and contains minerals such as potassium, phosphorous, and calcium. It also is a rich source of a variety of phytochemicals including carotenoids, flavonoids, anthocyanins, and lutein. Together, they contribute to a rich pharmacological profile that helps reduce free-radical damage and supports good health.

A recent article in the peer-reviewed *Journal of Food Processing and Preservation* (Satpal et al. 2021, 45) stated that pharmacological properties of the kiwifruit include antidiabetic, anti-tumor, anti-inflammatory, anti-ulcer, antioxidant, hypoglycemic (reduces blood sugar), hypolipidemic (reduces the amount of fat in the blood), and are also "well recognized for their medicinal and therapeutic properties against diseases associated with the cardiovascular system, diabetes, kidney problems, cancer, digestive disorders, bone, and eye problems."

New Zealand's kiwifruit industry began in 1934 in the town of Te Puke, near the Bay of Plenty, also known as the "Kiwifruit Capital of the World." China is the world's leading producer of kiwifruit today, followed by Italy, New Zealand, Greece, Iran, and Chile. Kiwifruit has also been grown in California since 1967.

Resources

"Chinese gooseberry becomes kiwifruit." *New Zealand History* website. Manatū Taonga—Ministry for Culture and Heritage. June 9, 2020.

"Kiwi." *Encyclopedia Britannica.* Accessed October 8, 2023.

"Kiwifruit Production in California." University of California, Davis. Accessed October 8, 2023.

Satpal, D., J. Kaur, V. Bhadariya, and K. Sharma. "*Actinidia deliciosa* (Kiwi fruit): A comprehensive review on the nutritional composition, health benefits, traditional utilization, and commercialization." *Journal of Food Processing and Preservation* 45, no. 6 (2021):e15588.

Wikipedia. "*Actinidia deliciosa.*" Accessed October 8, 2023.

Williams, Andy. "Health Benefits of Kiwi Fruit." The Paleo Gut website. Accessed October 8, 2023.

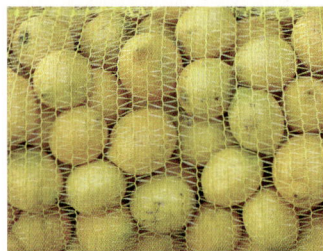

Lemon

Like oranges, lemons (*Citrus limon*) are part of a family of citrus fruits that include tangerines, pomelos, and grapefruit. Citrus is believed to trace its origin at least eight million years back to the southeastern Himalayan foothills, which include the eastern area of Assam (India), northern Myanmar, and western Yunnan (China). Anthropological evidence shows that the actual cultivation of citrus fruits goes back at least four thousand years.

The origin of lemons is not entirely clear. However, an exhaustive DNA study published in 2001 showed that most lemon varieties are derived from a single hybrid between the citron and another fruit that includes genes from both mandarin oranges and the pomelo, an ancestor of grapefruit. The early history of the lemon is difficult to trace, since it was often confused with the citron.

However, the first recipes that mentioned lemon appeared in a twelfth-century Egyptian treatise called *On Lemon: Its Drinking and Use* by Ibn Jumay, a Jewish physician in the court of Saladin, the first Sultan of Egypt and Syria. Ibn Jumay is credited with having found a way to preserve lemons with salt, and for promoting lemon's medicinal uses. Lemons held an important place in Arab culture, and were also highly valued in Persia.

The lemon travelled with Arabs along ancient trade routes, and was introduced into North Africa and Spain between 1000 and 1200 CE. Lemons soon became very popular in Italy and Sicily, and are still among Italy's most important crops. Christian Crusaders, who tried to conquer Jerusalem and its surrounding areas from Muslim rule between 1095 and 1291 CE, found lemons growing in Palestine, and later distributed them in parts of Europe. By 1494, lemons were cultivated in the Azores by early Portuguese settlers, and exported mostly to England. Lemons were said to have been introduced to the New World by Christopher Columbus in the 1490s.

Lemons first appeared at Mission San Gabriel in the San Gabriel Valley (part of Los Angeles County) as early as 1805. William Wolfskill, California's first commercial orange grower and developer of the famous Valencia juice orange, devoted a large portion of his property in southern California to growing lemons in the 1840s. Thanks to the opening of the Transcontinental Railroad and the development of modern refrigeration methods, lemons became an important crop in California by the early 1900s, soon being shipped all over the United States. Six major varieties of lemon tree—including the Eureka, Pink Variegated, Lisbon, Meyer, Primofiori, and Verna—are now grown in California, which is by far the largest lemon producer in the United States. India is the world's biggest grower of lemons, followed by China, Mexico, Argentina, and Brazil.

Lemon juice is a popular ingredient in many pastries and desserts, including cakes, tarts, and lemon meringue pie. Its distinctive astringent flavor is also used to enhance many poultry, fish, and vegetable dishes. Lemonade is a popular warm weather beverage, and juice from the lemon itself is commonly added to tea and water, whether carbonated or still.

Like other citrus fruits, lemons are rich in vitamin C, which supports the body's immune system and helps protect body cells from free-radical damage. Vitamin C also promotes healthy skin and enables the body to absorb iron and thus prevent anemia. The citric acid found in lemons may prevent kidney stones, while lemon juice has antibacterial and antifungal properties. Recent scientific studies in *Plants* have found that "proven therapeutic activities of *C. limon* include anti-inflammatory, antimicrobial, anticancer and antiparasitic activities." Although lemons are too astringent to eat like oranges, fresh lemon juice mixed with water is a pleasant way to obtain both the nutritional and medicinal benefits of lemon.

Resources

Alexander, Rebecca. "Lemon: A Global History." Elizabeth C. Miller Library. University of Washington. November 27, 2013.

Bailey, Natasha. "Most of the Lemons in the US Come from This State." TastingTable.com. November 3, 2022.

Glusen, O., and M. L. Roose. "Lemons: Diversity and Relationships with Selected Citrus Genotypes as Measured with Nuclear Genome Markers." *Journal of the American Society for Horticultural Science* 126, 3 (2001): 307–17.

Spitzzeri, Paul R. "Working the Land: Lemons in Greater Los Angeles." *The Homestead Blog*. The Homestead Museum website. November 28, 2016.

Klimek-Szczykutowicz, M., A.Szopa, and H. Ekiert. "*Citrus limon* (Lemon) Phenomenon-A Review of the Chemistry, Pharmacological Properties, Applications in the Modern Pharmaceutical, Food, and Cosmetics Industries, and Biotechnological Studies." *Plants (Basel)*9, 1 (2020):119.

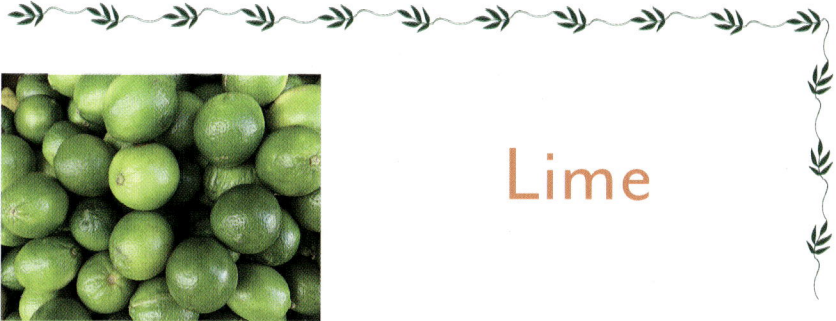

Lime

The lime (*Citrus aurantiifolia*) is a close relative of the lemon. Although their appearance is different, their nutritional and medicinal values are similar, although limes have more acidity and sugars than lemons do. Both have been enjoyed over the centuries in many of the same ways, such as a spritz for beverages and to add zest to food. Like the lemon, limes trace their ancestry to the southeastern Himalayan foothills at least eight million years ago.

Plant geneticists have suggested that only three "true" citrus types exist: the citron (*Citrus medica*), mandarin oranges (*Citrus reticulata*), and the pummelo or pomelo (*Citrus maxima*). Many of the varieties of oranges, lemons, grapefruit, and limes that we enjoy today trace their ancestry to ancient hybrids of two or more of these citrus plants. Limes form a diverse group including acid (or sour) limes and acid-free (or sweet) limes. The most popular lime varieties are Mexican lime; West Indian lime; Egyptian lime; Persian lime; and the Key lime, which helped make Key lime pie—and Florida's Key West—famous.

Limes thrive in humid tropical and subtropical regions of the world. Lime cultivation probably originated in the Malay Archipelago (now Malaysia) and India. The name "lime" is believed to have been derived from the Malay (Austronesian) word *limaw*. Lime cultivation spread to

Micronesia and Polynesia during what is known as the Austronesian Expansion, which took place between 3,500 and 5,000 years ago. Lime cultivation later reached the Mediterranean region via spice trade routes, beginning in about 1200 BCE. Arab traders are believed to have introduced limes to Persia, northern Africa, and Spain during the Middle Ages. In order to prevent scurvy on long voyages, British sailors were given lemons and limes during voyages. This is how they acquired the nickname "limey," which was actually considered an insulting term at the time.

Limes were introduced to the Florida Keys in 1838, where they eventually became known as Key limes. Commercial lime growing developed in Florida in the late 1800s and early 1900s, but was always relatively small. After the Great Miami Hurricane of 1926, most of the lime groves were destroyed. Some Florida farmers then planted Persian (or Tahitian) limes, which are more tolerant to frost, primarily in Miami–Dade county. Production continued until the 1980s, when citrus canker—a type of bacteria—decimated the lime groves, and commercial production ceased. Today, most of the limes consumed in the United States are imported from Mexico.

Like lemons, limes are widely used to enhance both the flavor and nutritional value of various beverages, including water and seltzer; they are also used in margaritas, highball cocktails (usually made with gin), and tropical rum drinks like the daiquiri. Lime juice is also a common ingredient in many traditional Thai, Vietnamese, and Mexican dishes— including guacamole. Limes are used in baking to make American Key lime pie, and are made into marmalade in Australia.

Like other citrus fruits, limes contain high amounts of vitamin C, as well as small amounts of the B vitamins. They also contain minerals—especially calcium, magnesium, phosphorous, potassium, and iron. Vitamin C supports the body's immune system and helps protect body cells from free-radical damage.

Consuming limes also promotes healthy skin and enables the body to absorb iron—thus preventing anemia. Food scientists believe that the citric acid found in limes may prevent kidney stones, while lime juice has antibacterial and antifungal properties. Nutritionists at the Cleveland Clinic (consistently ranked as one of the best hospitals in the United States) recommend that we consume fresh lime juice mixed with water at least once daily, preferably in the morning. This not only insures proper hydration, but helps limit our craving for sugary drinks during the day. In addition to the benefits of drinking water itself, adding fresh lime (or lemon) juice adds the nutritional and medicinal benefits of citrus to our daily diet as well.

Resources

"*Citrus aurantiifolia* (lime)." CABI Digital Library. November 20, 2019. https://www.cabidigitallibrary.org/doi/10.1079/cabicompendium.13438

Cleveland Clinic. "Is Lime Water Good for You?" healthessentials. December 12, 2022.

Harper, Douglas. "Lime." Online Etymology Digital Library. Accessed September 22, 2023.

"Lime." *Wikipedia*. Accessed September 22, 2023.

Plattner, Kristy. "Fresh Market Limes." Economic Research Service. United States Department of Agriculture. September 26, 2014.

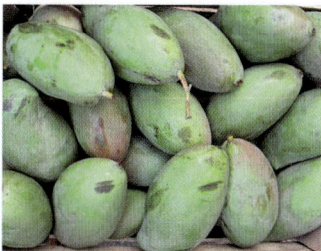

Mango

Like the guava, papaya, and pineapple, the mango (*Mangifera indica*) is one of the world's most important tropical fruits. Botanically known as a *drupe*, the mango consists of an outer skin, edible flesh, and a central stone enclosing a single seed, like the plum, peach, and cherry do.

Recent DNA research has revealed two distinct groups of mango varieties, with commercial varieties tracing their origin to India and indigenous varieties originating in Southeast Asia. The mango is part of the Anacardiaceae family, which includes cashews and pistachios.

Known as the "King of Fruits"—the mango is the national fruit of India, Pakistan, and the Philippines—mangos have been cultivated for over four thousand years within a large area in the Indo-Burmese and Southeast Asian regions. Cultivation spread to other parts of the world beginning around 300 CE, when mango seeds traveled from Asia to the Middle East and eastern Africa with the spice trade. The Portuguese were the first to establish a mango trade from Calcutta (now Kolkata) in the sixteenth century, and Spanish explorers brought mangos to South America and Mexico in the 1600s. European traders brought mango seeds to Brazil during the mid-1700s, and they were brought to Barbados soon after. The French introduced mangos to the Dominican Republic in 1782, and from there they were introduced to Jamaica by the British. Commercial production of mangos began with the introduction of the Haden variety of mango to Miami in 1863.

Traditional varieties have largely been produced through grafting, while mango crossbreeding has become dominant since its introduction to the United States, Australia, and China.

In India, the Jain goddess Ambika is traditionally represented as sitting under a mango tree, and mango blossoms are used to worship Saraswati, the Hindu goddess of knowledge, music, flowing water, abundance and wealth, art, speech, wisdom, and learning. Mango leaves decorate archways and doors in Indian houses during weddings and celebrations connected to Shri Ganesh, the Hindu "Elephant god" of New Beginnings and the Remover of Obstacles.

The mango has a long history as a medicinal food in India's Ayurvedic medical tradition. According to the School of Ayurvedic Diet and Digestion, based in North Carolina:

The smooth, fleshy feel of mango (a sign of demulcent quality) soothes inflamed tissues and prevents dry type constipation. Mangoes' diuretic qualities can be used to cleanse the kidney, while beta carotene's stimulating qualities purify the blood and liver. (Immel, Joyful Belly)

Mangos are often enjoyed raw, although prepared mango has long been a major part of many world cuisines, especially in Asia. In India, mangos are used in chutney (mango chutney) and are added to dahls to provide more flavor. Mango lassi—made with yogurt—is one of India's most popular drinks. In Vietnam, green mangos are sliced and made into salad. Fresh mango is often added to cooked oatmeal and granola, and is used to make juices, smoothies, ice cream (and ice cream topping), and pies. Mango is also enjoyed dried, either by itself or as an ingredient in fruit bars.

Fresh mango contains a wide variety of vitamins and minerals, but provides only vitamin C and folate in significant amounts. Mangos also contain high amounts of dietary fiber, which is linked to improving bowel regularity, supporting weight control, and reducing LDL or "bad" cholesterol. Mangos also contain a particular type of antioxidant called *mangiferin*, which has been found to possibly lower the risk of certain types of cancer, including those of the brain, breast, cervix, colon, and skin. According to dietitian Dr. Carly Sedlacek (2023) of the renowned Cleveland Clinic, "Eating mangoes and other produce in place of processed foods is an effective way to lower your overall cancer risk."

Although the fruit of the mango tree is indeed healthy, the leaves of the tree are considered toxic and can kill cattle or other grazing livestock. For this reason, mango growers and livestock owners are advised to avoid locating grazing areas near mango groves, and to not feed production discards to animals.

Mangoes are widely cultivated in tropical and warmer subtropical areas in the world. India, China, Indonesia, Pakistan, and Mexico are the five major producers. Within the United States, a limited number of mangos are grown in Florida, Hawai'i, California, and Puerto Rico. In a recent year, the global production of mango was 46.5 million tons, which ranks it as the fifth most produced fruit crop worldwide. Most of the mangos consumed in the United States are imported, with more than 80 percent coming from Mexico.

Resources

Cleveland Clinic. "Mango-licious: The Top 6 Health Benefits of Mango." healthessentials. July 3, 2023.

de Candolle, Alphonse. *Origin of Cultivated Plants*. New York: D. Appleton and Company, 1908, 202–203.

Immel, John. "Mango: Health Benefits and Uses." Joyful Belly. Accessed September 22, 2023.

National Mango Board. "Mango History and Production." Mango.org. Accessed September 22, 2023.

University of California, Davis. "Mangos." Western Institute for Food Safety and Security website. Accessed September 22, 2023.

Wang, P., Y. Luo, K. Huang et al. "The genome evolution and domestication of tropical fruit mango." *Genome Biology* 21, no. 60 (2020).

Wikipedia. "Mango," Accessed September 22, 2023. https://en.wikipedia.org/wiki/Mango.

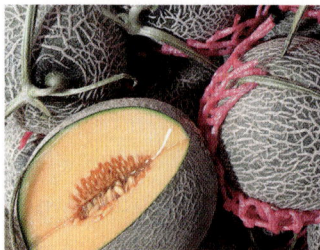

Melon

Most people—including this author—have always considered melons (*Cucumis melo*) to be a fruit, but they are actually a member of the gourd family (of which the cucumber is also a member), and are therefore classified as a *vegetable*. Seven distinct types of melon are grown throughout the world, with the best-known varieties being the cantaloupe, muskmelon, honeydew, casaba, Crenshaw, and Persian.

Plant scientists are confused about exactly where melons originated. The oldest wild relatives of the modern melon are said to be indigenous to Africa, with the first melons cultivated there some three thousand years ago. But there is also evidence that melons date back at least five thousand years, to China, Egypt, and Persia at around the same time. Recent molecular phylogenetic analysis suggests that the melon likely originated in India. Hence, the confusion.

During the 1400s, the first melons were brought from Armenia to the papal state of Cantaluppe, near Rome, from which the cantaloupe melon got its name. But, strangely, the melon we call "cantaloupe" is actually a muskmelon. Muskmelons are identified by the "netting" that covers most of their rind, while cantaloupes have prominent ribs and almost no netting—they are also sweeter and more fragrant than muskmelons. Most "true" cantaloupes are grown in France, where they've been cultivated for some seven hundred years.

Melons arrived in the New World during the second of Christopher Columbus's voyages in 1493, and were first grown in Haiti in 1494. They also spread throughout Latin America during the Spanish Conquest, beginning in the 1500s, and were introduced to California by Spanish explorers and missionaries by 1683.

A number of Native American tribes in New Mexico, including the Acoma, Cochiti, Isleta, Navajo, Santo Domingo, and San Felipe, maintain a tradition of growing their own melon varieties that were derived from melons originally introduced by the Spanish centuries ago. American farmers who trace their ancestry to Europe began to grow melons—especially casaba and honeydew varieties—in the late seventeenth century, and melons have been grown throughout much of the United States since that time. The first commercial hybrid melon was introduced in the United States by Burpee Seeds and Plants in 1955.

Hybrid melons are now the main types of melon grown in the United States today.

Due to their high water and sugar content, melons are tasty and very pleasant to eat, especially on hot summer days. They are primarily enjoyed fresh as a dessert fruit; they can also be sliced and dehydrated, and are a popular addition to a variety of fruit smoothies. In tropical countries, freshly made melon juice is a tasty and nutritious drink. Melons can also be puréed with a small amount of honey and lime juice and poured into molds to freeze and enjoy as frozen pops.

Cantaloupes contain high amounts of vitamins A and C. They are also a good source of potassium and folate.

While honeydew melons are not a great source of vitamin A, they are rich in vitamin C. Honeydews also contain dietary fiber, potassium, folate, and vitamin B_6 (pyridoxine). A recent study on melons carried out by researchers in India showed angiotensin-converting enzyme (ACE) inhibition activity, suggesting their potential usefulness in reducing hypertension. In addition to ACE inhibition, melons have high water content and also contain potassium, making them excellent choices for helping maintain hydration and healthy blood pressure levels.

One intriguing aspect of recent scientific research on melons is the discovery that both melon seeds and especially melon peel possess powerful antioxidants that have effective biological activity against the growth of human tumor cells. Since both melon seeds and peel are generally discarded, scientists are exploring new ways to utilize them more effectively.

China is the world's largest melon grower, followed by Türkiye, India, Iran, Afghanistan, and the United States. Most of the commercially grown melons in the United States are from California, Arizona, Texas, Georgia, and Florida.

Resources

Harvesting History. "The Melon and the Watermelon—A Little History and Some Growing Instructions," Growing Instructions. Accessed September 10, 2023.

Manchali, S., K. N. Chidambara Murthy, Vishnuvardana, B. S. Patil. "Nutritional Composition and Health Benefits of Various Botanical Types of Melon (*Cucumis melo* L.)." *Plants (Basel)* 10, 9 (2021):1755.

Mayo Clinic Health System. "Melons Pack a Nutritional Punch." *Speaking of Health.* August 28, 2018.

Rolim, P. M., G. P. Fidelis, C. E. A. Padilha et al. "Phenolic profile and antioxidant activity from peels and seeds of melon (Cucumis melo L. var. reticulatus) and their antiproliferative effect in cancer cells." *Brazilian Journal of Medical and Biological Research* 54, no. 4 (2018): e6069.

Texas A&M University. "Melons." Horticulture Update. Texas Cooperative Extension. April 2005.

Torres Quezada, Emmanuel. "Basic melon (*Cucumis melo* L.) physiology and morphology." Virginia Cooperative Extension. Virginia Tech. June 9, 2023.

Wikipedia. "Melon," Accessed September 30, 2023.

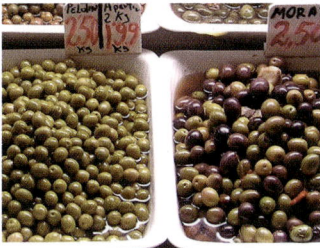

Olive

The olive is one of humanity's most ancient foods. Wild olives (*Elaeagnus angustifolia*) grow throughout the Mediterranean region, tropical and central Asia, and in various parts of Africa. Cultivation of the olive (*Olea europaea*) began about six thousand years ago in what is now Crete and Syria. Living olive trees that are thousands of years old have been found in Portugal, Crete, and the Sea of Galilee region.

The olive has been the symbol of peace, wisdom, glory, fertility, power, and purity since pre-Biblical times. The olive tree is one of the first plants mentioned in the Bible, and is one of the most significant. For example, the olive plant and olives are mentioned over thirty times in both the New and Old Testaments; it was an olive leaf that the dove brought to Noah to demonstrate that the flood was over.

From Crete and Syria, olive cultivation eventually spread to what are now Greece, Spain, Tunisia, Morocco, and other Mediterranean countries, and were an important part of each regions' culinary specialties. The Spaniards introduced olive tree cuttings to colonial Peru in the mid-sixteenth century, and from there Franciscan monks took olives to Central America and then north through the missions of Mexico. In 1769, the first olive cuttings were planted in California (which was then part of Spain) at the San Diego Mission, where the plants thrived. California farmers started planting acres of olive trees in response to the high demand for olive oil in the 1800s.

Olives are diverse and versatile. In addition to olive oil, which is widely used in cooking and as a salad dressing, olives can be made into spreads and tapenades, tossed in salads, or can be added to a wide variety of soups, stews, and sauces. There are literally dozens of olive varieties. They include the Kalamata and Amfissa (Greece); Nym, Picholine, and Niçoise (France); Castelvetrano, Liguria, Gaeta, and Cerignola (Italy); Gordal and Manzanilla (Spain); Alfonso (Chile); Beldi (Morocco); and Mission (United States). Their various flavors have been described as sweet, sour, salty, bitter, pungent, and complex.

As an integral part of the famous Mediterranean Diet, olive oil is an unsaturated fat that has been associated with lower rates of heart disease and regulating blood sugar. A study involving 26,000 women, published in the *Journal of the American Medical Association*, found that the Mediterranean diet could cut the risk of developing cardiovascular disease by up to 28 percent as compared with a control diet. Olive oil is also a good source of vitamins E and K.

Olives contain a wealth of antioxidant and anti-inflammatory micronutrients, some of which are unique to olives. The most important categories include simple phenols, terpenes, flavones, hydroxycinnamic acids, anthocyanidins, flavonols, and hydroxybenzoic and hydroxyphenylacetic acids. Recent studies indicate that these micronutrients may help reduce inflammation and prevent diseases of the heart and blood vessels, neurodegenerative disorders, type 2 diabetes, Alzheimer's disease, and even cancer.

The largest olive producing countries are Spain, Italy, Morocco, Türkiye, and Greece. More than 95 percent of olives in the United States are grown in California, primarily in the state's Central Valley.

Resources

Ahmad, S., M. V. Moorthy, O. V. Demler et al. "Assessment of Risk Factors and Biomarkers Associated with Risk of Cardiovascular Disease Among Women Consuming a Mediterranean Diet." *JAMA Network Open* I, 8 (2018): e185708.

Haifa Negev Technologies. "Crop Guide: Olives." Haifa Group website. 2021.

Howard, Hannah. "A Beginner's Guide to Olives: 14 Varieties Worth Seeking Out." *Serious Eats.* July 14, 2022.

Iowa State University. "Olives." Agricultural Marketing Resource Center website. February 2023.

"Where It All Began: The Story of California Ripe Olives." California Olive Committee website. Accessed October 3, 2023.

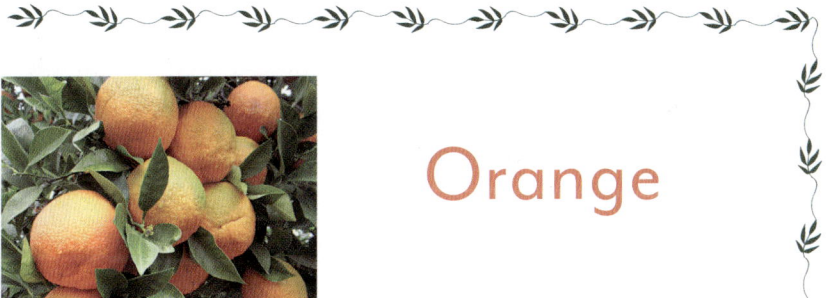

Orange

Oranges are a part of a family of citrus fruits that includes several major cultivated species, including *Citrus sinensis* (sweet orange), *Citrus reticulata* (tangerine and mandarin), *Citrus limon* (lemon), *Citrus grandis* (pomelo), and *Citrus paradisi* (grapefruit).

Citrus fruits are believed to trace their origin to the southeastern Himalayan foothills. A fossil specimen dating from the late Miocene epoch (11.6–5.3 million years ago) in China provides evidence for the existence of a common citrus ancestor within the province of Yunnan approximately eight million years ago. Anthropological evidence shows that human cultivation of citrus fruits goes back at least four thousand years.

The genetic origin of the sweet orange—whose many varieties make up most of cultivated oranges today—is not clear, although some botanists speculate that sweet oranges may have evolved from hybridization of two or more primitive citrus species (probably the pomelo and mandarin orange) at least 2,300 years ago, when sweet oranges were recorded in Chinese literature dating back to 314 BCE.

Cultivation of sweet orange varieties spread throughout China and the rest of Southeast Asia. They moved west along the Silk Road and other commercial trade routes—including one started by the Genoese—and eventually reached Europe during the 1400s. Orange cultivation quickly spread throughout Italy and other Mediterranean regions. Other sweet orange varieties were brought to Portugal from India in 1498 by the explorer Vasco da Gama. The sour or bitter orange (*Citrus aurantium*) is another hybrid that originated in either southern China or northern Vietnam. Early texts report that bitter oranges were eventually brought from India to Oman, and then to Iraq, Syria, Palestine, and Egypt by Arab traders sometime during the tenth century CE.

The Mandarin orange variety (*Citrus reticulata*), the last major orange to travel westward, was brought from China to England in 1805. It was later introduced to Italy and was widely cultivated there by 1850. Cultivation of Mandarin oranges spread quickly to other Mediterranean regions including those in Europe, Asia, and Africa.

Christopher Columbus brought the first orange seeds to the New World in 1493, and the first orange trees were planted in what is now Haiti on the island of Hispaniola. Spanish settlers introduced oranges to Florida between 1535 and 1565, and trees were growing in St. Augustine by 1579. Spanish missionaries brought orange trees to Arizona in 1707 and to San Diego in 1769. The first orange grove was planted at the San Gabriel Mission in 1804; the first commercial orange orchard was established in 1840 near present-day Los Angeles. The popular Navel orange was developed in the 1870s, and is the result of a mutation believed to have occurred sometime between 1810 and 1820 from an orange tree located in Bahia, Brazil.

There are dozens of orange cultivars. In addition to the Navel, some major cultivars include the blood, Cara Cara, "Encore" mandarin, Jaffa, Koji, Mineola, Nagpur, Sagada, Tangor, and Valencia. Over the past ten or twenty years, small orange varieties like the clementine (a hybrid of mandarin and sweet oranges) have become popular snack foods that are seedless, sweet, and easy to peel.

Orange juice has long been a breakfast favorite, although eating an individual orange at breakfast is considered by many nutritionists a better choice, since it contains more dietary fiber, fewer calories, and less sugar than a typical serving of orange juice. Small amounts of orange juice can be added to seltzer to make a healthy and refreshing drink, and oranges can be added to other fruits or vegetables in salad, added to stir-fried dishes, or made into marmalade.

Like other citrus fruits, oranges are high in vitamin C and other antioxidants, which not only support the immune system but promote healthy skin, reduce the risk of heart disease, and may even help prevent colon and other types of cancer. Oranges are also rich in carotenoid, which makes them orange in color. Foods high in carotenoids may reduce the risk of cancers of the head, neck, and prostate. Some carotenoids in oranges are converted into vitamin A, which supports eye health, improves night vision, and may help prevent age-related macular degeneration. Oranges are also a good source of other phytochemicals including D-limonene, a compound that is believed to help reduce the risk of lung, skin, and breast cancer.

Overall, oranges are the most cultivated fruit in the world, and are grown in 124 countries. The world's largest producers are Brazil, China, India, the United States, and Mexico. In the U.S., Florida and California are the two major orange growers: California grows more navel and other "eating" oranges, while Florida grows more oranges that are made into juice.

Resources

"Carotenoids: Everything You Need to Know." healthline. September 18, 2018.

"Health Benefits of Eating Oranges." *The Times of India.* April 11, 2022.

Lim, Lisa. "The orange's origins: how it travelled from East to West and its name evolved." *The South China Morning Post.* February 7, 2023.

"The Origin of Oranges." StoryMaps. Accessed December 1, 2023.

Xu, Q., L. L. Chen, X. Ruan et al. "The draft genome of sweet orange (*Citrus sinensis*)." *Nature Genetics* 45 (2013): 59–66.

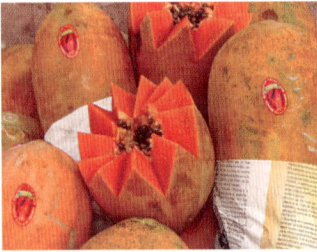

Papaya

The papaya (*Carica papaya*) is one of the world's most popular tropical fruits. Although papaya cultivation has spread throughout the tropics—including Hawai'i, central Africa, India, Australia, and eastern Asia, they are indigenous to southern Mexico (especially what are now the states of Chiapas and Veracruz) and western Central America. Some researchers also consider papaya indigenous to what is now the state of Florida. It is said to have been introduced before 300 CE by predecessors of the Calusa people, who lived on Florida's southwest coast, near the Everglades. Spanish explorers are believed to have introduced the papaya to the Philippines during the sixteenth century, and the fruit soon spread to India and then on to Europe.

Papayas are most commonly eaten raw as a dessert, as well as juice or as part of blended fruit drinks. They are also a popular ingredient in sorbet, ice cream, cakes, and pies. Firmer fruits can be cooked like a root vegetable or baked. In Southeast Asia, green papaya is enjoyed both cooked and raw as an ingredient in salad. In some parts of Asia, the young leaves of the papaya are steamed and eaten like spinach. In Brazil and Paraguay, unripe papaya is used to make sweets or preserves.

Papayas, packed with nutrients, are a major source of vitamin C. They also contain folate, vitamin A, magnesium, copper, pantothenic acid (vitamin B_5), and dietary fiber.

Papaya has long been prized for its medicinal value, especially as a digestive aid. It has also been used to help expel intestinal worms, and even as a contraceptive. In the Brazilian Amazon, traditional healers have used the fruit as an antiseptic. Recent research has discovered that papayas contain a wide variety of beneficial phytochemicals including caffeic acid, myricetin, rutin, quercetin, α-tocopherol, papain, benzyl isothiocyanate (BiTC), and kaempferol.

Clinical studies have found that the health benefits of consuming papaya may include a reduced risk of heart disease, diabetes, and cancer; eating papayas can also help reduce blood glucose levels and blood pressure. In addition to encouraging people to make papaya part of one's diet, scientists are exploring how some of the phytochemicals in papaya can be incorporated into medicines, skin creams, and drinks. A popular food supplement known as fermented papaya preparation (FPP), for example, holds promise in fighting both melanoma and Alzheimer's disease.

The United States is the largest consumer of papayas worldwide. Yet, India is by far the world's leading producer (with an estimated six million tons of fruit harvested in a recent year), followed by the Dominican Republic, Brazil, Mexico, and Indonesia.

Resources

Kong, Y. R., Y. X. Jong, M. Balakrishnan et al. "Beneficial Role of *Carica papaya* Extracts and Phytochemicals on Oxidative Stress and Related Diseases: A Mini Review." *Biology (Basel)* 10, 4 (2021):287.

Sheu, Scott Han, "Papaya." American Indian Health and Diet Project. The University of Kansas.

Ware, Megan, and Mia Blake. "What Are the Health Benefits of Papaya?" Medical News Today. March 23, 2023.

Wikipedia. "Papaya," Accessed December 1, 2023.

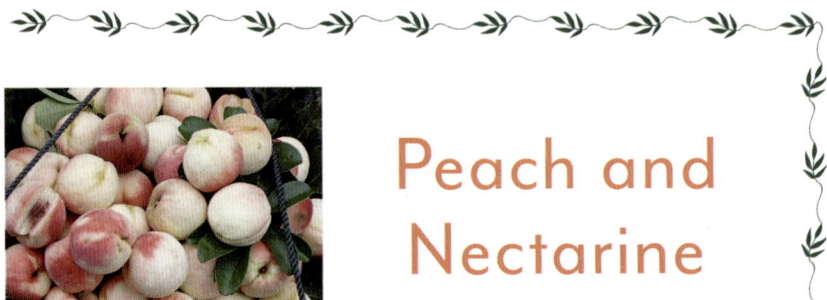

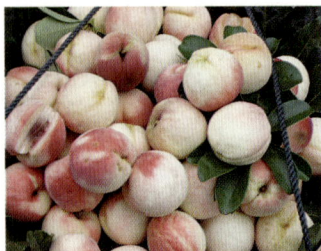

Peach and Nectarine

The peach (*Prunus persica*) is one of America's favorite summer fruits. There are two basic types: *clingstone* and *freestone*. With clingstone peaches, the flesh "clings" to the "stone" (or pit) of the peach, making the peach more difficult to eat, while the pit of the freestone peach "freely" separates from the flesh, making it perfect for quick consumption. Peaches also come in yellow or white varieties, with yellow peaches generally having more flavor.

The peach's botanical name (translated from the Latin as *Persian plum*) would lead people to think the peach originated in Persia, but it is actually indigenous to China. Peaches have been cultivated in China since 6000 BCE in what is now Zhejiang Province, just south of Shanghai.

Many people believe—erroneously—that the nectarine (*Prunus persica*) is a cross between a peach and a plum. Nectarines are actually a naturally occurring mutation of peaches. The two fruits are genetically identical except for one gene, which makes the skin of the nectarine smooth while the skin of the peach is slightly fuzzy. Nectarines are believed to have been domesticated in China some four thousand years ago. Their English name was likely inspired by the German *nektarpfirsich*, or "nectar-peach," in the 1600s.

Peaches have played a significant role in Asian legend, art, and literature. The Chinese have long believed that peaches are symbols of unity and immortality, and that they confer longevity on those who eat them. According to tradition, Chinese brides carry peach blossoms in their bouquets in the hope for a long and harmonious marriage. In Japan, one of the most popular stories for children is about Momotarō, or "Peach Boy." This legend, which is believed to date from the Muromachi period (1392–1573 CE), tells the story of a boy who was born from a peach and grew up to be a hero who fought evil demons. Momotarō is often considered a role model to Japanese children for his bravery and kindness.

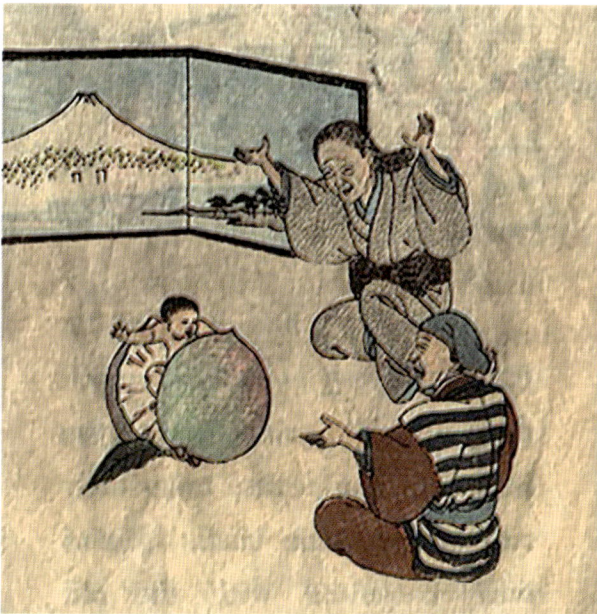

The birth of Momotarō, from *Momotarō or "Little Peachling."*
Kobuncha Publishing Company, Tokyo, 1885.

From China, the peach travelled west along the Silk Road to Persia, where it was widely cultivated—which is probably why it was named *Prunus persica*. Alexander the Great is said to have introduced peaches to Europe after his Macedonian army conquered Persia in 331 BCE. Peaches eventually arrived in England during the seventeenth century, where they were highly valued. However, most European peaches have been grown in the southern part of the continent, where the climate is milder.

Peaches were introduced to North America by Spanish monks around St. Augustine, Florida, in the mid-1500s. By 1607, peaches were growing in and around Jamestown, Virginia, and later began to be cultivated in what became the southern United States. The Elberta peach was introduced by horticulturist Samuel H. Rumph in Georgia during the 1870s. Described as "a clear seeded peach with yellow flesh and a crimson blush on its cheek," it became one of the most popular peach varieties in the United States.

Peaches are among the most delectable of fruits, and are usually eaten raw or baked into pies, cakes, or muffins. Peaches also can be eaten grilled or made into chutneys, jams, or relish; they are even a popular topping on ice cream. Dried peaches are a popular snack, whether alone or as part of trail mixes. They can also be enjoyed as freshly made juice or in fruit smoothies.

In Chinese mythology, peaches have been a symbol of immortality (or the wish for a long and healthy life) for thousands of years, and they have been a part of Traditional Chinese Medicine for centuries. Peaches are known for their ability to tonify *yin* (the so-called passive female quality in nature), help to promote the circulation of *qi* (life force), and to disperse cold. A medicine made from peach kernels is specifically used to treat blood stasis, or poor circulation.

Peaches contain moderate amounts of dietary fiber, protein, potassium, and vitamins A and C. Along with the vitamins, carotenoids—which give the peach its rich yellow-orange color—are powerful antioxidants and free-radical scavengers. A 2021 article in the peer-reviewed journal *Food Reviews International* adds:

> The phenolic compounds in peach-like quercetin, catechins, and cyanidin derivatives have been found to play important roles due to their antioxidant, antimicrobial, and anti-inflammatory properties. Evidence has risen about their preventive effects on multiple chronic and age-related diseases such as diabetes, obesity, hypertension, inflammation, cardiovascular, neurodegenerative, and oncologic (cancer-related) diseases. (Bento et al. 2020, 1703)

Peaches have been found to reduce cholesterol and help lower blood pressure; they also aid in digestion and reduce inflammation. Long-term inflammation can lead to heart disease and cancer, and has been linked to Alzheimer's disease. Nutritionists also teach that peaches strengthen the immune system and support healthy eyes and skin.

China is the world's largest grower of peaches and nectarines, followed by Spain, Italy, and the United States. The top four peach-producing states are California, South Carolina, Georgia, and New Jersey.

Resources

Bento, C., A. C. Gonçalves, B. Silva, and L. R. Silva. "Peach (*Prunus Persica*): Phytochemicals and Health Benefits." *Food Reviews International* 38, no. 2 (2020): 1703-34.

Cleveland Clinic. "All the Health Benefits of Eating Peaches." healthessentials. August 26, 2021.

"Countries by Peach and Nectarine Production." AtlasBig.com. Accessed December 2, 2023.

"Fascinating facts: peaches." The Royal Horticultural Society. Grow Your Own. 2023.

Iowa State University. "Peaches." Agricultural Marketing Resource Center website. February 2023.

Kajino, Atsuko, Wenming Bai, Norio Yoshimura, and Masao Takayanagi. "Identification of peach and apricot kernels for traditional Chinese medicines using near-infrared spectroscopy." *Vibrational Spectroscopy* 113 (2021): 103202.

"Nectarine." *Encyclopaedia Britannica.* August 18, 2023.

Okie, William Thomas. "The Fuzzy History of the Georgia Peach." *Smithsonian Magazine.* August 14, 2017.

University of Georgia. "Peaches." College of Agricultural and Environmental Sciences. Accessed December 2, 2023.

Pear

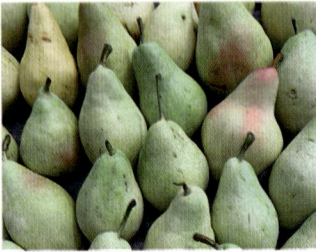

Pears (*Pyrus communis*) rank among world's most treasured fruits. Their refreshing, crunchy texture and sweet, yet delicate flavor have made them a favorite throughout the world. Like their cousin the apple (both are members of the rose [Rosaceae] family), pears are widely grown in the temperate regions of the world, and are enjoyed in similar ways.

Pears trace their genetic origin to the Tertiary period, between 65 to 55 million years ago, in the mountainous regions of southwestern China. Pear seeds gradually spread across mountain ranges both eastward and westward, probably by birds and other animals. Once in Europe, the pear had its dispersion toward the east from what are now northern Italy, Switzerland, and Germany to the former Yugoslavia, Greece, Moldova, and Ukraine; it also gradually spread west and south from China to what are now Japan, Korea, Bhutan, Uzbekistan, and Iran.

This eventually led to the independent development of Asian pears (*Pyrus pyrifolia*), including the Hosui and Nijisseiki varieties, and European pears (*Pyrus communis*), of which the Bartlett, Bosc, and

D'Anjou varieties are the most popular. Cultivation of European pears goes back more than three thousand years. The earliest cultivation of Asian pears can be traced back to about 3,300 years ago, with commercial orchards known to have existed for more than two thousand years in China.

The early Romans cultivated pears before the birth of Christ, and reported more than forty cultivars existing during the first century BCE. Early Roman writings also described methods of cultivation that were remarkably similar to how pears are grown today. By the mid-800s, French farmers had embraced pear cultivation, and by the sixteenth and seventeenth centuries France had become the world's largest producer of the fruit. Pear seeds were introduced by English and French settlers to British and French colonies in North America, and in 1629 there was record of its cultivation in New England. Other records indicate that Chinese immigrants introduced Asian pears to the West Coast of the United States during the 1800s. The crisp, juicy texture and apple-like flavors of Asian pears have led many to refer to this fruit as the apple-pear, although the Asian pear is not a cross between apple and pear.

Pears have a sweet yet subtle flavor, and are often used commercially to make processed foods like canned pears, baby food, pear nectar, vinaigrettes, and fruit and energy bars. Yet most people prefer to enjoy the pear *in natura* or dried, or as an ingredient in pies, cakes, jams, and ice cream.

Because they are low in calories, pears are a popular diet food. In addition to dietary fiber, pears contain generous amounts of vitamins A, B_1, B_2, B_3, and C, along with minerals such as potassium, phosphorus, calcium, magnesium, copper, and iron. Pears are also an excellent source of polyphenol antioxidants, which protect against oxidative damage. Regularly consuming polyphenols is thought to boost digestion and brain health, and to also protect against heart disease, type 2 diabetes, and even certain cancers. Nutritionists recommend that we eat the whole pear, minus the seeds, since the peel of the pear contains up to six times more polyphenols than the flesh. Pears are also recommended to treat constipation and intestinal inflammation. They have also been used in folk medicine as a cure for cystitis and kidney stones.

A recent article in the peer-reviewed journal *BMC Complementary Medicine and Therapies* (Hong et al. 2021, 219) highlighted the impressive medicinal effects of pears:

> From various in vitro, in vivo, and human studies, the medicinal functions of pears can be summarized as [having] anti-diabetic, -obese, -hyperlipidemic, -inflammatory, -mutagenic, and -carcinogenic effects, detoxification of xenobiotics [chemical substances found within an organism that are not naturally produced or expected to be present in the organism], respiratory and cardio-protective effects, and skin whitening effects.

China is the world's largest producer of pears, followed by the United States, Argentina, Italy, and Türkiye. In the United States, California, Oregon, and Washington are the major pear producers, followed by New York, Michigan, and Pennsylvania.

Resources

Hong, S. Y., E. Lansky, S. S. Kang, and M. Yang. "A review of pears (*Pyrus spp.*), ancient functional food for modern times." *BMC [BioMed Central] Complementary Medicine and Therapies* 21, no. 1 (2021): 219.

Iowa State University. "Pears." Agricultural Marketing Resource Center. February 2023.

Petre, Alina. "What are Polyphenols? Types, Benefits and Food Sources." healthline.com. July 8, 2019.

Powell, Arlie A., "Asian Pear Culture in Alabama." Auburn University. Accessed December 9, 2023.

Silva, G. J., Tatiane Medeiros Souza, Rosa Lía Barbieri, and Antonio Costa de Oliveira. "Origin, Domestication, and Dispersing of Pear (*Pyrus spp.*)." *Advances in Agriculture* (2014).

Wartenberg, Lisa. "9 Health and Nutrition Benefits of Pears." healthline. com. February 4, 2023.

Wu, Jun, et al., "Diversification and independent domestication of Asian and European pears." *Genome Biology* 19 (2018): 77.

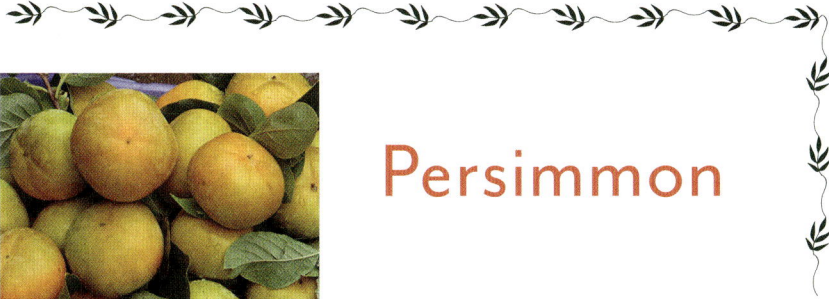

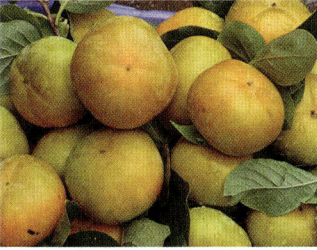

Persimmon

The first time I tasted a persimmon, I was in my early twenties—over fifty years ago. I had recently moved to Ojai, California, and my neighbor Rose welcomed me with a persimmon from a tree that was growing in her front yard. It was light orange, crunchy, and very sweet.

It appears there are two major commercial varieties of the persimmon. One is the American persimmon (*Diospyros virginiana*), which is indigenous to North America, and the Japanese persimmon (*Diospyros kaki*), which is native to China. The Latin name for persimmon (*Diospyros*) originates from the Greek *dióspuron*, which means "food of Zeus."

The American persimmon grows naturally in the eastern United States, from the Gulf States north to Pennsylvania and Illinois. The fruit is generally deep orange and red in color. The name persimmon comes from *putchamin*, a phonetic rendering of the name used by the Algonquin people. It can be translated to mean "choke fruit," probably in reference to the sour flavor of the unripe fruit. The earliest mention of persimmons is found in the journals of the Spanish explorer Hernando de Soto's expedition through parts of what is now the southeastern and south-central United States during the 1550s. He referred to them as a "tasty fruit," and as the source of a bread made by Native Americans.

The Japanese persimmon (known as *kaki*) grows extensively in both China and Japan, and tends to be light orange in color. It was introduced to France and other Mediterranean countries during the nineteenth century and was later brought to California, which is now the most important producer of Japanese persimmons in the United States. There are literally dozens of persimmon cultivars, with the Hachiya, Jiro, and Fuyu among the most popular.

China remains the world's major producer of persimmons, followed by Spain, Japan, South Korea, Azerbaijan, and Brazil. Persimmons imported into the United States are the Japanese varieties from Spain, Israel, Chile, and South Africa. American persimmons are exported from the United States, mostly to Canada and Mexico.

Fresh persimmons are often enjoyed peeled and cut up, firm or soft, and can also be used in salads. More astringent varieties are often frozen and eaten like ice cream. Persimmons are also used as an ingredient in cakes, cookies, and other baked goods, as well as in ice cream and preserves.

Native Americans prized the persimmon for its medicinal value. The inner bark of the tree and unripe fruit have been used by traditional healers in the treatment of fever, diarrhea, and hemorrhage. Persimmons have also been used in Traditional Chinese Medicine for improving the function of the lungs, stomach, spleen, and intestines. They have also been used by traditional Chinese doctors to treat a wide range of health problems including hypertension, hemorrhages, diabetes, insomnia, and atherosclerosis.

The fruit of the persimmon is astringent, and is a primary source of vitamin A, which supports eye health. It is also a good source of vitamins C, E, and K. Persimmons are rich in antioxidants and tannins, which kill off free radicals in the body. These free-radical scavengers in persimmons have been linked to reducing the risk of developing diabetes, lowering the chances of stroke, treating hypertension, and having anti cancer (especially anti-tumor) properties. Persimmons have also been found to have anti-inflammatory properties that have proven useful in treating arthritis and certain allergic reactions.

Resources

"American Persimmon." *Encyclopedia Britannica.* Accessed December 12, 2023.

"*Diospyros virginiana.*" NC State Extension. NC State University. Accessed December 12, 2023.

Direito, Rosa, João Rocha, Bruno Sepodes, and Maria Figueira. "*Diospyros kaki L.* (Persimmon) Phytochemical Profile and Health Impact to New Product Perspectives and Waste Valorization." *Nutrients* 13, no. 9 (2021): 3283. 10.3390/nu13093283.

Iowa State University. "Persimmon." Agricultural Marketing Resource Center website. March 2023.

Skalicky, Francis. "Facts of persimmons as interesting as folklore," *Springfield News-Leader.* October 5, 2018.

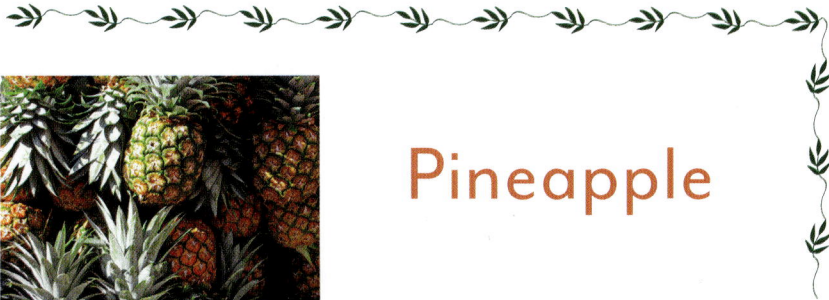

Pineapple

While its exact origins have yet to be determined, botanists agree that the pineapple (*Ananas comosus*) originated in South America, probably in the Iguassu Falls region where present-day Argentina, Paraguay, and Brazil meet. Archaeological evidence of pineapple consumption has been traced as far back as 1200–800 BCE in what is now Peru, and between 200 BCE–700 CE in Mexico, where it was cultivated by the Aztecs, Maya, and other Indigenous peoples.

The first European to encounter the pineapple was Christopher Columbus, during his visit to what is now the Caribbean island of Guadalupe in November 1493. Botanist Alphonse de Candolle reported that a pineapple was brought from Mexico to King Charles V of Spain, but he "mistrusted it, and would not taste it." The Portuguese took the fruit from Brazil and introduced it into India by 1550, while the Spanish introduced a pineapple cultivar to the Philippines at about the same time. The pineapple was finally introduced to Europe during the sixteenth century, and was grown in greenhouses as an exotic luxury fruit.

No one knows when the first pineapple (called *halakahiki*, or "foreign fruit," in Hawaiian) arrived in Hawai'i, but it was believed to have been introduced by Francisco de Paula Marín, a Spanish adventurer. He became both an interpreter and a trusted advisor to King Kamehameha I. He was also an accomplished horticulturist, and introduced both citrus fruits and mangoes to Hawai'i. In a simple diary entry from January 1813, he wrote: "This day I planted pineapples and an orange tree."

A sailor, Captain John Kidwell, is credited with establishing Hawai'i's pineapple industry, having imported and tested a number of varieties in the 1800s for commercial crop potential. But it wasn't until James Drummond Dole arrived on the islands in 1899 (a year after the United States annexed Hawai'i, which was previously a sovereign kingdom) that the pineapple was transformed from an exotic foreign fruit into an American household staple.

By 1923, his Hawaiian Pineapple Company (later, Dole Food Company) was the largest pineapple packer in the world. Between 1930 and 1940, Hawai'i dominated the canned pineapple industry, and at its mid-century peak eight pineapple companies were in operation, employing about three thousand people. After World War II, the canned pineapple industry spread to other parts of the world—especially Thailand and the Philippines—and the Dole cannery eventually closed its Hawaiian operations in 1991. Pineapples continue to grow in Hawai'i for the local market.

The pineapple has long been a symbol of hospitality in many parts of the world. It is believed that during one of Columbus' voyages to the West Indies, he found that natives who hung the fruit in front of their entrances were welcoming to strangers. Pineapples soon became a symbol of hospitality among the gentry in Europe, with the idea later spreading to Colonial America, where houses often had the pineapple's image displayed in common areas. It is also viewed as a symbol of "blooming" in Taiwan, and can be found on display when a new business or other enterprise opens for the first time.

The pineapple, one of the world's most popular fruits, is grown in many tropical countries. Pineapples are best eaten raw or prepared as juice. They are also enjoyed in dry form, and as an important ingredient in yogurt, cakes, candy, salads—and as a zesty pizza topping. I remember enjoying freshly peeled small pineapple on a stick in Taiwan and *jugo de piña* at traditional markets in Mexico.

In addition to being a good source of vitamin C, pineapples contain vitamins A, B_6, folate, E, and K, as well as essential minerals like calcium, iron, magnesium, phosphorus, potassium, and zinc. The pineapple has also been found to have medicinal value. In addition to being good for digestion, pineapples contain bromelain, a substance that reduces inflammation. A recent article in the peer-reviewed journal *Food Research International* stated:

> Pineapple contains considerable amounts of bioactive compounds, dietary fiber, minerals, and nutrients. In addition, pineapple has been proven to have various health benefits including anti-inflammatory, antioxidant activity, monitoring nervous system function, and healing bowel movement. (Ali et al., *Food Research International*)

Although they require some effort to prepare (washing the pineapple, removing the crown and skin, slicing the fruit from top to bottom, and removing the core), fresh pineapple ranks as the sixth most popular fruit in the United States, with the average per capita yearly consumption at 7.88 pounds.

More than 80 percent of the fresh pineapples consumed in the United States are imported from Costa Rica; other suppliers to the U.S. market include Mexico, Guatemala, Ecuador, and Thailand. In addition to Costa Rica, major world producers include the Philippines, Indonesia, Brazil, Thailand, and India. There are more than twenty-five commercial varieties of this fruit, with the most popular known as the *MD-2 cultivar* (called the "Golden Pineapple"), a hybrid developed for its sweetness, low acidity, and because it doesn't turn brown when refrigerated. Other varieties include the Hilo, the Pernambuco, the Red Spanish, and the popular Smooth Cayenne, which is grown extensively in the Philippines.

Resources

Ali, M. Mohd, N. Hashim, S. Abd Aziz, and O. Lasekan. "Pineapple (*Ananas comosus*): A comprehensive review of nutritional values, volatile compounds, health benefits, and potential food products." *Food Research International* 137 (2020).

Booth, Stephanie. "Health Benefits of Pineapple," Web MD. Accessed December 18, 2023.

de Candolle, Alphonse. *Origin of Cultivated Plants*. New York: D. Appleton and Company, 1908, 311.

"Per capita consumption of fresh fruit in the United States in 2021, by selected fruit type." Food & Nutrition. Statista.com. November 2022.

Rhodes, Jesse. "It's Pineapple Season, But Does Your Fruit Come from Hawaii?" *Smithsonian Magazine*. March 20, 2013.

"The History of the Pineapple." Dole Plantation website. Accessed December 18, 2023. https://www.doleplantation.com/resources.

"U.S.: APHIS seeks comments on pineapple imports from the Philippines." FreshFruitPortal.com. March 12, 2021.

Wiessman, Cale. "The Hidden History of the Housewarming Pineapple." *AtlasObscura*. November 14, 2022.

Wikipedia. "Pineapple," Accessed December 18, 2023.

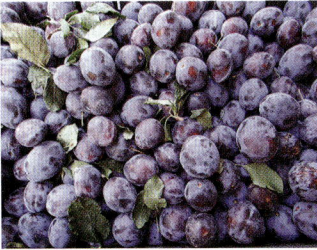

Plum

Plums are fleshy fruits that encase a single seed within a tough shell. Known mostly for their deep purple hues, plums actually come in a range of colors including white, yellow, green, and red. *The Plums of New York*, published in 1911, catalogs 1,500 varieties of Old World plums in that state, including the rare blue-skinned, green-fleshed Tragedy plum. There are now about 140 plum varieties commercially available in the United States, although most of the plums sold in American supermarkets are dark purple and red cultivars, as well as Italian prunes. Lesser-known plum varieties like the Myrobalan (cherry), Emperor, Victoria, Greengage, and Mirabelle can be found in farmers markets and at specialty greengrocers.

Origin stories of the plum suggest that remains of European plums (*Prunus domestica*), the most common plum species, have been found in archaeologic sites traced to the Caucasus Mountains during the Neolithic Age, which began some 12,000 years ago. Plums eventually were introduced to eastern Asia and Europe from the Caucasus and Caspian Sea regions by Mongols, Tartars, Turks, and Huns.

Japanese plums, also known as Chinese plums (*Prunus salicina*), originated in central China thousands of years ago, where the plum was enjoyed both as a food and used as a medicinal plant. Extensively developed in Japan, it was introduced to the rest of the world by Portuguese traders. Japanese plums eventually found their way to India, South Africa, the entire Mediterranean region, Mexico, South America, and certain areas of the United States.

There is also evidence that wild plums grew in what is now the northern United States, and have been a favorite food of Native Americans for thousands of years. These small native plums (*Prunus americana*) can still be found across much of North America, from New England to the Rocky Mountains.

European immigrants to the United States during the eighteenth and nineteenth centuries brought many varieties of plums, but mostly under the genus of *Prunus domestica*, which includes prunes, green-gages, and egg plums. They also brought varieties of *Prunus insititia*, a genus believed to have originated in Syria which includes damsons and bullaces.

The first named cultivars of European plums arrived in California in 1851, followed by Japanese plums in 1870. Most of the plums now grown in the United States (some 97 percent) are from California. China, Romania, Serbia, and the United States are the largest producers of plums worldwide. Chile provides most of the plums imported into the United States, especially during the winter months.

The American botanist and horticulturist Luther Burbank (1849–1926) developed 113 named varieties of plums from tress that were brought to the United States from Japan, including the popular Santa Rosa plum variety. California breeder Chris "Floyd" Zaiger (1926–2020) produced some of the most famous plum-apricot hybrids called *pluots*, which have become a popular summer fruit.

Plums are mostly eaten raw or dried (aka prunes), but can also be enjoyed in smoothies, cakes and pies, chutneys and jams. Creative chefs add plums to casseroles and stir-fried dishes. Plums are also pickled and preserved, especially in Asia. In addition to having been consumed as plum and prune juice, plums have long been a primary ingredient in alcoholic drinks. In her article about plums in the *Los Angeles Book Review*, Anca L. Szilágyi reported that varieties of plum brandy abound in eastern Europe, including the Romanian *tsuica*, often served before every meal; the Damson-derived *slivovitz* of Serbia; Hungary and

Transylvania's *pálinka*; and Albania's *raki*, which is made at home from small red plums. My Taiwanese friend Vincent buys small, green, fresh Japanese *ume* plums every fall and makes exquisite Japanese plum wine (*umeshu*) which he shares with family and friends. Umeshu is believed to have arrived in Japan from China some one thousand years ago, and was first used as a medicinal beverage to treat sore throat.

A standard-sized plum has 8.5 grams of carbohydrate, one gram of dietary fiber, and just thirty-five calories, making it a low-calorie food. Plums also contain vitamin C, vitamin A, and a variety of antioxidants and phytonutrients that promote cardiovascular health and reduce the risk of type 2 diabetes. Prunes (dried plums) have a reputation for promoting bowel regularity, and have been found to be a better laxative than psyllium to treat mild to moderate constipation.

Plums and prunes are also a good source of boron, a trace mineral that has recently been found to offer a wealth of health benefits: it is essential for the growth and maintenance of bone; greatly improves wound healing; beneficially impacts the body's use of estrogen, testosterone, and vitamin D; boosts magnesium absorption; raises levels of antioxidant enzymes; protects against pesticide-induced oxidative stress and heavy-metal toxicity; and improves the brain's electrical activity, cognitive performance, and short-term memory among elders.

A recent article published in the peer-reviewed *International Journal of Food Properties* addressed the abundance of phytochemicals in plums and their numerous health benefits:

> Plums are the abundant sources of predominant antioxidants and phenolic compounds [. . .] These antioxidants and bioactive compounds are effective in the treatment and prevention of gastrointestinal diseases, bone heath, and cardiovascular diseases and in maintaining the blood glucose level. Plums helps [*sic*] in the [*sic*] heart diseases prevention, as it is low in fat content and high in dietary fiber. It is also effective in the treatment of lung and oral

cancer. The consumption of plums boosts human health and prevents many diseases. (Ayub et al. 2023, 2388)

The world's leading plum grower is China, followed by Romania, Chile, Serbia, and Iran. The majority of plums grown in the United States—the world's seventh largest plum producer—are from California, followed by Washington, Oregon, Idaho, and Michigan. Most are "fresh" plums destined for supermarkets and greengrocers, while the remainder are grown for use as prunes, which have been recently renamed for marketing purposes as "dried plums." As a major grower of fresh plums, Chile exports a large portion of its summer crop to the United States and Canada during the winter months in North America.

Resources

"All About Japanese Plums." Minnetonka Orchards. September 14, 2022.

Ayub, H., M. Nadeem, M. Mohsin et al. "A comprehensive review on the availability of bioactive compounds, phytochemicals, and antioxidant potential of plum (*Prunus Domestica*). *International Journal of Food Properties* 26, no. 1 (2023): 2388–2406.

Damery, Jonathan. "Recalling Plums from the Wild." *Arnoldia*. 75, no. 3 (2018).

Iowa State University. "Plums." Agricultural Marketing Resource Center website. February 2023.

Karp, David. "Luther Burbank's Plums." *Horticultural Science* 50, 2 (2015): 189-94.

Oxender, Bethany. "Plums: A Sweet Fruit with a Juicy History." *Food & Nutrition* (2021).

"100 Best Drinks from Japan: #2 Umeshu." Food & Drink. All About Japan website. Updated January 30, 2018.

Pizzorno, Lara. "Nothing Boring About Boron." *Integrative Medicine: A Clinician's Journal* (Encinitas)14, no. 4 (2015): 35-48.

"Plum production by country–2024." World Population Review. 2024.

Szilágyi, Anca L. "Dark Fruit: A Cultural and Personal History of the Plum." *Los Angeles Review of Books*. October 6, 2016.

"What are Stone Fruits?" MasterClass.com. July 20, 2021

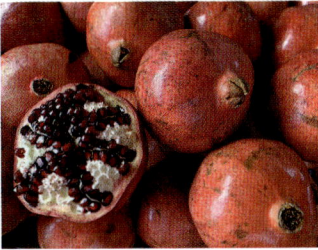

Pomegranate

The pomegranate (*Punica granatum*) is one of the world's most attractive fruits, with a rich red color topped by a "royal crown." Pomegranates have many soft seeds that are surrounded by crimson, pink, purplish, or white covers called *arils*, which are juicy and have a refreshing, sweet-sour flavor. Although it is considered one of humanity's most ancient fruits, its high concentration of antioxidants and other phytochemicals has recently propelled the pomegranate to "superfood" status.

The pomegranate originated in a region extending from modern-day Iran to parts of Afghanistan and southwestern Pakistan, and has been cultivated for at least five thousand years. They were grown in Persia by 3000 BCE, and also in the holy city of Jericho in what is now the West Bank. The Phoenicians introduced the fruit to what is now Tunisia and Egypt by 2000 BCE. Pomegranates also became naturalized in what are now Türkiye and Greece. Traders introduced the pomegranate to China by 100 BCE, and cultivation expanded throughout the country during the Ming (1368–1644) and Qing (1636–1912) dynasties. By 800 CE, the fruit had spread through the Roman Empire, including Spain. The Spanish brought the pomegranate to Mexico, Central America, and South America during the 1500s and 1600s.

Spanish settlers introduced the pomegranate to the California missions in 1768; California remains the biggest producer of pomegranates in the United States, with production centered in the San Joaquin Valley. Pomegranates thrive in Mediterranean climates, with cool winters and hot summers. More than twenty different pomegranate cultivars

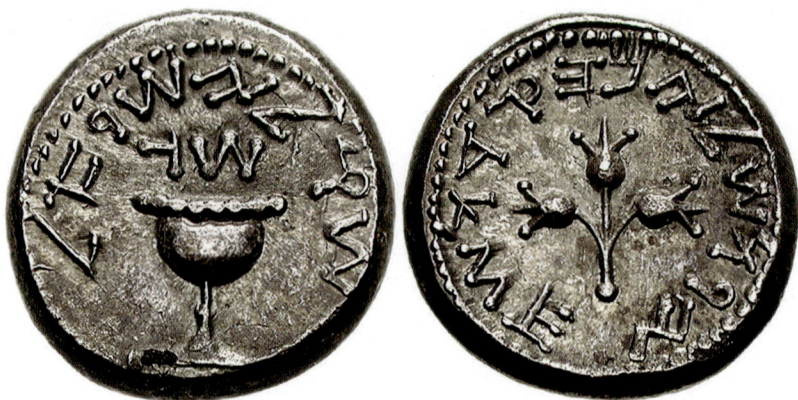

Shekel of Israel with Pomegranate Design,
dated year 3 (CE 68-69).
Courtesy of Classical Numismatic Group, Inc.

are grown today, mainly in India, Iran, Türkiye, China, and the United States.

The pomegranate has a rich cultural history. Early Jews and Christians considered the pomegranate tree to be a Tree of Knowledge, and images of the pomegranate were found in King Solomon's temple. Early Muslims believed that, in every pomegranate, one seed could be found that came from Paradise. To this day, fresh pomegranate juice is given to Muslim babies in the hope that the "Paradise seed" will be consumed by the baby.

In ancient Greece, the pomegranate was connected to both Aphrodite, the goddess of love, and to Hera, the goddess of marriage and childbirth. The Chinese poet Pan Yue (247–300 CE) called the pomegranate "the strange[st] tree under heaven with the most beautiful fruit in China." Pomegranate, or 石榴 (shí liú) in Chinese, has traditionally been considered to be one of the "five famous fruits"—along with the peach, apricot, plum, and quince—that have been essential to Chinese culture. Pomegranate's rich red color is believed to represent prosperity and happiness, and the fruit itself is symbolic of fertility and good fortune. Pomegranates were once given as a tribute to feudal emperors, and are now considered a thoughtful gift at weddings and other auspicious occasions. Pomegranate has played in an important role in ancient healing traditions including Traditional Chinese Medicine, and Ayurvedic medicine in India.

Pomegranates are best eaten fresh, although some make pomegranate into fresh juice, which can in turn be added to cocktails, mocktails, and smoothies. Pomegranate arils can also be added to cookies, cakes, and other pastries, as well as oatmeal and other cereals, salads, and grain bowls.

Pomegranates are rich in several nutrients, including vitamins E and C. The antioxidant content of pomegranate juice is among the highest of any foods, with the "Wonderful" cultivar displaying the highest among pomegranate varieties. Pomegranate juice contains polyphenol antioxidants (primarily ellagic acid and punicalagin) that may lower risk of heart disease and inhibit the growth of cancer cells. Studies have shown that eating pomegranates can promote heart health by reducing "bad" (low-density lipoprotein or LDL) cholesterol while increasing levels of "good" (high-density lipoprotein or HDL) cholesterol.

A variety of recent scientific evidence has shown that consuming pomegranate juice on a regular basis can improve memory, help relieve symptoms of osteoarthritis, reduce blood pressure, and increase fertility in men. Drinking pomegranate juice has also been found to help prevent and manage diabetes. Several studies have proposed the use of pomegranate, and especially its derivatives punicalagin and urolithins, as a potential nutritional strategy in slowing the progression of neurodegenerative disorders such as Alzheimer's disease.

Resources

Altman, Nathaniel. *Sacred Trees*. San Francisco: Sierra Club Books, 1994, 120.

Brewer, Grace. "5 things you didn't know about pomegranates." Royal Botanical Gardens Kew website. December 18, 2019.

Cleveland Clinic. "The Health Benefits of Pomegranates." healthessentials. June 13, 2022.

Ferreira, Mandy. "15 Health Benefits of Pomegranate Juice." Medical News Today website. January 12, 2023.

Iowa State University. "Pomegranates." Agricultural Marketing Resource Center website. March 2023.

Kandylis, P., and E. Kokkinomagoulos. "Food Applications and Potential Health Benefits of Pomegranate and its Derivatives." *Foods* 9, no. 2 (2020) :122.

Stein, Larry, Jim Kamas, and Monte Nesbitt. "Pomegranates." Texas A&M Agrilife Extension Service, 2015.

Stover, E., and E.W. Mercure. "The Pomegranate: A New Look at the Fruit of Paradise." *HortScience* 42,5 (2007): 1088-1092.

"What Is Pomegranate in Chinese Culture?" Son of China website. April 7, 2023.

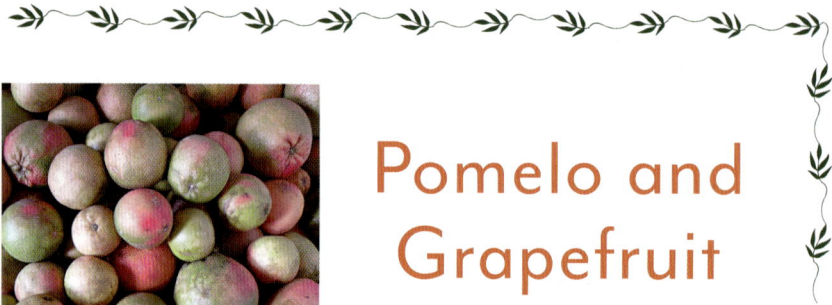

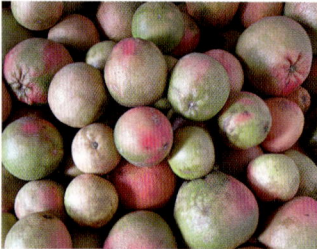

Pomelo and Grapefruit

Although the pomelo (*Citrus maxima*) is a popular citrus fruit in Asia and Latin America, it has only begun to become appreciated by North American food lovers. Indigenous to southern China, this yellow fruit with either yellow or pink flesh is the largest commercially grown citrus fruit in the world, and can be as large as a good-sized cantaloupe. Pomelos have thick peels and are less juicy than grapefruits; they also have a firm flesh with thick membranes and juice sacs, making them difficult to eat. Pomelos have white or pink flesh that contains lots of seeds.

The pomelo is considered one of the three original species of the genus *Citrus* (along with mandarin oranges and citron), and its evolutionary journey goes back millions of years. It is believed that the pomelo was introduced to China around 1,300 years ago, with cultivation gradually spreading throughout Southeast Asia, the Middle East, the Caribbean, and parts of Latin America. China remains the world's largest grower of pomelos (more than 53 percent of all pomelos are grown there), followed by Vietnam, the United States, and Mexico.

The grapefruit is the result of an accidental natural cross between the pomelo and the sweet orange. It originated on the island of Barbados during the eighteenth century. Both "parent" species had been introduced to the West Indies from China during the previous century. Like the pomelo, the grapefruit is known for its large fruit size, thick peel, and typical citrus fruit flavor with bitter tinges. Its flesh color ranges from yellow to pink and red, with the Ruby Red variety receiving the first grapefruit patent in 1928. In the United States, grapefruits are grown primarily in Texas and Florida. China is the world's largest producer of grapefruit, followed by Vietnam and Mexico.

Unlike lemons and limes, grapefruit are not astringent and can be enjoyed as oranges are. They can be cut in half and eaten with a grapefruit spoon, or peeled and slowly savored in sections, one by one. I have found this method the best way to enjoy both grapefruit and pomelo, although I remove the skin of each pomelo section by hand because it makes the sections difficult to chew. Both pomelo and grapefruit can also be enjoyed as juice, as a smoothie ingredient, or as an addition to fruit or vegetable salads.

The most common nutrients found in other citrus fruits are also components of both pomelo and grapefruit: vitamin C, provitamin A (carotenoids), thiamin (B_1), and riboflavin (B_2), along with carbohydrates, dietary fiber, organic acids, fatty acids, and a small amount of essential amino acids. Pomelo and grapefruit also contain antioxidants and other healthy phytochemicals (including limonoids, flavonoids, phytosterols, and polyphenols) that are common in most other citrus fruits. Both the pomelo and grapefruit contain *furanocoumarins*, a group of chemicals that have been found to have antioxidant, anti-inflammatory, and anti cancer properties. The health benefits of grapefruit were summarized in the textbook *Nutritional Composition and Antioxidant Properties of Fruits and Vegetables*:

> [G]rapefruit and its constituents have been studied for its free-radical scavenging, antimicrobial, and proliferation inhibition ability of several cancer cells using in vitro models. Further, the inhibition of atherosclerosis, oxidative stress, tumor growth, and hypolipidemic [lipid-reducing] activities have been demonstrated in both preclinical and clinical studies. These properties make grapefruit one of the most health beneficial citrus fruits. (Kotamballi et al. 2020, 393)

However, both the pomelo and grapefruit have chemical compounds that can block an enzyme that helps the body break down certain medicines, including those that lower cholesterol (statins), reduce high blood pressure, and fight allergies and immunosuppression. If this enzyme is blocked, too much medication can build up in the bloodstream, causing dangerously high levels. Pomelo and grapefruit do not adversely affect *all* such medications, so consult your physician before consuming pomelo or grapefruit or their juice if you are taking a statin or other medications.

Resources

"Fresh Pomelo." Tridge.com. Accessed January 5, 2024.

"Grapefruit Benefits." Johns Hopkins Medicine website. Accessed January 4, 2024.

Hung, W. L., J. H. Suh, and Y. Wang. "Chemistry and health effects of furanocoumarins in grapefruit." *Journal of Food and Drug Analysis* I (2017) 71–83.

Kotamballi, N., Chidambara Murthy, Alice Hepsiba et. al., Chapter 24 (Grapefruit) in Amit K. Jaiswal (ed.), *Nutritional Composition and Antioxidant Properties of Fruits and Vegetables*. New York: Academic Press, 2020, 393–404.

Matheyambath, A. C., P. Padmanabhan, and G. Paliyath. "Citrus Fruits" in *Encyclopedia of Food and Health*. New York: Academic Press, 2016, 136–140.

"Nutrition and Healthy Eating." WebMD. September 14, 2022.

Wikipedia. "Grapefruit." Accessed January 5, 2024.

Wikipedia. "Pomelo." Accessed January 5, 2024.

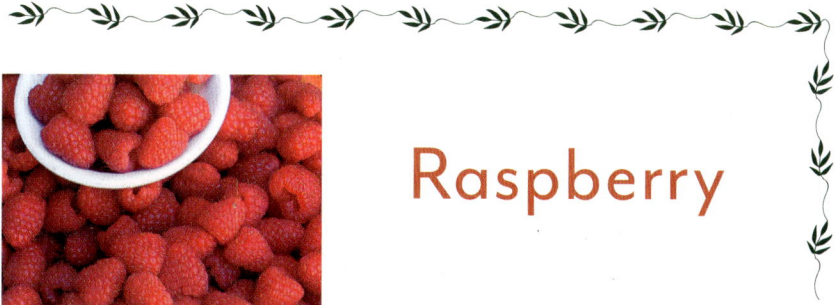

Raspberry

Like other berries, raspberries (*Rubus idaeus*) originally grew wild in forests, forming open stands both under tree canopies and in forest clearings. The fruit known as red raspberry is indigenous to high mountain altitudes in southern Europe and central Asia. Raspberries thrive in the Northern Hemisphere because they prefer growing through cool summers. The botanical name of the species refers to its early growth near Mount Ida in northwest Türkiye.

Other variants originated in North America, especially black raspberries (*Rubus occidentalis*). Although delicious, they are not as commercially available as red raspberries. I remember picking them as a child with my grandfather in upstate New York.

Native Americans used the black raspberry plant to treat a number of health problems: raspberry bark, leaves, and roots were prescribed for disorders of the intestinal tract, while raspberry leaf tea was used to increase urination, stop vomiting, and calm the nerves. Raspberry bark tea was used to treat dysentery and stomach aches.

When the Romans conquered most of Europe, they brought raspberries with them, eventually introducing the fruit to the British Isles. When Europeans colonized the Americas, they discovered the black raspberry but, preferring the red variety, the British began shipping the red fruit to New York in 1771. George Washington admired raspberries so much, he ended up growing over forty different varieties at his Virginia estate in Mount Vernon.

Raspberries are among the most popular of berries. They are known for their sweet, acidic flavor, and are most commonly eaten fresh, added to muffins and other baked goods, or made into delicious jams and jellies. They also make a great addition to breakfast cereals, pancakes, and fruit smoothies.

Like blueberries and blackberries, raspberries are a healthy food. In addition to dietary fiber, they are rich in vitamins C, A, B_1, B_2, B_3, and folic acid, along with the minerals iron, potassium, and manganese. Raspberries contain a wealth of beneficial phytochemicals, including anthocyanins and ellagitannins, both powerful antioxidants. Along with other berries, raspberries have attracted the attention of medical and nutritional researchers around the world, and are being investigated for their ability to prevent and treat cardiovascular diseases, diabetes mellitus, obesity, Alzheimer's disease, and cancer—especially of the colon and small intestine, and cancerous tumors in general.

Russia is currently the world's leading raspberry producer, followed by Mexico, Serbia, Poland, and the United States. California is the leading domestic producer of both red and black raspberries, followed by Oregon and Washington. Canada is also a major grower of raspberries, with most of their production located in British Columbia and Ontario.

Resources

Bailey, Natasha. "Most of the World's Raspberries Come from This Country." Cook, TastingTable website. Accessed November 11, 2023.

Burton-Freeman, B. M., A. K. Sandhu, and I. Edirisinghe. "Red Raspberries and Their Bioactive Polyphenols: Cardiometabolic and Neuronal Health Links." *Advances in Nutrition* 7, no. 1 (2016): 44–65.

"Health Benefits of Raspberries." WebMD. September 15, 2022.

Iowa State University. "Raspberries." Agricultural Marketing Resource Center website. February 2023.

"Raspberries," Minnesota Hardy, University of Minnesota.

Scully, Virginia. *A Treasury of American Indian Herbs—Their Lore and Their Use for Food, Drugs, and Medicine.* New York: Crown Publishers, Inc. 1970, 155, 236, 265.

"Which Country Produces the Most Raspberries?" Helgi Library. Accessed November 26, 2023.

Wikipedia. *"Rubus idaeus."* Accessed November 11, 2023.

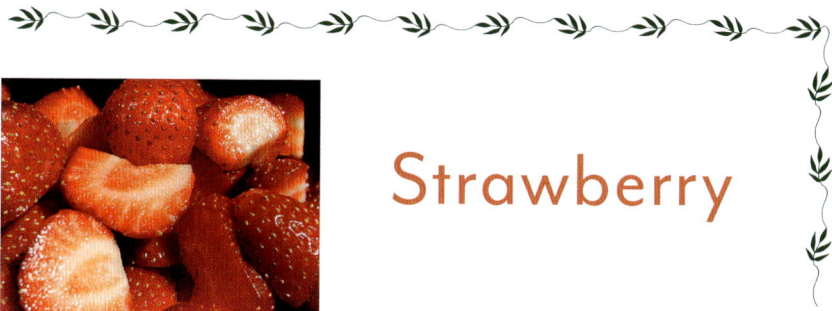

Strawberry

Photo by Marc-Lautenbacher

William Butler, the seventeenth-century English writer and physician, wrote, "Doubtless God could have made a better berry, but doubtless God never did." The strawberry (*Fragaria* spp.), with its vibrant red color and delicious, sweet flavor, remains one of our all-time favorite fruits.

Like blueberries, strawberries are indigenous to the United States, specifically what is now the state of Virginia. They were a treasured food among Native Americans, who mostly ate them raw but also mixed crushed berries and with cornmeal to bake into bread. Early European colonists soon discovered wild strawberries, which were so abundant, they saw no need to cultivate them. Early American colonists shipped strawberry plants to Europe, and they were growing in English gardens as early as 1629. Another strawberry variety, known as *futilla*, was discovered in Chile by European explorers.

Cultivation began in Europe soon after their introduction, but strawberry domestication didn't become widespread in the United States until the early nineteenth century. One of the first popular cultivars was the "Hovey" variety, introduced in 1838 by Charles Hovey, a Massachusetts-based fruit grower, breeder, and writer. New York state was an early center of strawberry production, and the advent of refrigerated railroad cars made distribution to other parts of the country economically viable. Production soon spread to Arkansas, Louisiana, Florida, Tennessee, and eventually to California. Today, some 75 percent of the North American strawberry crop is grown in California, which produces more than a billion pounds of strawberries a year. Another major source of strawberries consumed in the United States is Mexico, which exports millions of pounds of fruit grown primarily in Baja California and Central Mexico, including the states of Michoacán, Guanajuato, and Jalisco.

The versatile strawberry can be enjoyed in dozens of ways. While some like to eat them raw, either freshly picked or out of the box (careful washing is recommended), strawberries are a major ingredient in a wide variety of baked goods including breads, scones, and muffins, as well as more elaborate pastries like strawberry shortcake, tarts, cheesecake, trifles, and pies. Strawberries are also enjoyed in the form of ice cream and frozen pops, while strawberries dipped in chocolate have become a sought-after gourmet favorite. Strawberries add flavor and texture to both cooked and dry breakfast cereal, while strawberry jam and nut butter make a great combination when spread on bread. Dried strawberries are used commercially in trail mixes and energy bars. In Latin America, *fresas con crema* is a popular treat, while fresh strawberries, yogurt, and a touch of honey make a delicious and healthy evening snack. As beverages, strawberries are a popular ingredient in smoothies for children at breakfast, while their parents may prefer them in frozen daiquiris after dinner.

Like the blueberry, the strawberry has recently achieved status as a superfruit. Strawberries are high in dietary fiber, vitamin C, folic acid, and potassium. Few people know that strawberries contain more vitamin C than oranges: a cup of sliced strawberries contains 97 milligrams of vitamin C, or 108 percent of the recommended DV (daily value); a medium orange provides 83 mg of vitamin C, which is 92 percent of the DV.

Strawberries contain a wealth of antioxidants, such as *anthocyanin*, which protect the body against cell damage. Strawberries have also been found to boost brain power, strengthen the immune system, protect heart health (including reducing triglycerides and lowering LDL, or "bad" cholesterol), and help manage blood sugar. Ongoing research is studying how strawberries can be used therapeutically to treat oxidative stress driven pathologies, such as cancer, cardiovascular diseases, type 2 diabetes, obesity, neurodegenerative diseases, and inflammation.

An article in the peer-reviewed journal *Food & Function* summarized the healing mechanisms of this healthy and delicious fruit:

> Strawberries (*Fragaria X ananassa, Duch.*) are a rich source of a wide variety of nutritive compounds such as sugars, vitamins, and minerals, as well as non-nutritive, bioactive compounds such as flavonoids, anthocyanins, and phenolic acids. All of these compounds exert a synergistic and cumulative effect on human health promotion and in disease prevention. (Giampieri et al. 2015, 1386)

Strawberries are one of America's favorite snack foods. A cup of strawberries contains only fifty-five calories, making it a diet-friendly fruit.

Resources

de Candolle, Alphonse. *Origin of Cultivated Plants*. New York: D. Appleton and Company, 1908, 205.

Cleveland Clinic. "All the Reasons You Should Eat Strawberries." healthessentials. March 30, 2023.

Giampieri, F., T. Y. Forbes-Hernandez, M. Gasparrini et al. "Strawberry as a health promoter: an evidence based review." *Food & Function* 6, no. 5 (2015) 1386–98.

Trowbridge Filippone, Peggy. "A Brief History of the Strawberry." The Spruce Eats. Accessed November 11, 2023.

"Strawberry: A Brief History." Integrated Pest Management website., University of Missouri, May 21, 2012.

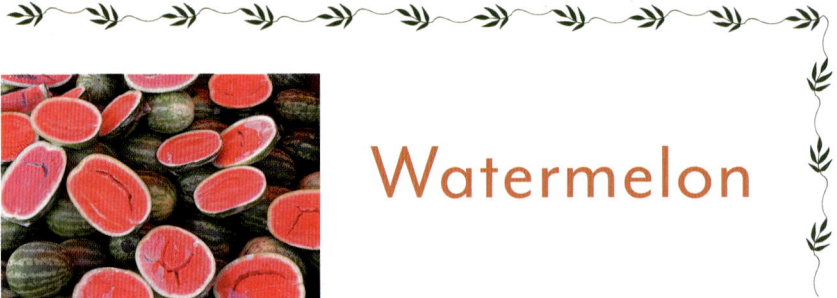

Watermelon

Watermelons (*Citruillius lanatus*) are known for their sweet flavor, crunchy texture, and high water content, which averages 92 percent. The watermelon is closely associated with the American South, and most believe that it originated there. In addition, most people consider the watermelon as a fruit—but it is actually a vegetable, like other melon varieties.

But archeologists have long believed that the ancestor of the modern watermelon traces its roots to one of several locations in Africa, including the north, west, and extreme south. Yet the results of a recent genomic (gene-based) study undertaken by European researchers from several universities found that the closest relative to the domesticated watermelon is the white-pulped Kordofan melon (*Citruillius lanatus*, subspecies *cordophanus*) that is indigenous to Sudan, in northeastern Africa. These findings are consistent with recently unearthed Egyptian tomb paintings that depict the consumption of raw watermelon as a dessert over 4,300 years ago in the Nile Valley. The early Israelites were also acquainted with watermelon, and called it *abbatitchim*, from which the Arabic term for the plant (*battich*) was derived.

Watermelons were introduced by traders to India and China by the seventh through tenth centuries. The Moors (Muslims of primarily Arab or Berber descent from North Africa) are said to have introduced watermelons to the Iberian Peninsula during the thirteenth century; cultivation spread throughout southern Europe from there. By the seventeenth century, watermelon was found growing in gardens throughout Europe, especially in the warmer parts of the continent.

European colonists—as well as victims of the slave trade from Africa—likely introduced watermelons to North America, including the southern United States. Watermelons were found growing in Florida as early as 1576 and in Massachusetts by 1629. Slaves belonging to Thomas Jefferson grew watermelons at his plantation in Monticello. They were also grown by Native Americans from Florida to the Mississippi Valley from the 1600s.

The science of watermelon cultivation has produced many varieties over the years: today, more than 1,200 watermelon varieties are grown in ninety-six countries around the world. One of the most important developments were seedless varieties, first introduced in 1950. In addition, botanists have developed small "icebox" hybrids that are both tasty and resistant to disease. The ever-inventive Japanese have even developed a watermelon in the form of a square, which can be found in specialty stores in Japan and sell for the equivalent of seventy-five to one hundred dollars each.

Mark Twain praised the watermelon as "the chief of this world's luxuries, king by the grace of God all over the fruits of the earth. When one has tasted it, he knows what the angels eat." While some readers may view his observations as slightly exaggerated, watermelon is one of our favorite and most refreshing summer treats. Watermelon is best enjoyed chilled and eaten either alone, as part of fruit salad, or combined with other melon varieties.

The early Greeks and Romans believed that watermelon had medicinal properties, and the Greek physicians Hippocrates and Dioscorides prescribed it as a diuretic and to treat children suffering from heatstroke. Later, the Roman naturalist Pliny the Elder (23/24–79 CE) described watermelon as a "cooling food" in his encyclopedia *Historia Naturalis*.

Although one cannot survive on watermelon alone, it is packed with important nutrients: high amounts of vitamins A and C, and significant amounts of vitamin B_6, potassium, and amino acids. It also contains a variety of antioxidants, such as lycopene, which help prevent cell damage that can lead to heart disease, diabetes, and premature aging. Another phytochemical found in watermelon is the amino acid *citrulline*, which has been reported to have both antioxidant and circulation-enhancing properties. Watermelons also contain *cucurbitacins*, a family of bitter-tasting compounds that have drawn interest among scientists due to their anticancer properties. Due to its high water content, eating watermelon is a great way to stay refreshed and hydrated on a hot summer day.

Americans love watermelons, and are eating more every year: annual per capita consumption in the United States reached 15.5 pounds by 2019. Most of the watermelons Americans eat are grown in Arizona, California, Delaware, Florida, and Texas. About a quarter of the watermelons sold in the United States are imported from Mexico and Central America. China is the world's largest watermelon producer, followed by Türkiye, India, and Brazil.

Resources

de Candolle, Alphonse. *Origin of Cultivated Plants*. New York: D. Appleton and Company, 1908, 263.

Iowa State University. "Watermelon." Agricultural Marketing Research Center website. Revised April 2024.

Renner, Susanne S. et al. "A chromosome-level genome of a Kordofan melon illuminates the origin of domesticated watermelons." *Proceedings of the National Academy of Sciences of the United States* 118, no. 23 (2021): e2101486118.

Sorokina, M., K. S. McCaffrey, E. E. Deaton et al. "A Catalog of Natural Products Occurring in Watermelon - *Citrullus lanatus.*" *Frontiers in Nutrition* 14, no. 8 (2021):729822. doi: 10.3389/fnut.2021.729822.

"The Wonders of Watermelon." Mayo Clinic Health System. July 27, 2021.

"Watermelon: A Brief History." Integrated Pest Management website. University of Missouri. July 17, 2020.

Wempen, Kristi. "The Wonders of Watermelon." *Hometown Health* blog. Mayo Clinic Health System website. July 27, 2021.

"World Watermelon Production by Country," AtlasBig.com. Accessed November 12, 2023.

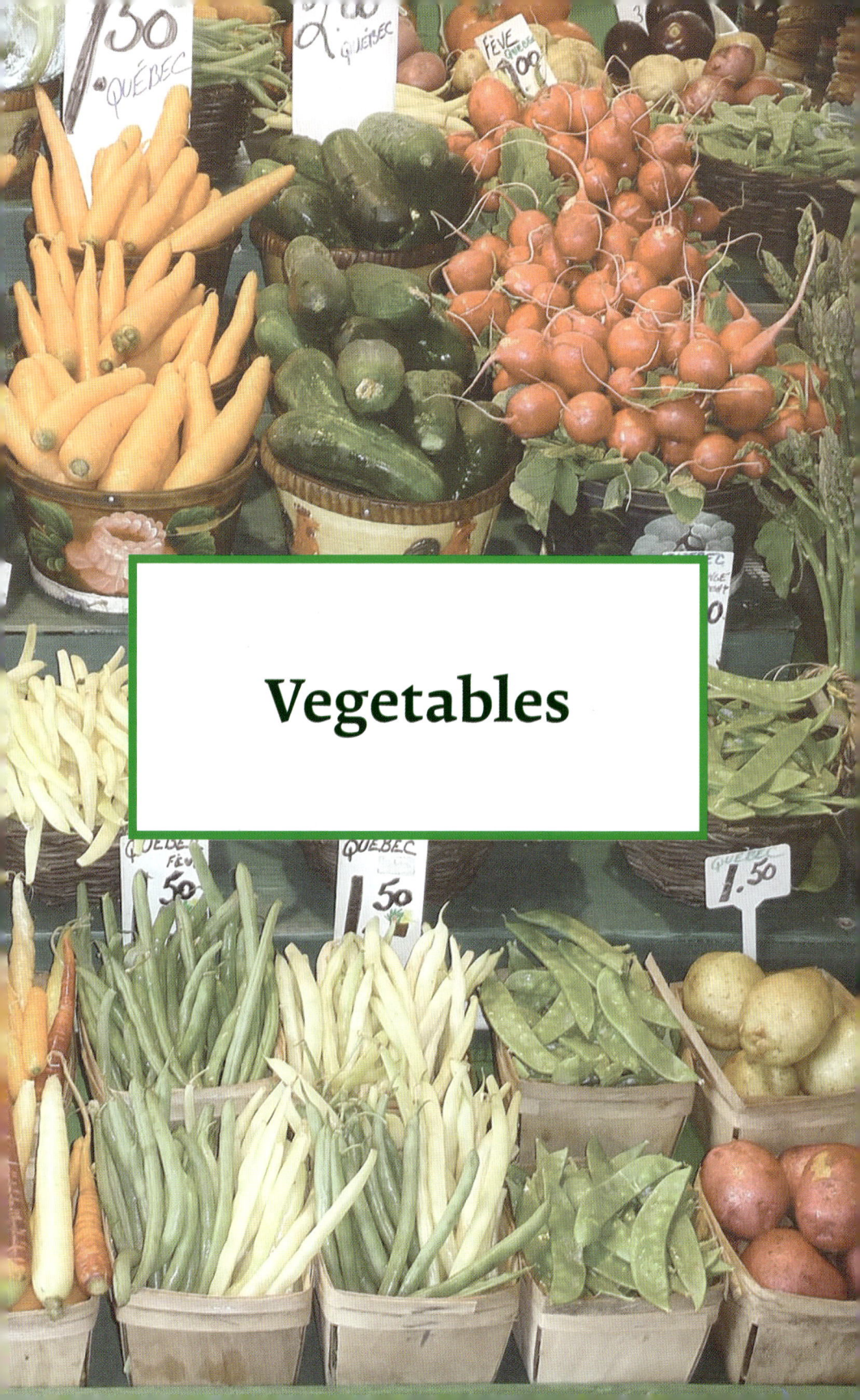

Vegetables

Vegetables have traditionally been defined, in general terms, as "parts of plants that are consumed by humans or other animals as food," which can include flowers, fruits, stems, leaves, roots, and seeds. An alternative definition of the term—which is the one used in this book—includes savory fruits such as tomatoes and cucumbers, flowers such as broccoli and cauliflower, and seeds like snap beans and green peas.

The term "vegetable" is derived from the Medieval Latin word *vegetabilis*, which refers to the "growing, flourishing" of a plant. This section will include fruits that are commonly eaten as vegetables, like peppers, cucumbers, and tomatoes.

Although herbs and spices are technically vegetables, eleven of the most popular of these are included in a dedicated section of this book, to honor their special uses in culinary preparations.

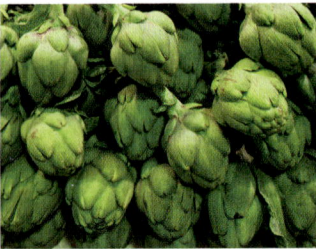

Artichoke

The artichoke (*Cynara cardunculus*) isn't the most popular food in North America, but those who have eaten artichokes often find them irresistible. The inner leaves and heart are delicate and have a sweet, earthy flavor. Both fresh artichokes and canned or bottled artichoke hearts are sold in supermarkets, and stuffed artichokes are sometimes a featured delicacy in upscale Italian and French gourmet stores and restaurants.

The artichoke is believed to have come from a wild cardoon, which is native to the western Mediterranean region, including southern Spain, northern Morocco, Madeira, and the Canary Islands. The cardoon is a member of the thistle family (Asteraceae) to which both sunflowers and lettuce also belong.

Recent molecular data show that the artichoke has extremely ancient roots: a wild ancestor of all Cynara species is said to have moved from the Mediterranean coast to the region of the Sahara Desert during the fourth glaciations of the Pleistocene Era, which took place some 2.5 million years ago. Examples of the artichoke's ancestor moved back to the Mediterranean basin (including southern Europe) around 18,000 years ago, and began to grow wild throughout the region.

Artichokes were considered a source of food and medicine by the ancient Egyptians, Greeks, and Romans. During the fourth century BCE, the Greek philosopher Theophrastus reported that artichokes were grown in Sicily. It was reported that the Egyptian king Ptolemy Euergetes (c. 280–222 BCE) recommended that his soldiers eat artichokes because they were considered a source of strength and courage. It is believed that artichoke cultivation began in what is now Italy during the fifth century BCE, and gradually made its way through Europe. The French–Swiss botanist Alphonse de Candolle wrote that artichokes were first introduced to England in 1548.

Spanish settlers are believed to have introduced the artichoke to California, where they were first grown in the early 1920s, near Half Moon Bay, a coastal city south of San Francisco. Large scale cultivation began in and around Castroville, Monterey County, in 1922. By 1927 there were over fifty growers, with 12,000 acres (4,900 hectares) of artichokes growing in Castroville and the Monterey Bay area. Castroville calls itself "The Artichoke Center of the World," and holds an artichoke festival every year. Marilyn Monroe was crowned Castroville's Artichoke Queen in 1948. Although some 80 percent of California's artichokes come from farms in Monterey County, they are also grown in Oxnard and Coachella, as well as in Mexico's Baja California. The artichoke was named California's official state vegetable in 2013. The "big three" artichoke-producing countries are Italy, Egypt, and Spain, while the United States ranks at number eight.

The part of the artichoke which we eat is actually the bud of a purple flower before it blooms. Artichokes can be served stuffed, although the simplest way to enjoy this unusual vegetable is to steam them on the stove or in a pressure cooker until tender. Each leaf, or petal, can be pulled off by hand, and the tender flesh scraped off using one's teeth. Once the leaves are removed, the fuzzy substance (called the choke) can be scooped out with a spoon until you reach the artichoke "heart." You can then remove the heart from the stem to eat on its own; or, for more flavor, the leaves and heart can be dipped in butter, olive oil, or a prepared dressing. Artichoke hearts can also be grilled, fried, or used as a pizza topping or salad ingredient. Precooked artichoke hearts are widely available in cans, while marinated artichoke hearts are usually sold in glass jars.

In addition to providing dietary fiber, potassium, vitamin C, magnesium, and folate, artichokes are rich in beneficial phytochemicals, with known nutritional and pharmacological properties such as polyphenols, sesquiterpene lactones, and terpenoids. These elements have been found to help regulate blood pressure, lower cholesterol, aid digestion, and improve liver function.

A 2015 article published in *Phytochemistry Reviews* highlighted the liver-protective qualities of artichokes, along with their ability to reduce harmful fats in the body and increase the production of bile from the liver, which enables the body to better release toxins. Artichoke extract, which contains high concentrations of chemical compounds found in the plant, is available as a dietary supplement.

Resources

de Candolle, Alphonse. *Origin of Cultivated Plants*. New York: D. Appleton and Company, 1908, 93.

de Falco, B., G. Incerti, M. Amato et al. "Artichoke: botanical, agronomical, phytochemical, and pharmacological overview." *Phytochemistry Reviews* 14 (2015): 993–1018.

"Health Benefits of Artichokes." WebMD. September 14, 2022.

"Our Story." Ocean Mist Farms website. Accessed November 20, 2023.

Rocchetti, G., L. Lucini, G. Corrado et al. "Phytochemical Profile, Mineral Content, and Bioactive Compounds in Leaves of Seed-Propagated Artichoke Hybrid Cultivars." *Molecules* 25, no. 17 (2020): 3795.

Smith, Noah. "When Marilyn Monroe Reigned as California's Artichoke Queen." *The California Sun*. Medium.com. Accessed November 20, 2023.

University of Oregon. "All About Artichokes." *The Urban Farm* blog. 2023.

Wikipedia. "Castroville, California." Accessed November 20, 2023.

"World Artichoke Production by Country." AtlasBig.com. Accessed November 20, 2023.

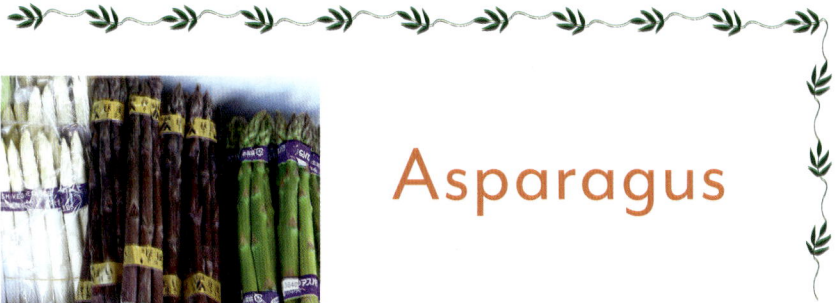

Asparagus

One of only three common perennial vegetables (that don't need to be replanted every year), this Mediterranean native is said to date back more than five thousand years. Ancient Egyptians—and later Greeks and Romans—likely used it for medicinal purposes. The Greeks considered asparagus to be a plant with aphrodisiac properties, and the Greek physician Hippocrates used asparagus to treat diarrhea and pains in the urethra. The Romans appreciated asparagus for its distinctive flavor, and often ate it fresh, as a stand-alone entrée, or with fish. They also dried it for winter use. In 200 BCE, the Roman author Cato the Elder wrote detailed directions for growing asparagus that are close to current recommendations.

Those who valued the unique flavor of asparagus went to extreme measures to grow and preserve it. Romans froze it high in the Alps, to serve to emperors on the Feast of Epicurus. Asparagus began to be more widely served to European heads of royalty beginning in the seventeenth century. King Louis XIV of France was said to have loved asparagus so much that he had greenhouses built to grow it year-round.

Asparagus was brought to North America by European settlers at least as early as 1655. Adriaen van der Donck, a Dutch immigrant to New Netherland (now the state of New York), mentions asparagus in his description of Dutch farming practices in the New World. Asparagus was also grown by British immigrants. In 1685, one of William Penn's advertisements for Pennsylvania included asparagus in a long list of crops that grew well in Colonial America.

There are a number of asparagus species, but only *Asparagus officinalis* is cultivated for food. Asparagus is a favorite spring vegetable, both for its early harvesting and its distinctive flavor. White asparagus is enjoyed primarily by Europeans, while green varieties are popular in the United States and China, where asparagus was first introduced about one hundred years ago. A purple variety can also be found in supermarkets and farmers markets, although it is not as widely available as the green varieties. The Chinese have grown to love asparagus, and China is now the world's largest asparagus producer.

Asparagus shoots are often prepared and served either as an appetizer or side dish. In Asian-style cooking, asparagus is often stir-fried, eaten as a side dish, or cooked with chicken, shrimp, or beef. It is also a valued ingredient in stews and soups. Although the tender shoots of the plant are the most delicious and easy to chew, the fibrous lower stalks can be liquefied in a blender to be used as a nutritious base for soups and stews. Pickled asparagus can be stored for long periods of time.

Asparagus is considered a highly nutritious food. It is not only low in calories, but is an excellent source of vitamins A and C—antioxidants that help the body fight off free radicals (oxygen particles body cells produce as waste). Free radicals can damage the DNA of nearby cells, leading to diseases like cancer and heart disease. Asparagus also provides significant amounts of dietary fiber, calcium, phosphorus, riboflavin, and iron.

By 2020, Americans were consuming over 500 million pounds of asparagus a year. While domestic production has declined over the years (harvesting asparagus is labor-intensive), per capita consumption is increasing. Growers in the United States produce 60–70 million pounds per year, mostly in Michigan, California, and Washington. Most of the asparagus consumed in the United States is imported, mainly from Mexico and Peru.

Resources

Burrows, Rhoda, and David Graper. "Growing Asparagus." Agronomy, Horticulture & Plant Science Department. South Dakota State University Extension website. Updated February 2019.

Geist, Linda. "Asparagus, the food of emperors, reigns supreme." University of Missouri Extension website. January 2, 2018.

Helin, X., P. Mingsheng, and F. Xiaotang. "Asparagus Production in China." *Acta Horticulture* 415 (1996), 41–44.

Iowa State University. "Asparagus." Agricultural Marketing Research Center website. Revised May 2024.

Myers, Clayton. "Happy National Asparagus Day! Get to Know Spring's Delicious Vegetable." USDA Blog. United States Department of Agriculture website. May 24, 2022.

Negi, J. S., P. Singh, G. P. Joshi et al. "Chemical constituents of Asparagus." *Pharmacognosy Review* 4, no. 8 (2010): 215–20.

"Our Asparagus." Les Cultures de chez nous website. Accessed November 20, 2023.

Wikipedia. "Asparagus." Accessed November 20, 2023.

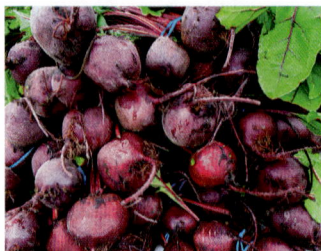

Beet

Now considered a superfood due to its abundance of antioxidants and other essential nutrients, the humble beet (*Beta vulgaris*) has been food for humans for almost four thousand years. Beets are believed to have originated from the "sea beet" that grew wild by the Mediterranean Sea, and beet remnants excavated from the Saqqara pyramid at Thebes date back to the 2600s BCE.

The ancient Greeks, Romans, and Egyptians cultivated beets, but consumed only the leaves as food—the roots were used in folk medicine to cure fevers and constipation, and were also considered an aphrodisiac. Some fifteen centuries ago, in what is now Iraq, Rav Ḥisda, a Jewish Talmudist, wrote: "A cooked dish of beets is beneficial for the heart, good for the eyes, and all the more beneficial for the intestines." Beets were also used by the Greeks as a sacred offering to Apollo, the Sun god of many attributes: light, healing, archery, music and art, knowledge, protection of herds and flocks, and protection of the young.

Beet cultivation spread from the Middle East to northern Africa and Europe by the early 1600s. Beets were often used as animal feed, but gradually became a cheap and nutritious food among Jews as both a soup ingredient and a substitute for meat. The ubiquitous borsht—a beet-based soup prized in Ukraine and Russia, as well as among Ashkenazi Jews everywhere—is said to have first appeared in what is now Ukraine and became popular from the sixteenth century onwards among Jews and non-Jews alike.

Beets are incredibly versatile and can be used and enjoyed in many ways, including raw, boiled, steamed, roasted, and pickled. In addition to borsht, beets are a popular salad ingredient, and are used in soups, stews, side dishes, and casseroles. Beet juice is considered one of the healthiest vegetable juices one can drink.

Sugar beets have been cultivated since the eighteenth century, after it was discovered that sugar could be isolated from the beet and consumed like cane sugar. By 1880, about half of the world's sugar supplies came from sugar beets.

In addition to antioxidants, potassium, and fiber, beets contain tryptophan and betaine, both substances that promote a feeling of well-being. They also contain high amounts of boron, a trace mineral that increases the level of sex hormones in the human body, revealing that the ancient folk belief that beets are an aphrodisiac wasn't far off the mark. Although they are often discarded, beet greens can be eaten like kale, collard greens, or spinach. They are highly nutritious and are an excellent source of vitamins A, C, and K.

Juice made from beets has been shown to be a potent medicine. A 2020 article in the peer-reviewed journal *Nutrition & Metabolism* highlighted the medicinal quality of beet juice, especially regarding diabetes, heart disease, and renal (kidney) health:

> Chronic and acute beetroot juice supplementation, as a cost-effective strategy, is proposed to hold promises in controlling diabetes and insulin hemostasis, blood pressure and vascular function, renal health and the possible effect on microbiome [friendly gut bacteria] abundance. (Mirmiran et al. 2020, 17)

In addition to highlighting beets as a food providing a wide variety of health benefits, the authors of the article (2020, 13) concluded that consuming beets has proven therapeutic value in the treatment of several major metabolic diseases: "Available data supported the health-promotional properties of beetroot and its byproducts as potential therapeutic treatments for various metabolic disorders including hypertension, diabetes, insulin resistance and kidney dysfunction."

Resources

Avey, Tori. "Discover the History of Beets." Food.PBS.org. October 8, 2014.

Castellano, Orge. "The Beet Goes On: How a humble root became a staple in Jewish cooking." *Tablet* magazine. July 5, 2023.

Levinson, Jessica. "Beets—The History, Myriad Uses, and Health Benefits of These Beloved Roots." *Today's Dietitian* 22, no. 2: 26.

Mirmiran, P., Z. Houshialsadat, Z. Gaeini et al. "Functional properties of beetroot (*Beta vulgaris*) in management of cardio-metabolic diseases." *Nutrition & Metabolism* 17, 3 (2020).

Broccoli

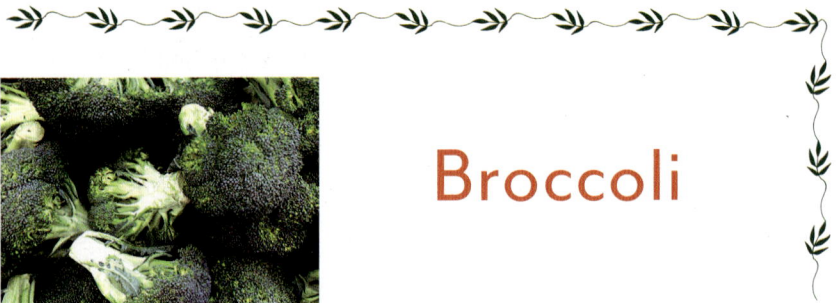

Despite former President George H. W. Bush's famous quote, "I do not like broccoli. And I haven't liked it since I was a little kid," broccoli is currently the sixth most popular vegetable in the United States. The word *broccoli*, first coined in the seventeenth century, comes from the Italian plural of the word *broccolo*, meaning "the flowering crest of a cabbage." Broccoli (*Brassica oleracea* var. *italica*) has its origins in primitive cultivated varieties first grown in the Roman Empire. It has been cultivated in Italy since ancient Roman times. The variety the most Americans are familiar with is green Calabrese broccoli, named after the Italian region of Calabria. There are also purple and white varieties of broccoli, which sometimes appear on supermarket shelves.

Like cauliflower, cabbage, brussels sprouts, and kale, cultivated broccoli descended from a type of wild cabbage (*Brassica oleracea*) through many years of selective breeding. The vegetable was first introduced into England around 1720. Unlike cauliflower, which was first grown in the United States in the seventeenth century, broccoli was introduced to the United States by Italian immigrants during the nineteenth century, and was grown primarily in family gardens. Commercial broccoli cultivation began in California in 1924; however, it did not become an economically successful crop in the United States until after World War II, when new and better hybrid varieties were developed by agronomists in both the United States and Japan.

My personal connection to broccoli: my brother and I grew up in the 1950s, and were picky eaters. During our preteen years, we demanded hamburgers, mashed potatoes, and broccoli for almost every evening meal. Because these foods were both nutritious and easy to prepare—and probably to keep us from whining—our mother accommodated us, and prepared a more varied and sophisticated dinner menu for herself and our father.

Broccoli is one of the most versatile of vegetables, and can be served as a cooked (preferably steamed, broiled, baked, or microwaved) side dish or in salads, casseroles, stews, stir-fried dishes, sauces, and soups. All of the plant can be eaten, although most Americans discard the stalk and leaves. Discerning chefs grind or blend the stalk to use later as a nutritious and tasty soup base.

Broccoli rabe (also known as *rapini*) is a relative of broccoli. It has ancient origins that trace back to the Himalayan foothills, and has long been considered a type of weed or "feral plant" that is derived fully or partially from domesticated crops. As opposed to large florets, rapini (*Brassica rapa* var. *ruvo*) has many spiked leaves that surround clusters of green buds that resemble small heads of broccoli. Its flavor has been described as bitter and pungent, and many find it quite delicious, especially when braised with olive oil and garlic. Rapini was given the name

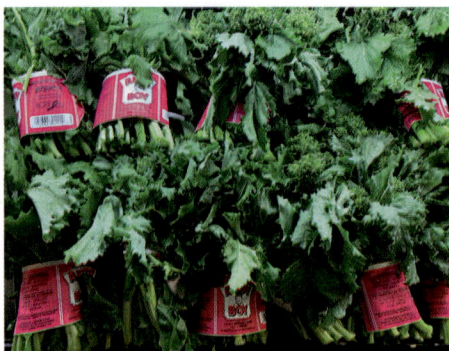

Broccoli rabe

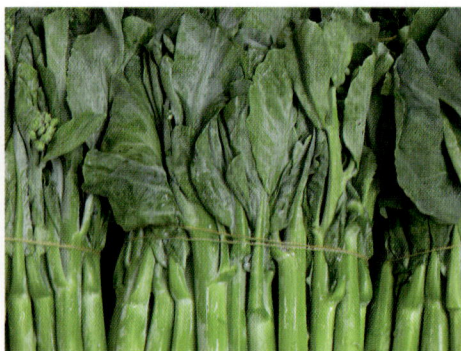

Chinese broccoli

broccoli rabe by D'Arrigo Brothers, a California-based grower and distributor of fresh produce. It is generally found in Italian produce markets, and commands a higher price than most other green vegetables.

Broccoli is a highly nutritious vegetable, providing calcium, iron, phosphorus, potassium, zinc, B vitamins, and vitamins E and K. Like cauliflower, kale, brussels sprouts, and cabbage, broccoli is a *cruciferous* vegetable that naturally produces bitter, sulfur-containing chemical compounds which the plant makes to protect itself from insect predators. These phytochemicals have been found to help regulate blood sugar and slow osteoarthritis, and have been linked to reducing the risk of developing cancer.

A recent article in *The Pharma Innovation Journal* detailed the many beneficial phytochemicals found in broccoli and how they contribute to good health. This included a long list of biological activities including antioxidant, anticancer, anti-obesity, antimicrobial, anti-diabetic, cardio-protective, and hepato- (liver) protective.

Indole-3-carbinol can also be found in abundance in broccoli. Since they continue to possess a number of anticancer qualities and their benefits, these components found in broccoli are well recognized to be extremely popular. It is extensively utilized to treat different types of cancer as well as other neurological diseases. [. . .] The medicinal potential of broccoli has been discussed in relation to its use in the treatment of cancer, diabetes, and other major diseases. Brassinin, isothiocyanates, indole-3-carbinol, and other phytochemicals similar to those found in broccoli have been shown to be very useful in the treatment of cancer. Glucosinolates, glucoraphin, and sulforaphane are a few more compounds that cause broccoli to produce more antioxidant activity. (Kamboj et al. 2023, 633)

The article also highlights laboratory findings that explore the medicinal value of broccoli sprouts due to the phytochemical sulforaphane, which has the potential to treat neurological conditions like Parkinson's and Alzheimer's disease.

Another paper published in the peer-reviewed journal *Cancer* (Basel) focused on the anticancer benefits of not only broccoli but cruciferous vegetables in general—all of which are explored in this book.

A multitude of studies has shown that ingestion of cruciferous vegetables (plants belonging to the *Cruciferae* family) may lower overall cancer risk, especially for breast, colorectal, bladder, lung, and prostate cancer. This is especially true with vegetables in the *Brassica* genus, including broccoli, brussels sprouts, cabbage, cauliflower, and bok choy. (Kaiser et al. 2021, 4796)

Some 90 percent of commercial broccoli grown in the United States is from California, with the rest grown primarily in Arizona, Texas, and Oregon. China is the world's largest producer of broccoli, followed by India, Spain, Italy, the United States, and Mexico.

Resources

A. Kamboj, S. Sharma, V. P. Singh et al., "Phytochemical and therapeutic potential of broccoli (*Brassica oleracea*): A review." *The Pharma Innovation Journal* 12, 6 (2023): 633.

A. E. Kaiser, M. Baniasadi, D. Giansiracusa et al., "Sulforaphane: A Broccoli Bioactive Phytocompound with Cancer Preventive Potential." *Cancers* (Basel) 13, 19 (2021): 4796.

Booth, Stephanie. "Health Benefits of Broccoli." WebMD. July 17, 2023.

Orzolek, Michael, William Lamont Jr., and Lynn Kime. "Broccoli Production." Penn State Extension website. June 20, 2005.

Kaiser, A .E., M. Baniasadi, D. Giansiracusa et al. "Sulforaphane: A Broccoli Bioactive Phytocompound with Cancer Preventive Potential." *Cancers* (Basel) 13, 19 (2021): 4796.

Kamboj, A., S. Sharma, V. P. Singh et al., "Phytochemical and therapeutic potential of broccoli (*Brassica oleracea*): A review." *The Pharma Innovation Journal* 12, 6 (2023): 633–38.

McAlvay, Alex C., Aaron P. Ragsdale, Makenzie E. Mabry et al. "*Brassica rapa* Domestication: Untangling Wild and Feral Forms and Convergence of Crop Morphotypes," *Molecular Biology and Evolution* 38, no. 8 (2021): 3358–3372.

Orzolek, Michael, William Lamont Jr., and Lynn Kime. "Broccoli Production." Penn State Extension website. June 20, 2005.

Smith, David. "Flower Development: Origin of the cauliflower." *Current Biology* 5, no. 4 (1995): 361–63.

Tarlach, Gemma. "The Deep Roots of the Vegetable that 'Took Over the World,'" *Atlas Obscura*. June 11, 2021

Wikipedia. "Broccoli." Accessed November 5, 2023.

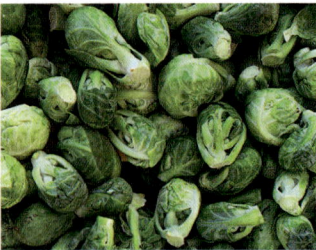

Brussels Sprouts

Brussels sprouts (*Brassica oleracea* var. *gemmifera*) are a many-headed subspecies of the common cabbage. As a member of the cabbage family, it is related to other cruciferous vegetables such as broccoli, kale, and cauliflower.

Considered one of the least appealing vegetables in North America just thirty years ago, brussels sprouts are now enjoying a renaissance. In the past, brussels sprouts had a bitter flavor and were often overcooked in boiling water until they were mushy and greenish-brown. As a result, few people would eat them. This began to change in the 1990s, when scientists in the Netherlands figured out what made the vegetable (known as *spruitjes* in Dutch) bitter. Using old seeds from a gene bank, they experimented with hybrids that would not only taste less bitter, but would also yield greater harvests.

The result was a much better-tasting vegetable that attracted the attention of commercial chefs in the United States, who prefer stir-frying, roasting, grilling, broiling, and baking brussels sprouts to endless boiling. Today the demand for brussels sprouts is booming, and four times as much land in the United States is used to grow brussels sprouts than in 1990.

Despite its name, brussels sprouts did not originate in Brussels, but are believed to have first appeared in the Mediterranean region; its forerunners were cultivated in ancient Rome. The vegetable as we know it was first propagated in northern Europe during the fifth century CE, and introduced to the Flanders countryside in Belgium—of which Brussels is a part—eight hundred years later. It is believed to have been named in honor of Brussels, where the vegetable enjoyed widespread popularity. Its French name is *choux de Bruxelles*, or "Brussels cabbage." The earliest written reference to brussels sprouts in English was in 1747, when author Hannah Glasse gave the following cooking advice:

Cabbage, and all Sorts of young Sprouts must be boiled in a great deal of Water. When the Stalks are tender, or fall to the Bottom, they are enough; then take them off, before they lose their Colour. Always throw Salt into your Water before you put your Greens in. Young Sprouts you send to Table just as they are [. . .]. (FoodTimeline website)

Brussels sprouts were first introduced to Louisiana by French settlers during the eighteenth century, and the first plantings of the vegetable began in California's Central Coast in the 1920s, where most domestic brussels sprouts are still grown today. California is the main producer of brussels sprouts in the United States, followed by the state of Washington and New York. The largest producer of the vegetable in Europe is the Netherlands, followed by Great Britain and Germany. Brussels sprouts are also grown in Baja California in Mexico, with most of the crop exported to the United States.

Brussels sprouts are always eaten cooked. They make a perfect side dish (especially when sautéed or roasted), or can be added to soups, stews, casseroles, and stir-fried dishes.

Brussels sprouts are highly nutritious. In addition to dietary fiber, they are rich in Vitamins C and K, and provide moderate amounts of B vitamins, especially vitamin B_6 and folate. They are also good sources of iron, manganese, phosphorous, and potassium.

Like other cruciferous vegetables, brussels sprouts contain *sulforaphane*, a phytochemical under basic research for its potential to support heart health, protect against cancer, prevent and manage diabetes, and improve digestion. According to an article published by the MD Anderson Cancer Center at the University of Texas (Austin), sulforaphane neutralizes toxins due to their antioxidant activity, reduces inflammation, blocks mutations in DNA that can lead to cancer, and may slow tumor growth. Another benefit of eating foods rich in sulforaphane is that they are readily available at greengrocers and supermarkets. Steaming, stir-frying, or roasting these foods retains most of their nutrients.

Resources

Anderson, Heather. "Sulforaphane benefits: How leafy veggies like broccoli and Brussels sprouts may help reduce your cancer risk." MD Anderson Cancer Center. The University of Texas (Austin). April 2020.

"Brussels sprouts." FoodTimeline website. Accessed November 5, 2023.

Charles, Dan. "From Culinary Dud to Stud: How Dutch Plant Breeders

Built Our Brussels Sprouts Boom." *The Salt*. National Public Radio. October 30, 2019.

Coyle, Daisy. "Sulforaphane: Benefits, Side Effects and Food Sources." healthline. February 26, 2019.

Wikipedia. "Brussels sprout." Accessed November 5, 2023.

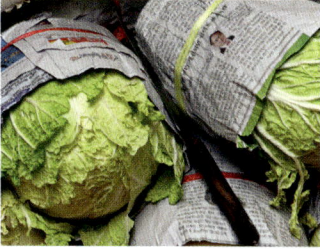

Cabbage

Although widely considered an inexpensive and somewhat boring staple food for centuries, an article published in *The New York Times* in March 2024 described cabbage as "having a star turn on the American culinary scene," pointing out how cabbage has become a featured attraction at many gourmet restaurants throughout the country. The article added that "cabbage fever" has been compared to the hoopla over bacon during the 1990s.

There are three major types of cabbage (*Brassica oleracea* var. *capitata*): green, red, and savoy. Cabbage belongs to the same plant family as many other vegetables including broccoli, mustard, collards, kale, cauliflower, brussels sprouts, and turnips. Nineteenth-century researchers believed that the cabbage originated in Europe due to the many varieties documented by early Greek and Roman writers.

Recent genomic and archeological evidence has revealed that the Brassicaceae appeared in the Iranian–Turanian region as a tropical-subtropical genus as far back as the Eocene era—around 37 million years ago—which is believed to be the ancestral region of the Brassica family of plants. According to ancient Sanskrit texts, crops of the genus Brassica were used in India as far back as 3000 BCE. Other archeological evidence and historic writings have led researchers to believe that cabbages were first cultivated in the Middle East.

Other research has shown that cabbage (along with cauliflower) evolved from kales introduced from Europe to the Middle East, possibly transported along the tin-trade routes during the Bronze Age (3300–1000 BCE) and later reintroduced to Europe. Some researchers maintain that the Romans introduced cabbage to the rest of Europe, although it seems probable that the Celts introduced it (along with kale) even earlier. The word "cabbage" is an Anglicized form of the French *caboche*, meaning "head." In any event, the cabbage became an important crop in much of Europe by the Middle Ages.

Cabbage has been an important medicinal plant in Europe since ancient Greek and Roman times. It was used as an antidote to mushroom poisoning and as a treatment for hangovers and headaches. It has also been used to relieve the symptoms of sunstroke and to reduce fevers. European folk healers prescribed cabbage leaves to soothe swollen feet and to treat childhood croup. They also used cabbage to treat a wide range of health problems including sore throat, rheumatism, colic, hoarseness, and even melancholy. Cabbage's anti-inflammatory activity has been valued by traditional healers to treat wounds and skin irritations.

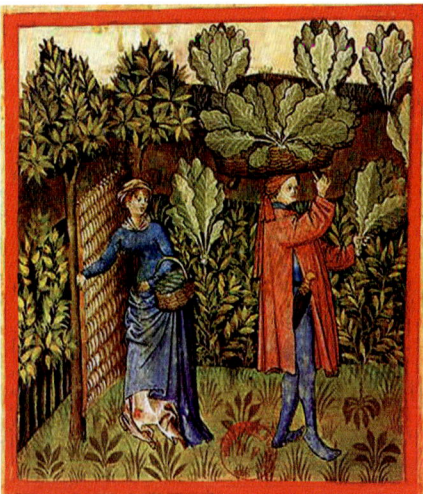

Harvesting Cabbage in Europe, fifteenth century. *From* Tacuinium Sanitatis *via Wikipedia.*

Cabbage has a long history in Traditional Chinese Medicine. Chinese varieties were recognized for their ability to regulate the flow of qi (life force), cool the body, strengthen the kidneys, improve brain function, and cleanse the blood of toxins. Traditional Chinese doctors have prescribed cabbage to treat a wide variety of health problems including arthritis, joint pain, muscle aches, tendonitis, swollen joints, low back pain, shortness of breath, lethargy, dementia, worms, constipation, anxiety, depression, anemia, allergies, hot flashes, and coughs. A story about Empress Dowager Cixi's experience with the napa variety of cabbage (*Brassica pekinensis*) took place during the final years of the Qing Dynasty, which lasted from 1636–1912.

It was said that the Empress Dowager Cixi of the Qing Dynasty at around 1900 became very ill in her old age and was having respiratory failure, high fever, lack of energy, and was unable to eat or drink, urinate, or move her bowels. No doctor or medicine was able to help her. Upon the advice of a monk she was fed only Chinese cabbage juice and soup, which saved her life. She was nursed back to health by eating mostly food made with Chinese cabbage to replace her usual diet of delicate, expensive, highly refined, meaty, and rich foods. After her recovery, she praised Chinese cabbage as the king of all vegetables. (Chan, Chinese Medicine Living website)

Cabbage was introduced to North America by the French explorer Jacques Cartier in 1541–42, who planted it in what is now the Canadian province of Québec during his third voyage to the New World. It was likely introduced to what is now the United States by early European settlers, although there is no written record of it until 1669. In the eighteenth century, cabbage was being grown by Native Americans as well as by newly arrived European colonists.

The familiar, round-headed cabbage, the oldest of the hard types of cabbage, was the only variety described during the sixteenth century. Flat-headed, egg-shaped, and conic-shaped varieties appeared later on. Most of the varieties grown in the United States today originated in Germany and the Low Countries, which include Belgium, the Netherlands, and Luxembourg.

Two types of cabbage indigenous to China, relatives of "Western" cabbage, have been cultivated there for over 1,600 years. Chinese cabbage (*Brassica pekinensis*) is called napa in English, *wongbok* in Japanese, *baechu* in Korean, and *dà báicài* ("large white vegetable") in Mandarin. It is light green in color and cylindrical in shape. Chinese cabbage is grown primarily in China, Taiwan, Japan, and Korea, where it is fermented to produce *kimchi*. The other cabbage variety, *Brassica chinensis*, is widely known as *bok choy*. It is dark green and does not grow as a "head," looking more like celery or mustard than cabbage. Bok choy is grown primarily in southern China and Southeast Asia. These and other varieties of Chinese cabbages are now being grown in North America, and are sold mostly in Asian grocery stores and in some Western supermarkets as well.

Most people think that cabbage is only eaten as coleslaw and sauerkraut, but cabbage is far more versatile. It can be grilled, stuffed, baked, sautéed, or added to stir-fried dishes, salads, soups, and casseroles. But cabbage is a part of almost every national and ethnic cuisine, including those from China, India, Mexico, France, and Eastern Europe. In Russia and Ukraine, where cabbage consumption is the greatest, cabbage soup is the ultimate winter comfort food, while in Korea, fermented kimchi is served at literally every meal.

Like other cruciferous vegetables, cabbage is a very healthy food. In addition to dietary fiber, cabbage contains small amounts of protein and large amounts of vitamins C and K, along with potassium, which helps reduce blood pressure. It contains *anthocyanins*, which are antioxidants that reduce inflammation; long-term inflammation is connected to heart disease, cancer, rheumatoid arthritis, and other serious medical conditions. Cabbage also contains high amounts of

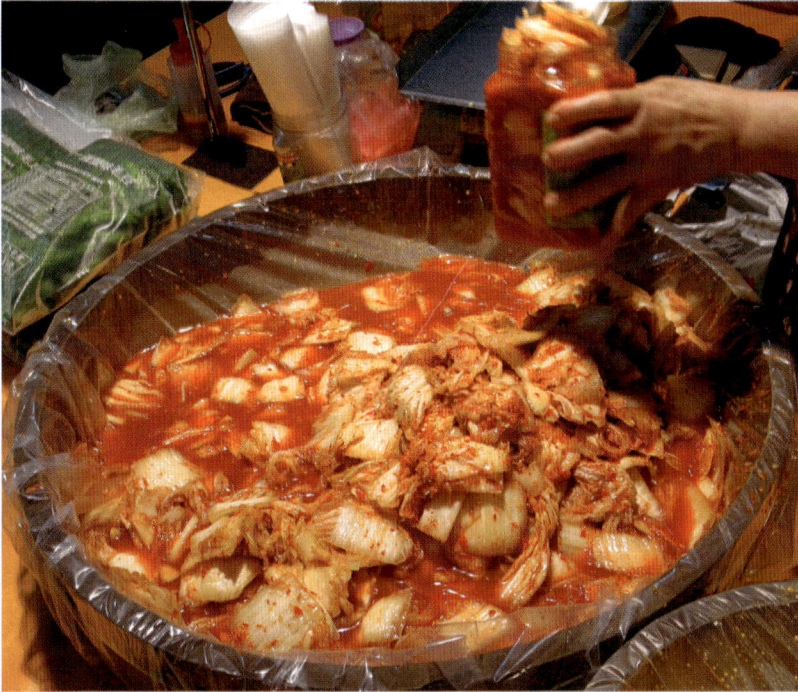

Cabbage prepared as kimchi.

polysterols, which are plant compounds that block the body's absorption of "bad" cholesterol—on top of that, they also help keep bowel movements regular. Fermented cabbage, like in kimchi and sauerkraut, support "good" intestinal bacteria and strengthen the immune system.

The majority of cabbage grown in the United States is used in commercial processing for coleslaw (45 percent) and sauerkraut (12 percent), followed by fresh head cabbage (35 percent) and other fresh-cut products (5–10 percent). The major cabbage-growing states are California, Arizona, Texas, and Michigan. China is the world's leading producer of cabbage, followed by Russia, South Korea, and Ukraine.

Resources

Cai, Chengcheng, Johan Bucher, Freek T. Bakker et al. "Evidence for two domestication lineages supporting a middle-eastern origin for Brassica oleracea crops from diversified kale populations." *Horticulture Research* 9 (2022).

"Cabbage (Juan Xi Cai)." The White Rabbit Institute of Healing website. Accessed November 5, 2023.

Chan, Vicki. "Chinese Cabbage–The King of All Vegetables." Chinese Medicine Living website. February 6, 2014.

Cleveland Clinic. "8 Health Benefits of Cabbage." healthessentials website. September 22, 2022.

de Candolle, Alphonse. *Origin of Cultivated Plants*. New York: D. Appleton and Company, 1908, 84–85.

Iowa State University. "Cabbage." Agricultural Marketing Resource Center website. October 2021.

"Of Cabbages and Celts." Texas AgriLife Extension Service. Texas A&M System. Accessed November 5, 2023.

"Our Cabbages Originated in the Middle East (and with the warming climate, that is a very good thing)." Wageningen University & Research website. March 14, 2022.

Severson, Kim. "The Morning: Cabbage Is Having a Moment." *The New York Times*. March 10, 2024.

Stefan, Iona, and Andrea Ona. "Cabbage (*Brassica oleracea L.*). Overview of the Health Benefits and Therapeutical Uses." *Hop and Medicinal Plants* 28 (2020).

Vegetables 2020 Summary. Washington, D.C.: United States Department of Agriculture, 2021, 28–29.

Wikipedia. "Cabbage." Accessed November 5, 2023.

Wikipedia. "Chinese cabbage." Accessed November 5, 2023.

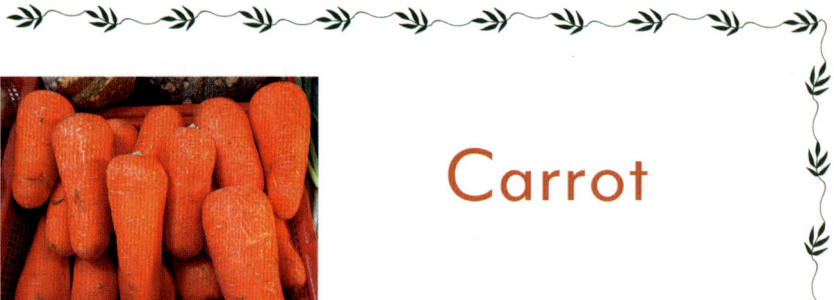

Carrot

Carrots (*Daucus carota*), one of humanity's most important root vegetables, are cultivated all over the world. Based on historical documents and genetic research, central Asia is believed to be one origin of cultivated carrots, which are mainly classified into "Eastern" carrots and "Western" carrots based on the color of their root. Most Eastern carrots are purple or yellow, and are thought to have originated in today's Afghanistan, while the origin of Western carrots, whose roots are orange, red, or white is still uncertain. Orange carrots are more popular, and are the carrots most Westerners are familiar with.

Wild carrots started off as either white or pale yellow, but changed to purple and yellow when *homo sapiens* first domesticated the vegetable almost five thousand years ago in the Persian Plateau area.

These domesticated carrots were later split into two main classes: the Asiatic (Eastern) group, which was cultivated in the Himalayan foothills, and the Western group, which grew largely in the Middle East and Türkiye. Yellow carrots in the Western group probably mutated into more orange hues, which farmers then selectively planted.

It is believed that orange-carrot seeds were first introduced to Europe by Islamic traders moving between the Ottoman Empire's North African territories and the Iberian Peninsula as far back as the fourteenth century. Dutch farmers began to cultivate carrots in the sixteenth century, and Dutch merchants then spread the orange produce across the continent; they were especially well received in what are now France, Germany, and England. Orange types, first grown in the Netherlands during the seventeenth century, were brought to North America by early settlers. Carrots have long been viewed as good for health, and the recent interest in healthy diets has increased carrot consumption. The introduction of "baby-cut" or "baby" carrots in the late 1980s placed the carrot among America's most popular healthy snack foods.

The carrot, a versatile vegetable, can be part of many popular diets including vegan, vegetarian, keto, paleo, and more. Carrots can be made into a delicious and highly nutritious juice, and are often enjoyed raw in salads or eaten with hummus as a dip. They can also be steamed, boiled, or roasted to be served as a side dish. Carrots also work well in soups, stews, and stir-fried dishes. While perhaps not the healthiest way to eat them, carrots also make a delicious loaf or carrot cake.

Cultivation of carrots for medicinal purposes began two to three thousand years ago. They were used to treat a wide range of health problems including stomach ulcers, abscesses, bladder, liver and kidney problems, to aid in childbirth, and even as an aphrodisiac.

Carrots are widely praised by nutritionists due to their richness in dietary fiber, vitamins (especially beta-carotene, vitamin C, and vitamin K), and other nutrients, including potassium. Other phytochemicals include phenolics and polyacetylenes. Together, these chemicals aid in the reduction of the risk of cancer and cardiovascular diseases, due to their antioxidant, anti-inflammatory, plasma lipid modification and anti-tumor properties. *Carotenoids* in particular, which are also found in tomatoes and peppers, have been found to help prevent cancer, cerebrovascular disease (CVD), human immunodeficiency virus (HIV), and cataracts. They also give carrots their rich orange color. *Anthocyanins* found in carrots have been reported to have many health benefits, including prevention of cardiovascular diseases, anticancer activity, control of diabetes, and improvement of vision.

A recent review article published in the journal *Foods*, based on more than 130 scientific research papers, books, and book chapters about carrots concluded:

> The biological activities of some of the phytochemicals found in carrots, namely phenolic compounds (particularly chlorogenic acid), carotenoids, polyacetylenes, and ascorbic acid (vitamin C), have indicated their potential to improve human health due to their anti-cancer, antioxidant, anti-inflammatory, antibacterial, plasma lipid modification, and serotogenic [improvement in nerve function] effects. (Ahmad et al. 2019, 424)

The four major carrot growing countries are China, Russia, Uzbekistan, and the United States. In the United States, the four biggest carrot producing states are California, Washington, Michigan, and Wisconsin.

Resources

Ahmad, T. M. Cawood, Q. Iqbal et al. "Phytochemicals in *Daucus carota* and Their Health Benefits-Review Article." *Foods*8, 9 (2019): 424.

Chepkemoi, Joyce. "The World's Top Carrot Producing Countries." WorldAtlas.com. Accessed November 15, 2023.

McAvoy, Ted. "Commercial Production and Management of Carrots." Bulletin no. 1175. University of Georgia Extension website. Accessed November 15, 2023.

Plackett, Benjamin. "Are carrots orange because of a Dutch revolutionary?" Livescience. September 5, 2020.

Que, F., X. L. Hou, G. L. Wang et al. "Advances in research on the carrot, an important root vegetable in the Apiaceae family." *Horticultural Research* 6, no. 69 (2019).

Vegetables: 2019 Summary. United States Department of Agriculture, February 2020.

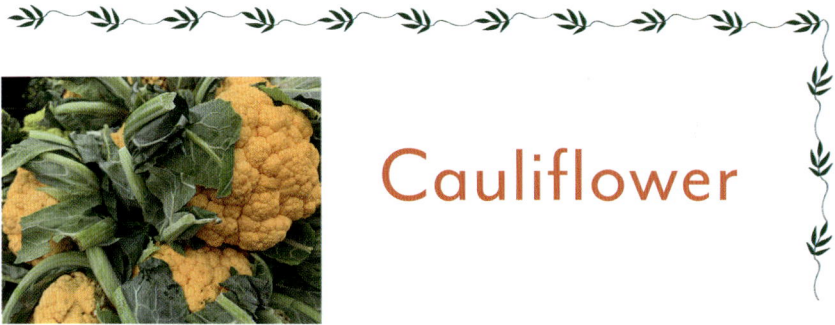

Cauliflower

For many years, Westerners considered the cauliflower (*Brassica oleracea* var. *botrytis*) to be among the most boring of vegetables, to be boiled and eaten as a side dish to meat. Drawing from childhood memories of being forced to eat cauliflower at summer camp, it was one of the few foods my father would not allow in the house. As a result, I didn't taste cauliflower until I was in college.

Yet, creative chefs around the world have recently discovered that this vegetable is among the healthiest, tastiest, and most versatile around. As a result, the popularity of cauliflower has skyrocketed. *Time* magazine even recently named cauliflower the "it" vegetable:

> The versatility of cauliflower has boosted its popularity. It can be mashed and buttered like potatoes, sautéed in spices for a curry, or toasted in buffalo sauce and fried to make meatless chicken wings. (Gajanan, *Time*)

The vegetable's name comes from the Latin *caulis*, for cabbage, and *floris*, for flower. Like its cousin broccoli, the cauliflower is a descendant of a type of wild cabbage that has been developed through centuries of selective breeding. Its tightly bunched white florets are connected by a thick core, often with a few light green leaves surrounding it.

It is believed that cauliflower was first cultivated in the eastern Mediterranean region and Asia Minor over two thousand years ago. The ancient Greeks and Romans were among the first to grow cauliflower, which was later introduced to other parts of Europe by Arab traders. Cauliflower eventually spread to India and China via the Silk Road, where it is now considered an essential part of both countries' cuisines.

The cauliflower was first introduced to the United States during the seventeenth century, and was cultivated in California since the early twentieth century. Today, some 90 percent of the cauliflower grown in the United States comes from California. Most cauliflower has white florets, but interesting varieties (often available at specialty grocers or at farmers markets) contain florets that are either green, orange, yellow, or purple.

Cauliflower is among the most versatile of vegetables. Its popularity increased nearly threefold in the United States during the 2010s, and continues to grow at a rapid pace. A key to cauliflower's popularity is the vegetable's versatility: its richness can be enjoyed in an Indian curry, a North African stew, a Chinese stir-fry, or as a creamy and comforting

soup. Cauliflower can also be added to broiled or stir-fried vegetable plat-
ters, steamed or sautéed as a side dish, baked in a casserole, served raw with
a dip, or eaten raw or steamed in a salad. Cauliflower has even become a
gluten-free "rice," and is being used as an ingredient in pizza crust. Mashed
cauliflower is a low-carb alternative to mashed potatoes. While most consumers discard the core of the cauliflower head, chefs recommend that
all of this nutritious veggie be used. The core can be chopped or mashed,
then frozen for use as a future ingredient in soup or a casserole.

Like its broccoli cousin, cauliflower is highly nutritious: it is packed
with vitamins C, B$_6$, K, and folate. One small head of cauliflower has
more than 125 milligrams of vitamin C—nearly twice as much as a
medium orange. Cauliflower is also a good source of dietary fiber, is low
in carbohydrates and calories, and is a cholesterol-free food. Cauliflower
contains a number of "good for you" phytochemicals (especially *isothiocyanates* and *glucosinolates*). A May 2022 article appearing in the peer-
reviewed journal *Antioxidants* (Basel) reported:

> In fact, cauliflower is considered as one of the most important
> Brassicas due to its healthy properties. These health benefits are due
> to the fact that this vegetable contains a substantial amount of dietary
> fiber, and a substantial number of vitamins; minerals; and bioactive
> compounds, such as glucosinolates, isothiocyanates, and polyamines.
> These health-promoting compounds have been found to be effective
> in protecting against many chronic human diseases, including several
> kinds of cancer. (Collado-González et al. 2022, 958)

Another research paper published in the same journal the previous year mentioned that the highest content of phytochemicals and the
highest antioxidant capacity in cauliflower were found in the leaves and
stems, two parts of the vegetable that are usually discarded. They were
also found to be rich in nutritive compounds including minerals, proteins, and amino acids. Although consumers can save both the (carefully

washed) leaves and stems to use in soups, casseroles, or juice, the authors suggested that these neglected parts of the cauliflower be utilized by the food industry as additives for developing new and functional foodstuffs.

China is currently the world's largest producer of cauliflower, followed by India, Spain, Mexico, and Italy. Cauliflower is grown in gardens throughout most of the United States and Canada. In addition to California, most of the cauliflower that's commercially grown in North America comes from Oregon and Arizona.

Resources

Collado-González, J., M. C. Piñero, G. Otalora et al. "Enhancement of Bioactive Constituents in Fresh Cauliflower By-Products in Challenging Climate Conditions." *Antioxidants (Basel)* 11, 5 (2022): 958.

Drabińska, N., M. Jeż, M. Nogueira. "Variation in the Accumulation of Phytochemicals and Their Bioactive Properties among the Aerial Parts of Cauliflower." *Antioxidants (Basel)* 10, 10 (2021): 1597.

Gajanan, Mahita. "Why Cauliflower Is the New 'It' Vegetable." *Time*. July 14, 2017.

Lambert, Tim. "A History of Vegetables." Local Histories website. Accessed November 15, 2023.

O'Neill, Tony. "Uncovering the Roots: The Fascinating History of Cauliflower," Simplify Gardening. May 28, 2023.

Smith, David. "Flower Development: Origin of the Cauliflower." *Current Biology*, 5, no. 4 (1995): 361–63.

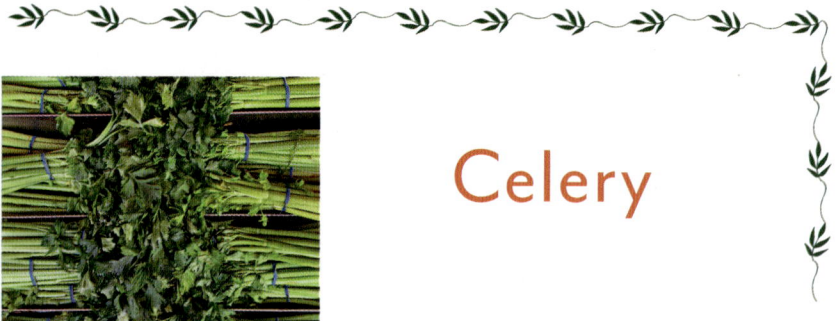

Celery

Celery (*Apium graveolens*) is a member of the parsley family. The plant grows wild in wet environments, and has become one of the most popular garden vegetables in both Europe and North America.

Archaeological remains from Switzerland have suggested that humans were transporting celery seeds as early as 4000 BCE. Another variety of celery, called "Nan Ling," was present in China as early as the fifth century CE.

Celery was first cultivated in the Mediterranean region some three thousand years ago. It was first used as a seasoning, but printed records from France dating from 1623 show that it was later consumed as an actual food. Celery's common name comes from the French word *céleri* and the Italian word *seleri*. Both were derived from Greek word *selinon* (σέλινον), meaning "parsley." Reference was made to selinon in Homer's *Odyssey*, which dates from the seventh to the eighth century BCE.

By the middle part of the eighteenth century CE, celery was enjoyed by affluent northern Europeans as both a food and a seasoning, and its use spread rapidly. Celery was probably introduced to North America by European colonists; by 1806, four cultivated varieties were being grown in the United States. Widespread celery cultivation began near Kalamazoo, Michigan, in the late 1800s, which helped make Michigan the nation's largest celery producer until the 1950s. "Pascal" celery dominates commercial production today, and is easily found in every North American supermarket.

Most people eat the celery stalk only, as a raw stand-alone food or paired with dips or hummus for an easy snack. Diced celery can enhance flavors of other foods and add texture to soups, stews, stir-fried dishes, and casseroles. Celery leaves can be chopped and used as a garnish. Celery juice is popular either alone or combined with other vegetables like beets or carrots.

Celery is a popular diet food because its high fiber content provides a feeling of fullness without the calories. In addition, celery is rich in several vitamins including A, B_2, B_5 (pantothenic acid), B_6, C, and K. It also provides calcium, magnesium, and phosphorus. Finally, celery is a good source of antioxidants—including caffeic acid, ferric acid, tannin, saponin, and kaempferol—that reduce inflammation and both treat and lower the risk of a wide range of health conditions. A landmark 2017 article appearing in the peer-reviewed *Journal of Evidence-Based Complementary and Alternative Medicine* highlighted these phytochemicals in celery, and addressed celery's wide spectrum of documented healing properties:

> Celery can prevent cardiovascular diseases, jaundice, liver and lien [spleen] diseases, urinary tract obstruction, gout, and rheumatic disorders. Research on rats shows that ethanol extracts of celery leaves increases spermatogenesis and also improves their fertility. Celery reduces glucose, blood lipids, and blood pressure, which can strengthen the heart. Experimental studies show that celery has antifungal and anti-inflammatory properties. Moreover, its essential oils have antibacterial effects. Its seeds are useful in the treatment of bronchitis, asthenopia [eyestrain], asthma, chronic skin disorders including psoriasis, vomiting, fever, and tumors. The root of the celery is diuretic and it is used for the treatment of colic. (Kooti and Daraei 2017, 1029)

The United States and Mexico are the world's leading growers of celery. Within the United States, most of the commercial celery crop is grown in California, Arizona, Florida, and Texas.

Resources

Iowa State University. "Celery." Agricultural Marketing Resource Center website. Revised May 2024.

Jacewicz, Natalie. "Celery: Why?" *The Salt*. National Public Radio. June 13, 2016.

Johnson, Greg, "Celery Volume Booms." Produce Blue Book Services website. June 5, 2020.

Kooti, Wesam, and Naheed Daraei. "A Review of the Antioxidant Activity of Celery (*Apium graveolens L*)." *Journal of Evidence-Based Complementary and Alternative Medicine*. 4 (2017):1029–1034.

Trinklein, David. "Celery: A Brief History." Integrated Pest Management website. University of Missouri. November 1, 2011.

Wergin, Allyn. "Celery: Not Just for Veggie Trays." *Hometown Health Blog.* Speaking of Health. Mayo Clinic Health System website. June 2, 2023.

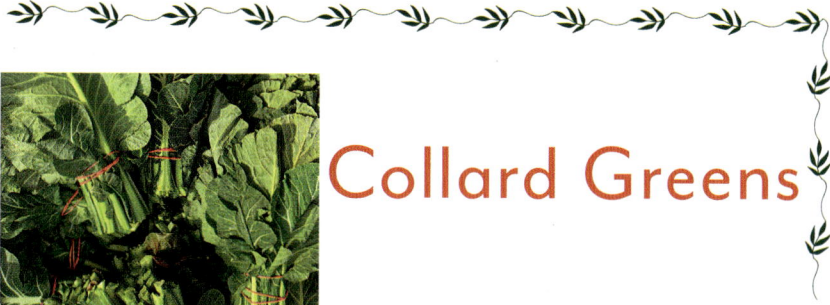

Collard Greens

Collard greens (*Brassica oleracea* var. *viridis*) date back to prehistoric times. As the oldest leafy green in the cabbage family, they developed from wild cabbage species indigenous to an area near Greece, by the Mediterranean Sea, as well as in Anatolia (now part of Türkiye). Collards were likely first domesticated five thousand years ago. They became a staple crop in both Greece and Rome as far back as the first century CE, and were also cultivated extensively in what are now Montenegro, central Croatia, and Herzegovina. Cultivation of collard greens eventually spread throughout eastern and southern Africa, and collards became especially popular in the highlands of Kenya and surrounding regions.

It is believed that collard greens were introduced to North America in the early 1600s through Jamestown, Virginia, on boats carrying African slaves. Collards were one of the most common plants grown in plantation kitchen gardens, and cooking methods used for many collard dishes were based on African customs dating back to pre-slavery times. Collards remain a popular side dish in the southern United States, and many recipes have been passed on over generations. There is an American superstition that the green collard leaves represent money, and that eating them on New Year's Day will ensure financial prosperity throughout the year.

Eating collard greens may not make you wealthy, but this highly adaptable, green, leafy vegetable is definitely rich in nutrition and health benefits. In addition to being a good source of dietary fiber, collards provide generous amounts of iron, manganese, magnesium, and calcium, plus vitamins A, B_6, C, E, and K.

Antioxidants and other phytochemicals in collard greens have been found to provide anti-inflammatory properties; they also promote healthy skin and hair, lower "bad" cholesterol, support liver health, and contain cancer-fighting properties. Collards contain a good amount of dietary fiber, which, along with vitamins B and K, support digestion and help regulate blood sugar levels in the body. Vitamin K may lower the risk of osteoporosis and bone breakage.

Collards are best prepared boiled, sautéed, or steamed in order to preserve their nutritional content. They can be cooked with garlic, herbs, and spices, or added to a wide variety of stir-fried dishes, soups, and casseroles. In addition to that of the American South, collards make up an important part of the cuisines of northern India, eastern Africa, Zimbabwe, Portugal, and Brazil. *Caldo verde*, a popular Brazilian and Portuguese soup, is based on collard greens.

The leading collard-growing states in the United States are South Carolina (collards are its official state vegetable) and Georgia.

Resources

Seidel, Allison. "Collard Greens." Food Source Information. Colorado State University website. Accessed November 16, 2023.

Tufts University. "Collard Greens." New Entry Sustainable Farming Project website. Accessed November 16, 2023.

Yang, Elsie. "7 Proven Health Benefits of Collard Greens, According to Nutritionists." *Prevention*. September 29, 2020.

Wikipedia. "Collard (plant)." Accessed November 16, 2023.

Corn and Maize

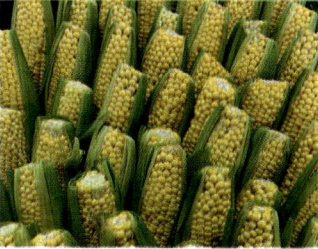

Corn is one of many foods gifted from Mesoamerica to the world. Indigenous farmers in the Tehuacán Valley in eastern Mexico first cultivated a wild ancestor of the first corn plant (a spiky grass called *teosinte*) some ten thousand years ago. Although this ancient plant featured very small cobs, the genetic difference between it and modern-day corn was very small. Corn has been a primary source of nutrition for members of many Indigenous groups in Mexico and Central America, including the Aztecs, Mayans, Mixtecs, Zapotecs, and Chinantecs.

Known in Mexico as *elote* (from the Nahuatl word *élotl*) corn has also played an important role in ceremonies, myths, and legends. Speakers of Nahuatl refer to corn as *tlaolli*, or "our sustenance." Corn has provided the foundation for no fewer than six hundred different Mexican foods including tortillas, tacos, tamales, quesadillas, sopes, chalupas, tostadas, enchiladas, and chilaquiles; it is also used to make traditional beverages such as pozol, atole, and chichi. Over the years, Indigenous farmers selectively bred teosinte for favorable traits, and it gradually became the type of corn we know today. Overall, sixty different varieties of corn are grown in Mexico—the most diverse national collection of corn in the world.

As early Indigenous Mexicans migrated north into what is now the southwestern United States, and south down the coast to Peru, they brought their carefully bred corn seeds with them. Corn arrived in the Eastern Woodlands (an area extending from the Atlantic Ocean to the eastern Great Plains, and from the Great Lakes region to the Gulf of Mexico) about one thousand years ago. As cultivation spread among Native American communities, the breeding of corn continued to improve. Corn was an early food source for early American colonists, and is said to have been consumed at the first Thanksgiving in 1621 by residents of the Plymouth Colony in Massachusetts.

It is believed that corn was unknown in Europe until explorer Christopher Columbus encountered it during his visit to Cuba in 1493, and brought it back to Spain. Corn was introduced to Italy and France in 1494, northern Europe by 1571, Egypt in 1525, and Africa, India, and China by the end of the sixteenth century, where it was widely planted. Although farmers grew corn in the United States for centuries as food for both humans and livestock, the first commercial hybrid corn seeds were developed in the early 1930s with the support of Henry A. Wallace, an Iowa farmer, and President Franklin Delano Roosevelt's secretary of agriculture from 1933–1940. Today, almost all of the corn planted in the United States is of hybrid varieties.

While there are more than one hundred varieties of cultivated corn throughout the world, only three basic types of corn are grown commercially in the United States. *Field corn* is commonly grown as livestock feed and for making ethanol, an alternative to gasoline. *Yellow corn* (also known as sweet corn) is the most popular type of corn sold in supermarkets and farm stands in the United States today. It is a mutation of field corn (*Zea mays*). Varieties of this corn were first grown in Pennsylvania during the mid-1700s, with the first commercial variety introduced in 1779. Sweet corn is usually harvested before it is fully mature, while its sugar content is still high. *White corn* is the type most widely grown in Mexico and Central America, and, aside from being consumed directly as corn, it is the major ingredient in traditional tortillas. In the United States, white corn is considered a "niche" crop, and is mostly used to make corn chips and other snacks.

Only three percent of the corn grown in the United States is eaten by humans; the rest is fed to livestock or exported. Corn is grown throughout the fifty U.S. states, but most of the sweet corn sold commercially comes from Florida, Washington, Georgia, New York, or Oregon.

Many people ask: "Is corn a vegetable or is it a grain?" According to the United States Department of Agriculture, it is both:

> Corn that is harvested when fully mature and dry is considered a grain. It can be milled into cornmeal and used in such foods as corn tortillas and cornbread. Popcorn is also harvested when it matures and is considered to be a whole grain. On the other hand, fresh [sweet] corn (e.g., corn on the cob, frozen corn kernels) is harvested when it is soft and has kernels full of liquid. Fresh corn is considered a starchy vegetable. (*AskUSDA*, United States Department of Agriculture)

When it comes to food, fresh corn can be enjoyed on the cob or as an ingredient in soups, stews, salads, casseroles, and stir-fried dishes. As mentioned earlier, corn is a primary ingredient in hundreds of traditional Mexican dishes. A gluten-free grain, corn can be made into cornmeal to be enjoyed as grits, cornflakes, or boiled to make *polenta*, an Italian specialty; when finely ground into flour, it is a popular ingredient in donuts, pancakes, muffins, and baby food. Corn starch is a thickening agent for liquids, and corn oil is widely used for frying. High-fructose corn syrup is a cheap alternative to cane sugar, and is used to sweeten almost every canned and packaged food imaginable. Corn also has many industrial uses, such as in making cosmetics, whiskey, and fuel (ethanol).

With the exception of high-fructose corn syrup, corn is a healthy food. In addition to dietary fiber, corn provides vitamins C, B, E, and K, along with magnesium and potassium. Corn also contains carotenoids like lutein and zeaxanthin, which support eye heath and may help prevent cataracts. Popcorn (preferably oil-free and unsalted) has been found to help prevent diverticulitis. Tea made from corn silk has long been used by folk healers to treat minor urinary tract infections.

A chapter in the textbook *Corn: Production and Human Health in Changing Climate* discusses the numerous phytochemicals in corn and their therapeutic potentials:

> The principal phytochemicals present in corn seed and corn silk include polyphenols, phenolic acids, flavonoids, anthocyanins, glycosides, carotenoids, and polysaccharides of biological importance, reducing compounds and some water-soluble vitamins. The presence of these phytochemicals makes corn a medicinal plant which shows various biological activities particularly the antioxidant, antimicrobial, antidiabetic, anti-obesity, antiproliferative [inhibits tumor cell growth], hepatoprotective [liver protective], cardioprotective, and renal-protective [kidney-protective] activities. (Nawaz et al. 2018, 49)

The United States is the world's leading producer (and exporter) of corn, followed by China, Brazil, and Argentina.

Resources

"History of Corn: From Ancient Grain to Modern Maize," *Cornstalk* blog. Nebraska Corn Board website. 2023.

"Is Corn a Grain or a Vegetable?" AskUSDA. United States Department of Agriculture. November 4, 2022.

Iowa State University. "Niche Corn Opportunities." Agricultural Marketing Resource Center website. April 2022.

Iowa State University. "Sweet Corn." Agricultural Marketing Resource Center website. April 2022.

Mota Cruz, Cecilio, Caroline Burgeff, and Francisca Acevedo Gasman. "Maíces." Biodiversidad Mexicana. Updated December 12, 2022.

Nawaz, Haq. Muzaffar Saima, Aslam Momna, and Ahmad Shakeel. Chapter 4. "Phytochemical Composition: Antioxidant Potential and

Biological Activities of Corn." In *Corn - Production and Human Health in Changing Climate*. London: InTechopen, 2018, 49–68.

Shanahan, Andrew. "History of Corn." Student Papers. North Dakota State University. Accessed November 20, 2023.

Smith, C. Wayne, et al. eds. *Corn: Origin, History, Technology and Production*. New York: Wiley & Sons, 2004, xii–xiii.

Watson, Stephany. "Corn." WebMD. 2022.

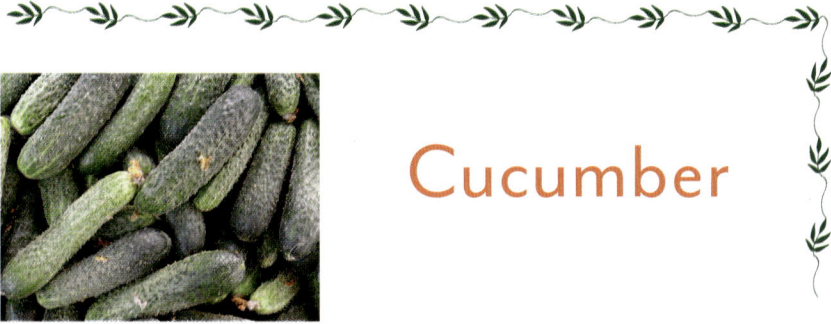

Cucumber

The cucumber (*Cucumis sativus*) is one of America's top five garden vegetables. Valued as a diet food because of its low-calorie content, cucumbers have been found in recent studies to contain significant amounts of phytonutrients that provide a wide range of health benefits.

Cucumbers belong to the Cucurbitaceae family, which also includes watermelon, muskmelon, pumpkins, and squash. Cucumbers originated in India and descended from a wild variety that had a bitter flavor. Wild cucumber can still be found in India and northwestern Thailand, where it is sold in local markets. The cucumber is considered one of our oldest vegetables, having been cultivated for over three thousand years. Cucumbers were introduced to China by 200 BCE, and spread west to Asia Minor and Africa.

Three major cucumber groups evolved over the centuries. They include the Eurasian variety, which are enjoyed raw and often added to salads; East Asian cucumbers, which are used primarily to make pickles; and Xishuangbanna, a Chinese variety that looks like a gourd but has a tasty orange flesh—it dates from the Han dynasty (202 BCE–9 CE; 25–220 CE) and remains popular in China.

Cucumbers were cultivated in Egypt since pre-Biblical times. Numbers 11:5 reads: "We remember the fish, which we did not eat in Egypt freely; the cucumbers and the melons, and the leeks and the onions, and the garlick." The ancient Greeks also cultivated cucumbers, and the Romans did as well. The Roman emperor Tiberius (42 BCE–37 CE) liked them so much, he ate them every day. When he traveled, he had cucumbers accompany him, which were grown in special pots. The Romans are credited with innovative ways of growing cucumbers, such as making frames with translucent panes—not unlike the cold frames farmers use today.

Charlemagne (747–814 CE), Holy Roman Emperor and the King of the Franks and Lombards, had cucumbers grown in his gardens in Italy. Cucumber cultivation later spread to western Europe and arrived in England during the reign of Henry VIII. His first wife, Catherine of Aragon, liked to include them in salads.

Christopher Columbus introduced cucumbers to Haiti in 1494, and Spanish explorer Hernando de Soto found them growing in Florida in 1519, from seeds probably brought from Haiti. By 1806, no fewer than eight cucumber varieties were growing in Colonial America.

Now, there are dozens of cucumber varieties. As a child, cucumber was my favorite vegetable—but we ate only one variety, the one available in supermarkets with the boring name "American slicing." I later discovered crisp Kirby cucumbers, a short and stubby variety that's often used to make pickles but is also delicious eaten raw. When visiting Japan, I discovered a long, thin variety with a rough, bumpy skin. Known as *kyuri*, this crisp and tasty cucumber has been enjoyed in Japan for centuries, and is increasingly available in Asian markets in North America and Europe. Persian cucumbers are also crisp and delicious, and the long, thin "English" or "European" cucumber is a popular import often grown in a hothouse.

Cucumbers contain about 95 percent water, which make them both refreshing and good for hydration. They are also high in important nutrients including vitamin K—important for bone health—vitamin B complex, and C, plus essential minerals like calcium, copper, iron, phosphorous, potassium, and magnesium.

Recent research has found that cucumbers are loaded with phytochemicals (especially antioxidants) that are good for health. They contain high amounts of *Cucurbitacon B* (CuB) that may be useful in fighting liver, breast, lung, and prostate cancers. CuB also has been credited with maintaining healthy blood vessels and preventing arteriosclerosis.

Cucumbers are low in calories and sugar, are useful for maintaining healthy weight and managing blood sugar, and may have potential in preventing and managing diabetes. They also have a cleansing action within the body, removing accumulated pockets of waste materials and chemical toxins. Their high fiber and water content aid bowel movement regularity, while pickled cucumbers contain friendly bacteria that support gut health. While some cucumbers have thicker skin that some people prefer to peel, small and thin imported varieties have tender skin, and thus contain more fiber and nutrients than varieties eaten peeled. Fresh cucumber juice is widely used for nourishing the skin, soothing irritations and reducing swelling. Cucumber also has the power to alleviate sunburn pain.

China is the world's leading cucumber producer, followed by Türkiye, Russia, Ukraine, and Mexico. Michigan, Florida, and Georgia are the most important cucumber-growing states in the United States. Like many other fruits and vegetables, most of the cucumbers imported to the United States are from Mexico.

Resources

de Candolle, Alphonse. *Origin of Cultivated Plants*. New York: D. Appleton and Company, 1908, 266.

Chomicki, G., H. Schaefer, and S. S. Renner. "Origin and domestication of Cucurbitaceae crops: insights from phylogenies, genomics and archaeology." *New Phytologist* 226 (2020): 1240–1255.

Cleveland Clinic. "6 Health Benefits of Cucumbers." healthessentials. April 3, 2023.

Mukherjee, P. K., N. K. Nema, N. Maity, and B. K. Sarkar. "Phytochemical and therapeutic potential of cucumber." *Fitoterapia*84 (2013): 227–36.

University of California, Davis. "Most US Fresh Cucumbers Are Imported from Mexico." *Rural Migration Blog.* February 28, 2022.

University of Missouri. "Cucumber: A Brief History," Integrated Pest Management website. March 3, 2014.

Vidhi, J. "Cucumber: Origin, Production and Varieties | India." Biology Discussion website. Accessed November 16, 2023.

Wikipedia. "List of Countries by Cucumber Production." Accessed November 17, 2023.

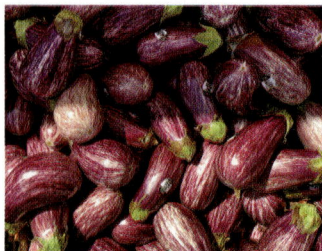

Eggplant

The eggplant (*Solanum melongena*) is a member of the genus *Solanum* (containing around 1,400 species), which is a member of the nightshade family. Eggplant (known as *aubergine* in the United Kingdom and France) is related to potatoes, tomatoes, peppers, and tobacco.

Early studies led scientists to believe that eggplants were first domesticated in China and India, possibly from the wild nightshade species *thorn* or *bitter apple*. It was also believed that there were two sites of independent domestication: one in southern Asia and the other in eastern Asia. However, recent investigations have found that the wild species related to the cultivated eggplant existed in the savannahs of northeastern Africa some two million years ago. Plants then dispersed eastward to tropical Asia, as well as to southern and western Africa. In Asia, the dispersal gave rise to a species that plant scientists call

Solanum insanum. It is from this wild species that the today's eggplant was later domesticated.

Spanish Moors are believed to have brought eggplant to southern and eastern Europe from India in the 1400s, while European explorers introduced the vegetable to the Americas in the 1500s. Thomas Jefferson was said to have carried eggplant seeds to his home in Virginia from France in the late 1700s. However, eggplants were not an immediate success in the United States because people were suspicious of its being a member of the nightshade family, of which poisonous Deadly Nightshade (along with non-poisonous tomatoes and potatoes) are members.

Most commercial eggplant varieties are purplish-black in color and tend to be oval or teardrop in shape; globe eggplants tend to be large, while Italian eggplants are smaller. Chinese eggplants, which are widely available in Asian markets in Europe and North America, tend to be purple in color and are long and slender. Baby or miniature eggplants are also available in Indian and southern Asian markets. Other varieties are egg-shaped, and may be white or orange in color. The name "eggplant" was first used to describe white cultivars, which resemble chicken eggs.

Eggplants have been an important part of traditional Chinese, Japanese, Indian, Thai, Italian, Turkish, and Middle Eastern cuisines for centuries. Some of the most famous eggplant dishes are baignan bhartha (India), baba ganoush (Türkiye and the Middle East), eggplant parmigiana and eggplant rollatini (Italy), eggplant moussaka (Greece, Middle East, Egypt), eggplant with garlic sauce (China), green and red curry (Thailand), and soy-glazed eggplant donburi (Japan). Eggplants are well adapted to Western tastes and are widely used in soups, stews, and stir-fried dishes, or can be cut into slices to be grilled, baked, or fried. When cooked, eggplants have a rich, meaty interior that makes them a good stand-in for meat.

Though delicious, eggplants have not been considered a nutritional powerhouse, although they do contain a wide range of dietary fiber, carbohydrates, proteins, vitamins (especially vitamins A, B, C, and folate), minerals (including trace amounts copper, zinc, iron, and potassium), and several other bioactive compounds, such as phenolic acids. White eggplant has been used in India's ancient Ayurvedic system of medicine to treat diabetes and asthma.

Recent laboratory and clinical research show that eggplant is a very healthy food and is loaded with beneficial phytochemicals. According to an article about the biochemical content of eggplant, published in the peer-reviewed journal *Applied Sciences* in 2021:

> Due to this biochemical composition, eggplant may possibly be used in the treatment of anemia, atherosclerosis, and fatty degeneration. [. . .] Its antioxidant property potentially reduces the risk of various types of cancer, protects against cardiovascular diseases, and prevents acute respiratory infections. Further, eggplant fibers help in digestion by removing toxins and harmful materials from the stomach and reducing colon cancer. Plant polyphenols present in eggplants can help protect cell membranes and boost the brain's memory function. (Sharma and Kaushik 2021, 7078)

China is the world's largest eggplant producer, followed by India, Egypt, Türkiye, and Indonesia. New Jersey (The Garden State) has the most acreage devoted to eggplant cultivation in the United States, followed by California, Georgia, and Florida.

Resources

Chewy Media. "The Eggplant: A Little History and Growing Instructions." Harvesting History. Accessed November 20, 2023.

Sharma, M., and P. Kaushik. "Biochemical Composition of Eggplant Fruits: A Review." *Applied Sciences* 11 (2021): 7078.

Iowa State University. "Eggplant." Agricultural Marketing Resource Center website. August 2021.

"Tracing the evolution of the aubergine." Natural History Museum (London). August 30, 2018.

Watson, Stephanie. "Health Benefits of Eggplant." WebMD. August 8, 2021.

Wikipedia. "Eggplant." Accessed November 20, 2023.

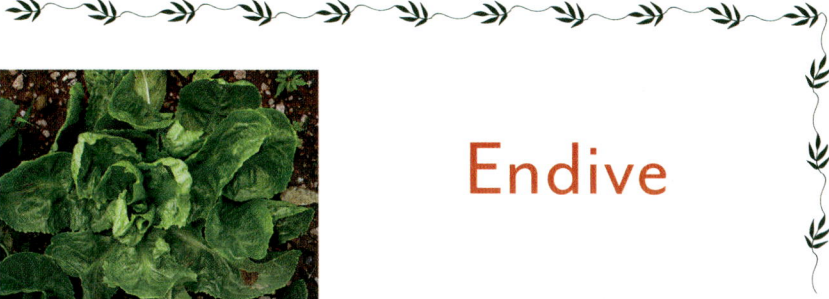

Endive

Photo by Natalie Schmalz

The endive (*Cichorium endivia*) is a crunchy and slightly bitter-tasting salad green that has been popular in Europe since the 1800s. While less known in North America, culinary interest in this nutritious vegetable has been growing, and it has been dubbed both "elegant" and "sophisticated" by gourmets and gourmands alike. There are two distinct varieties of endive: curly endive (var. *crispum*, commonly called just "endive"), Belgian endive and escarole (var. *latifolium*). Endive has curled, fringed leaves while escarole leaves are smooth, broad, and less bitter than endive.

Due to its connection with chicory, the origin of endive is southern Asia, probably India, and some food historians regard it as being indigenous to northern Africa. It was well known to the ancient Egyptians, who used it in salads and as a cooked vegetable. Endive was also cultivated by the ancient Greeks and Romans, enjoying in a variety of culinary preparations.

During the Middle Ages, endive cultivation spread across Europe. The spread of endive cultivation was closely linked to the movement of people, trade networks, and the exchange of agricultural practices throughout the continent. The plant was brought to the New World by early European settlers, and the first references of this crop in America come from 1803.

One story concerns the accidental discovery of endive in Belgium: In 1830, a farmer named Jan Lammers stored some chicory roots in the cellar on his farm near Brussels just before leaving to serve in the army during the Belgian Revolution (1830–31) which led to the establishment of the Kingdom of Belgium. He was planning to dry and roast them, as chicory was (and still is) a popular coffee additive and substitute. But when Lammers returned home, he discovered that his chicory roots had sprouted small, greenish-white leaves that were tender, crunchy, and very tasty.

Endive is most often added to salads, although its firm, boat-like shape makes it well suited to be paired with dips. It can also be grilled or roasted with olive oil and seasonings to make a tasty side dish. Chopped endive can be added to soups, stews, stir-fries, and casseroles.

Like many green leafy vegetables, endive is rich in dietary fiber, vitamin A, and folate, which supports heart health and helps reduce cholesterol. It also contains generous amounts of potassium, which is linked to the proper functioning of the kidneys, liver, nervous system, and heart.

One of the phytochemicals found in endive is the flavonoid *kaempferol*. This antioxidant has both anti-inflammatory and antibacterial properties, and has been found to help protect the body from heart disease and diabetes, as well as cancers of the colon, liver, and skin. The following excerpt, from the textbook *Dietary Interventions in Gastrointestinal Diseases* (Watson and Preedy 2019, 279), highlights the numerous medicinal benefits of consuming kaempferol-rich foods:

Numerous preclinical studies have shown that kaempferol and some glycosides of kaempferol have a wide range of pharmacological activities, including antioxidant, anti-inflammatory, antimicrobial, anticancer, cardioprotective, neuroprotective, antidiabetic, antiosteoporotic [fights osteoporosis], estrogenic/antiestrogenic, anxiolytic [reduces anxiety], analgesic [pain-reducing], and antiallergic activities.

China and the United States are the world's biggest growers of endive, followed by Spain, Italy, and India. California is the major grower of Belgian endive in the United States, while California, Arizona, and Florida are leading growers of escarole and curly endive.

Resources

"Endive, *Cichorium endivia*/Compositae." Fruits & Vegetables. Fruitashortalizas website. Accessed November 20, 2023.

"Endive Market Summary." Produce Bluebook website. Accessed November 20, 2023.

"The History of Endive Cultivation." Savory Suitcase website. November 17, 2023.

North Carolina State University. "*Cichorium endivia*." North Carolina Extension Gardener website. Accessed November 20, 2023.

Tan, Sharlene. "What Are the Health Benefits of Endive?" WebMD. May 20, 2022.

Watson, R., and V. Preedy, eds. *Dietary Intervention in Gastrointestinal Diseases*. Cambridge, MA: Academic Press, 2019, 277–87.

Wikipedia. "Chicory." Accessed November 20, 2023.

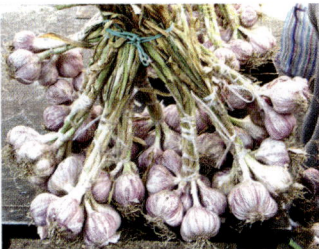

Garlic

Garlic (*Allium sativum*) is a member of the onion (Amaryllidaceae) family, and is classified in the same genus to which onions, leeks, chives, and shallots belong. Garlic appears to be a genomic variant of an ancient species of onion that grew wild in Central Asia almost one hundred thousand years ago. Most researchers agree that garlic has been used as a medicinal plant and food source for over seven thousand years, making it one of the world's most ancient vegetables.

Ancient Egyptian and Indian cultures referred to garlic as far back as 3000 BCE, and there is clear historical evidence that it was used by the Babylonians in 2500 BCE and by the Chinese at least as far back as 2000 BCE, which likely predated the semi-legendary Xia dynasty (2100–1766 BCE).

Garlic has always been regarded as both a food and a medicine. For example, during the reign of the Egyptian pharaohs, garlic was fed to the slave laborers who built the great pyramids, as it was believed to increase their strength and stamina, as well as protect them from disease. When the tomb of Egyptian Pharaoh King Tutankhamun was excavated in 1922, cloves of garlic were discovered among his valuable treasures.

In early China and Japan, garlic was prescribed to aid digestion, cure diarrhea, and help rid the body of intestinal worms. It also was used to alleviate depression. In ancient India, a medical text titled *Charaka Samhita* recommended garlic to treat heart disease and arthritis. In ancient Greece, Hippocrates—"the father of medicine"—advocated the use of garlic as a cleansing agent, as well as to treat lung problems and to eliminate abdominal growths. In his book *Historia Naturalis*, the Roman naturalist Pliny the Elder recommended garlic to treat gastrointestinal disorders, animal bites, joint disease, and seizures. Texts from early Chinese history show that garlic was widely used as a medicine as early as 2000 BCE. In addition to its medicinal properties, garlic was highly valued for its culinary uses and its effectiveness as a food preservative.

Like the onion, garlic was likely introduced to Europe by the

Romans. While a close cousin of garlic grew in North America centuries before Europeans arrived, garlic as a culinary staple didn't become known in the Americas until the seventeenth century when French, Spanish, and Portuguese explorers brought garlic from Europe. Several hundred years passed before garlic cultivation dramatically increased. The arrival of immigrants to the United States in the 1920s from Poland, Germany, and Italy, among other places, created a demand for what is now considered a culinary essential.

Like onions, garlic is a versatile food. It can be roasted whole or eaten raw (best prepared in a garlic press or finely chopped) in salads, sauces, and dressings. When cooked, it can elevate the flavor of almost any recipe, including sauces, roasts, casseroles, pasta dishes, marinades, stir-fries, and soups. *Sopa de ajo*, a traditional garlic soup from Mexico, is as delicious as it is nutritious.

Although garlic's medicinal properties have been known for millennia, its healing attributes have recently been found to be due to sulfur-containing compounds called *thiosulfinates*, as well as other beneficial phytochemicals.

A recent article about the chemical constituents and pharmacological activities of garlic appeared in the peer-reviewed journal *Nutrients*. The authors (Batiha et al. 2020, 872) identified a number of important phytochemicals in garlic, including several sulfur-containing phytoconstituents (alliin, allicin, ajoenes, and vinyldithiins), and flavonoids such as quercetin. They also addressed the many documented therapeutic abilities of the phytochemicals found in garlic:

> Allium species and their active components are reported to reduce the risk of diabetes and cardiovascular diseases, protect against infections by activating the immune system, and have antimicrobial, antifungal, anti-aging as well as anti-cancer properties, which [was] confirmed by epidemiological data from human clinical studies.

In addition to consuming garlic as part of one's daily diet, garlic is widely recommended as an herbal supplement to help boost the immune system—it makes a great addition to one's diet during cold and flu season. It also has been found to help prevent heart disease by reducing unhealthy levels of LDL ("bad") cholesterol and high blood pressure. The allicin found in garlic has been proven to increase testosterone. Because traditional Chinese healers believe that it also "builds heat" in the body, Buddhist monks are prohibited from eating garlic because it is believed to increase sexual desire.

According to the United Nations Food and Agriculture Organization (FAO), about 1.6 million hectares (3.95 million acres) of farmland globally produced some 30.7 million metric tons of garlic in a recent year. Garlic is grown on a large scale in more than one hundred countries. The world's most important garlic producer is China, followed by India, Bangladesh, Egypt, and Spain. California is the leading garlic producer in the United States, with most farms centered around the city of Gilroy in Santa Clara County, which bills itself as the "Garlic Capital of the United States."

Resources

Batiha G., El-Saber, A. Magdy Beshbishy, G. Wasef et al. "Chemical Constituents and Pharmacological Activities of Garlic (*Allium sativum* L.): A Review." *Nutrients* 12, 3 (2020): 872.

"A Brief History of Garlic." Gilroy Garlic website. June 8, 2021.

Ford, Thomas G., Michael Orzolek, Lynn Kime et al. "Garlic Production." Penn State Extension. June 17, 2015.

Li, Ninyang, Xueyu Zhang, Xiudong Sun et al. "Genomic insights into the evolutionary history and diversification of bulb traits in garlic." *Genome Biology* 23, no. 188 (2022).

Simon, Philipp W. "The origins and distribution of garlic: How many garlics are there?" Madison, WI: Agricultural Research Service. U.S. Department of Agriculture. March 3, 2020.

"Top 10 World's Garlic Producing Countries." *The Science Agriculture.* Accessed November 22, 2023.

Trinklein, David. "Garlic: A Brief History." Integrated Pest Management website. University of Missouri. September 1, 2015.

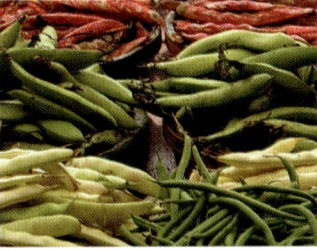

Green Bean

Like spinach, my first introduction to green (or string) beans was at my elementary school's cafeteria, where canned and overcooked string beans were often part of our lunch. They were rarely served at home—mostly because my father had a similar experience to mine when he was in school and didn't like them, no matter how they were served. I became reacquainted with string beans as a young adult, at a Chinese restaurant. They were bright green, crisp, lightly stir-fried, and sautéed in garlic and herbs. Delicious!

The green bean (*Phaseolus vulgaris*) is a close relative to kidney, navy, and pinto beans. Like its relatives, the green bean contributes to environmental sustainability due to its biological *nitrogen fixation*, which has a beneficial effect on both soil and weed control. Green beans are essentially bean pods containing soft, immature seeds that we eat whole as vegetables. This is in contrast to kidney or pinto beans, which are harvested from their pods before they are cooked and prepared as legumes. Early varieties of green beans had fibrous "strings" that ran the length of the pod. They were often difficult to chew, and varieties were later developed that were "string-free."

The common bean is thought to have originated in Mexico more than one hundred thousand years ago, but recent genomic research found that beans were actually domesticated separately at two different geographic locations: Mexico (where it was likely cultivated concurrently with maize by the Aztecs) and the southern Andes (by the Incas) some eight thousand years ago. The Aztecs called the bean *ayacotl,* and even used it as a form of currency.

Like many other indigenous American vegetables and fruits, the green bean was introduced to Europe—especially the Mediterranean countries—by Christopher Columbus when he returned from his second voyage to the New World in 1493. Indigenous communities in North America brought their seeds to other areas, and by 1492 green beans had spread northward to what is now the American Southwest, and eastward to what are now Florida and Virginia. Like the Aztecs and other Indigenous Mexican peoples, Native Americans in what is now the United States also grew green beans with corn: the beans would use the corn as a pole and grow up them. American farmers began breeding the green bean in around 1890 because they were interested in developing bean varieties with "stringless" pods. The first stringless bean was bred in 1894 by Calvin N. Keeney in New York State, who developed eighteen other varieties of "snap" beans between 1884 and 1911. Today, most modern green bean varieties do not have strings.

String or green beans are known by a number of names including snap beans, French beans, and *haricots verts.* Over the centuries, more than one hundred varieties have been developed, including Blue Lake, Kentucky Blue, Romano, and Trionfo beans. However, yellow, or "wax," beans are the best-known variety of string beans.

Green beans can be steamed, grilled, roasted, or lightly sautéed to retain their color and nutrients. Green beans are mostly enjoyed as a side dish, but are also added to stir-fries, casseroles, soups and stews, pasta and rice dishes. They are also used in salads such as three-bean salad, green bean and pasta salad, and *salade Niçoise.*

Green beans are good for you. In addition to dietary fiber, green beans contain vitamin C, vitamin A, and several of the B vitamins including folate, thiamine, and niacin. They also provide calcium, iron, magnesium, phosphorus, potassium, and zinc. In addition, green beans contain antioxidants like flavonols, quercetin, and kaempferol. Along with vitamin C, these antioxidants fight free radicals in the body, which helps to reduce cell damage and may lower the risk of heart disease, diabetes, and certain types of cancer.

A 2013 study of phytochemicals in green beans, conducted at the University of Granada in Spain, was published in the peer-reviewed journal *Phytochemical Analysis*. Utilizing high-performance liquid chromatography coupled with time-of-flight mass spectrometry, the researchers found a total of seventy-two different phytochemicals in green beans, with fifty-four being reported for the first time.

A chapter in the textbook *Nutritional Composition and Antioxidant Properties of Fruits and Vegetables* highlighted the major phytochemicals found in this "powerhouse" vegetable:

> Along with their chlorophyll content, green beans also provide a host of other phytonutrients like carotenoids, phenols, and flavonoids. All these phytonutrients function both as antioxidant and anti-inflammatory agents in our body's metabolism. (Chaurasia 2020, 293)

The author also addressed the medicinal value of these phytochemicals in reducing the risk of a wide variety of chronic illnesses including cardiovascular diseases, high blood pressure, arthritis, diabetes, Alzheimer's disease, and cancer.

Wisconsin, Florida, New York, and Michigan are the major green-bean-producing states in the United States. The leading global producers of green beans are China, Indonesia, India, and Türkiye.

Resources

Abu-Reidah, I. M., D. Arráez-Román, J. Lozano-Sánchez et al. "Phytochemical characterisation of green beans (*Phaseolus vulgaris* L.) by using high-performance liquid chromatography coupled with time-of-flight mass spectrometry." *Phytochemical Analysis* 24, no. 2 (2013): 105–16.

Chaurasia, Savita. Chapter 17, "Green Beans" in Amit K. Jaiswal, ed., *Nutritional Composition and Antioxidant Properties of Fruits and Vegetables.* Cambridge, MA: Academic Press, 2020, 290–96.

"Green Bean Production in the United States." Stockingblue website. November 23, 2017.

"Green Beans." The Bresov Project website. Accessed November 17, 2023.

"Green Beans Characteristics." Botanical Online. Accessed November 17, 2023.

"Guide to Green Beans: 10 Common Types of Green Beans." MasterClass. com. September 17, 2021.

"Health Benefits of Green Beans." WebMD. November 28, 2022.

Oregon State University, Corvallis. "Green Beans." Oregon Agriculture in the Classroom Foundation. Accessed November 17, 2023.

Orzolek, Michael. "Snap Bean Production." Penn State Extension website. June 20, 2005.

Schmutz, J, P. McClean, S. Mamidi et al. "A reference genome for common bean and genome-wide analysis of dual domestications." *Nature Genetics* 46 (2014): 707–713.

Wikipedia. "Green Bean." Accessed November 17, 2023.

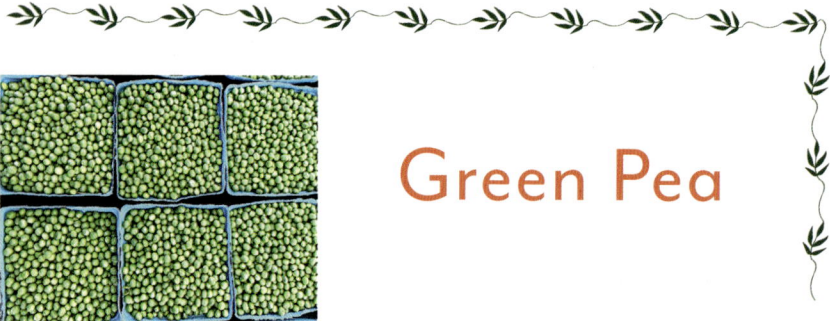

Green Pea

The green pea (*Pisum sativum*) gets its English name indirectly from the Latin *pisum*. In Anglo Saxon, the word became *pise* or *pisu*; later, in English, it was *pease*.

The centers of origin of *Pisum sativum* are the high central plateau and mountains of Ethiopia; the Mediterranean; and central Asia, from northwestern India through what is now Afghanistan. In these areas, wild peas of related species have been found, along with a remarkable diversity of cultivated forms. Humans have likely been eating peas for approximately 9,500 years, and cultivating them for 8,500 years. Greek and Roman writers mentioned peas, but specific varieties were not described until the sixteenth century.

The green pea was first grown only for its dry seed, and some varieties are still grown as dry seeds for split pea soup. Varieties known up until about a thousand years ago had seeds that were much smaller, dark-colored, and otherwise different from what people grow in their gardens today.

Although botanist Alphonse de Candolle mentions that evidence of garden peas was found in lake dwellings in Switzerland and Savoy, in what is now France, dating back to the Bronze Age (3300–1200 BCE), they were not widely grown in Europe until the eighteenth century. Toward the end of the seventeenth century, they were a rare delicacy and only the rich could afford them. "This subject of peas continues to absorb all others," Françoise d'Aubigné, Marquise de Maintenon, a French noblewoman who was secretly married to King Louis XIV, wrote in 1696. "Some ladies, even after having supped at the Royal Table, and well supped too, returning to their own homes, at the risk of suffering from indigestion, will again eat peas before going to bed. It is both a fashion and a madness." (Texas A&M University 2023)

The English later developed several varieties of peas, which later became known as "English peas" in America. The popularity of green peas spread to North America during the 1700s, and Thomas Jefferson grew more than thirty varieties at Monticello, his estate in Virginia. One of the most popular modern varieties of green pea is the *snow pea*, a cultivar with flat pods and thin pod walls that was first named in 1825. Popular in Chinese restaurants throughout North America, this crisp pea variety is eaten whole—pods and all—in sautéed form or added to stir-fried dishes.

Peas were one of the first vegetables studied by plant scientists, with the German-Czech biologist and monk Gregor Johann Mendel (1822–1884) being the best known. Green peas remain an important subject of study by plant geneticists today; there are important collections of pea germplasm with one thousand or more pea varieties located in fifteen different countries. Both Mendel and other plant geneticists have long been fascinated by peas due to their rapid growth cycle, their ability to naturally self-pollinate or be easily cross-pollinated. They also produce a large number of offspring, and they have clearly definable traits as compared to other plant species as a whole.

Green peas picked fresh from the garden are best eaten raw, either alone or in salads. Yet most people purchase green peas canned or frozen. They make a popular side dish, and are often added to soups, stews, stir-fries, casseroles, and dumplings. Peas are an important addition to many of the world's cuisines, including those of Greece and Türkiye, as well as eastern Asian countries like China, Taiwan, Japan, Thailand, and the Philippines. Green peas are also highlighted in one of India's most famous dishes, *aloo matar*, a curry made with peas and potatoes. Dried split peas, with their indigestible skins rubbed off, were developed in the late nineteenth century and are the main ingredient in traditional pea soup, popular in the United States, northern Europe, Russia, Iran, Iraq, and India.

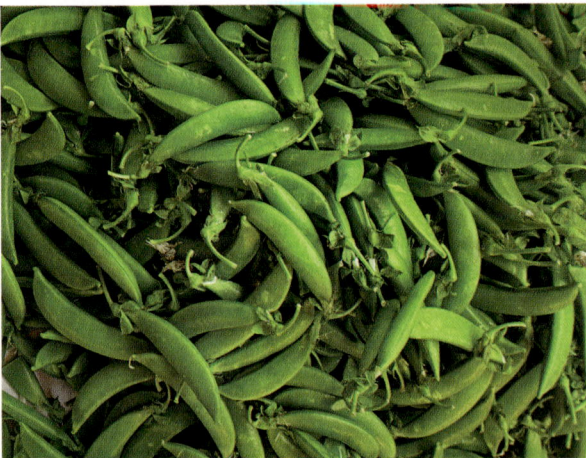

Green peas in their pods.

Like other legumes, green peas are packed with nutrition. In addition to protein and dietary fiber, green peas contain generous amounts of the major B vitamins (B_1, B_2, B_3, B_6, and folate), vitamin C, and vitamin K. They are also excellent sources of iron, manganese, phosphorous, and zinc. In addition to promoting bowel regularity, the high fiber content in green peas supports the growth of beneficial gut microbes. Eating more fiber is also associated with a reduced risk of obesity, type 2 diabetes, heart disease, high cholesterol, and cancer.

Green peas are rich in phytonutrients like carotenoids and flavonols, which protect the heart and support cardiovascular function. Green peas contain *saponins*, which have been shown to help protect against some forms of cancer. They also contain a variety of antioxidants such as polyphenols and phenolic acids, which prevent free-radical damage to cells.

A comprehensive review of the green pea was recently published in the July 2023 issue of the peer-reviewed journal *Foods*. In addition to documenting their rich nutritional and phytochemical profiles, the authors addressed the health values of green peas:

> Owing to the multiple bioactive ingredients in peas, the pea and its products exhibit various health benefits, such as antioxidant, anti-inflammatory, antimicrobial, anti-renal fibrosis, and regulation of metabolic syndrome effects. (Wu et al. 2023, 2527)

The authors recommended that pea proteins and pea fiber should be explored in developing meat alternatives. They also pointed out that while pea pods and hulls were good sources of dietary fiber and polyphenols, they are usually discarded, and called on food scientists to find ways to convert these by-products into functional foods. Addressing food shortages in various parts of the world during the recent COVID-19 pandemic, they suggested that the sprouts and microgreens derived from pea by germination may be an alternative choice for temporarily solving the shortage of domestic vegetables.

Most of the green peas grown in the United States come from Minnesota, Washington, Wisconsin, Oregon, and New York. The world's biggest producer of green peas is China, followed by India, the United States, France, and Egypt.

Resources

de Candolle, Alphonse. *Origin of Cultivated Plants*. New York: D. Appleton and Company, 1908, 328.

"Garden Peas and Spinach from the Middle East." Aggie Horticulture. Texas A&M University. Accessed November 17, 2023.

"Minnesota leads nation in sweet corn, green pea production." Farm Progress website. Accessed November 17, 2023.

U.S. Department of Agriculture. "Pea." Natural Resources Conservation Service. Plants USDA website. Accessed November 17, 2023.

Wikipedia. "Pea." Accessed November 17, 2023.

Wu, D. T., W. X. Li, J. J. Wan et al. "A Comprehensive Review of Pea (*Pisum sativum* L.): Chemical Composition, Processing, Health Benefits, and Food Applications." *Foods* 12, 13 (2023): 2527.

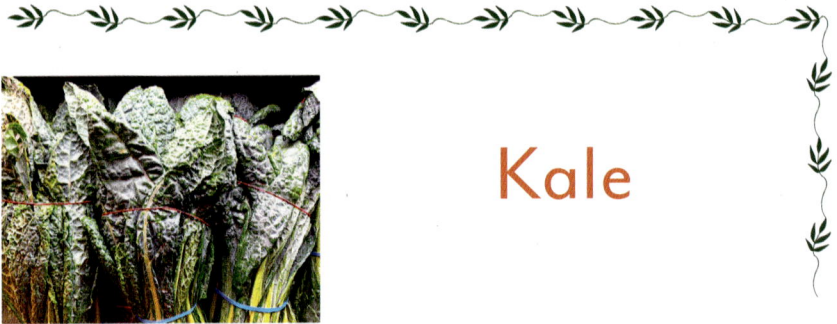

Kale

Kale (*Brassica oleracea* var. *sabellica*), which is closely related to cabbage, cauliflower, broccoli, and brussels sprouts, is grown for its edible shoots and young leaves. It likely originated along with other varieties of the species in western Europe. Recent genetic investigations reveal that cabbage and cauliflower varieties stem from kales introduced from western Europe to the Middle East, and were possibly transported over the tin-trade routes during the Bronze Age (300–1000 BCE), to be reintroduced into Europe later on. Today, the cultivation of kale is widely distributed throughout the world, including many varieties such as green, Siberian, Tuscan, Starbor, Red Russian, curly leaf, Scotch, and tree kales.

According to descriptions of kales by the Greek scholar Theophrastus (370–285 BCE), the Greeks grew kale and collard greens more than two thousand years ago, which they cultivated (and ate) as though they were the same plant. One type of kale, now known as Sabellian kale, is said to be the ancestor of most modern varieties today. Pre-Christian Romans also cultivated kale—known as "coles" (cabbage) at the time. Coles were described in the first, third, fourth, and thirteenth centuries CE by European writers. Due to influence from Old Norse, "cole" eventually became known in Scottish English as "kale."

It is believed that the Romans introduced kale to Britain and France, although some historians believe they were taken there somewhat earlier by the Celts. In much of Europe, kale was the most widely-eaten vegetable until cabbage became more popular during the Middle Ages. The first mention of kale (coleworts) in America was in 1669, although some speculate that kale could have been introduced earlier. It was both a human food and also fed to farm animals.

Kale is considered one of the most nutritious of vegetables. It is high in vitamins A and C, is a good source of dietary fiber, calcium, and iron, and also contains 103 health-promoting phytochemicals—thirty-three of which are unique to kale—including glucosinolates (GLSs), isothyocianates (ITCs), carotenoids, and a variety of phenolic and organic acids. Recent epidemiological studies suggest that consumption of kale is associated with reduced risk of developing cancer and cardiovascular diseases.

An article published in the peer-reviewed journal *Molecules* in 2021 highlights the major phytochemicals found in kale, along with their health benefits:

The main phytochemicals found in kale with health benefits [*sic*] are glucosinolates, polyphenols, and carotenoids. Consumption of kale has been reported to relieve symptoms of gastric ulcers, treat diabetes mellitus, rheumatism, bone weakness, ophthalmologic [eye-related] problems, hepatic disease, anemia, and obesity. Additionally, similar to other cruciferous vegetables, kale showed antioxidant and anti-carcinogenic potential. (Nemzer et al. 2021, 2515)

Due to its numerous health benefits, kale has become a very popular vegetable in recent years, with American kale production increasing by 100 percent between 2007 and 2012 alone; this trend has continued into the 2020s. The easiest way to enjoy kale is by steaming or sautéing the leaves with garlic and seasonings, or adding them to stir-fried dishes. Kale is also a popular smoothie ingredient, and the leaves can be baked by themselves to make kale chips.

Kale is a hearty plant, and is easily grown in backyard gardens. California and Georgia are the leading producers of kale in the United States. A large portion of kale production is certified organic, which is believed to help strengthen its commercial appeal to health-conscious consumers.

Resources

Cai, Chengcheng, Johan Bucher, Freek T Bakker et al. "Evidence for two domestication lineages supporting a middle-eastern origin for *Brassica oleracea* crops from diversified kale populations." *Horticulture Research* 9 (2022).

Harper, Douglas. "Kale." Online Etymology Dictionary. Accessed December 2, 2023.

Jagdish. "How to Grow Kale in the USA . . ." Agri Farming website. Accessed December 2, 2023.

Kavanagh, Una. "Food for Thought: A Short History of Kale." her. March 19, 2014.

Nemzer, B., A. Fadwa, and A. Nebiyu. "Extraction and Natural Bioactive Molecules Characterization in Spinach, Kale and Purslane: A Comparative Study" *Molecules* 26, no. 9 (2021): 2515.

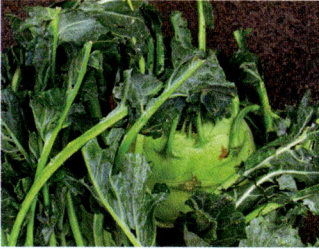

Kohlrabi

Kohlrabi (*Brassica oleracea* var. *gongylodes*) is an attractive, exotic-looking vegetable related to several members of the cabbage family including common cabbage, brussels sprouts, kale, broccoli, and cauliflower. These all came from a common parent, simply known as "wild cabbage," originating somewhere in the eastern Mediterranean.

The name "kohlrabi" is derived from the German: *kohl* meaning cabbage and *rabi* meaning turnip. Kohlrabi has a turnip-like enlargement of the stem above ground. There are white, purple, and green-skinned varieties, but all have creamy, pale flesh. They taste like a cross between a turnip and a cucumber, and can be enjoyed both raw or cooked.

Kohlrabi was first cultivated in northern Europe during the 1300s in what are now Germany and France. It was later grown in Austria and Switzerland. The first description of this cold-climate hardy vegetable was by the Italian botanist Pietro Andrea Mattioli in 1554. By the end of the sixteenth century, kohlrabi was well known in Italy, Spain, Libya, and the eastern Mediterranean. It is said to have been first cultivated commercially in Ireland in 1734, and in England in 1837, where it was used mainly as cattle fodder until the twentieth century. It is believed to have been grown by American farmers as far back as 1806.

The bulbous stem of kohlrabi is often eaten raw in salads, and can be grated and added to coleslaw. The leaves can be cooked as you would collard greens or kale, and can also be added to stir-fried dishes. The bulb can be pureed and combined with onions for a soup base. Kohlrabi plays an important role in the cuisines of Kashmir, Cyprus, Vietnam, and other parts of eastern Asia.

Kohlrabi is both a low-calorie and low-sodium food. It is a good source of dietary fiber, vitamin C, iron, magnesium, potassium, and selenium. Kohlrabi is rich in folate, an important nutrient for pregnant women because it can help prevent some birth defects. The fiber in kohlrabi helps reduce both blood glucose levels and LDL cholesterol. It also supports the growth of bifidobacteria and lactobacilli in the gut, which help protect the body from obesity and heart disease.

A chapter dedicated to the nutritional and medicinal values of kohlrabi was included in the textbook *Brassica Germplasm: Characterization, Breeding and Utilization*, published in 2018. The authors discuss the wide variety of healthy phytochemicals in kohlrabi, including carotenoids, polyphenols, and flavonoids, which protect the body from free-radical damage that can lead to heart disease, diabetes, and cancer; and alkaloids, which possess proven analgesic, anti-malaria, anti-asthma, and anticancer properties. The authors also highlighted clinical studies which showed that kohlrabi can increase body metabolism and improve digestion—thereby helping to control weight—strengthen bones, prevent anemia, boost energy levels, regulate blood pressure, and improve vision.

While most of the world's kohlrabi crop is grown in China and India, Russia, South Korea, and the United States are also major producers.

Resources

"Health Benefits of Kohlrabi." WebMD. November 24, 2022.

"Kohlrabi and Brussels Sprouts Are European," Texas AgriLife Extension Services, Texas A&M University. Accessed January 4, 2024. https://aggiehort.tamu.edu/archives/parsons/publications/vegetabletravelers/kohlrabi.html

"Kohlrabi, Brassica oleracea var. Gongylodes / Cruciferae (Brassicaceae)." Fruits & Vegetables. Frutas-hortalizas website. Accessed January 4, 2024.

Mabry, Makenzie E., Sarah D. Turner-Hissong, Evan Y. Gallagher et al.

"The Evolutionary History of Wild, Domesticated, and Feral *Brassica oleracea* (Brassicaceae)." *Molecular Biology and Evolution* 38, no. 10 (2021): 4419–4434.

Mahr, Susan. "Kohlrabi." Wisconsin Master Gardener website. University of Wisconsin Extension. April 15, 2005.

Sorescu, Ana-Alexandra, Alexandrina Nuta, and Rodica-Mariana Ion. "Pale-Green Kohlrabi, a Versatile Brassica Vegetable" in *Brassica Germplasm - Characterization, Breeding and Utilization*. London: InTechOpen Publishing, 2018.

Wikipedia. "Kohlrabi," Accessed January 4, 2024.

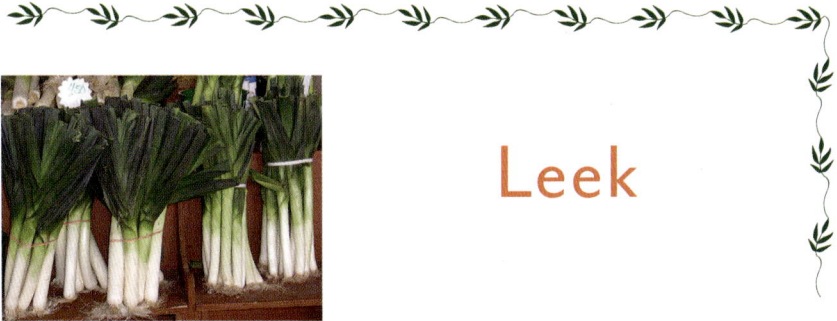

Leek

I first encountered leeks in a suburb of Montreal during the 1970s, where my friend Philippe grew them on his family's farm. He gave me several dozen leeks to bring back to New York, where my aunt and mother eagerly received them. They divided their bounty and marinated them; my mother also used some of the leeks to make a delicious potato leek soup. Leeks have a mild "oniony" flavor, but a sweeter flavor than onions and a texture all their own. The leek has become one of my favorite vegetables.

The leek (*Allium porrum*) is a member of the Liliaceae (lily) family and a cousin of both onion and garlic. Originally from western Asia and the eastern Mediterranean, leeks have been consumed by humans since ancient times. Wild leeks were used as food during the early Bronze Age (around 4000 BCE) and were probably first domesticated around 2000 BCE. They were part of the diet of early Egyptians, and were also used as offerings to the gods. They were believed to have aphrodisiac properties, which likely aided their popularity.

The ancient Greeks cooked leeks in soups and stews, and Hippocrates prescribed leeks as a cure for nosebleeds. The philosopher Aristotle credited the clear voice of the partridge to a diet of leeks. Leeks were also enjoyed by the early Romans, who used them both as a food and as medicine. The Roman emperor Nero supposedly ate leeks every day to make his voice stronger. The Romans are thought to have introduced leeks to the United Kingdom, where they were able to flourish because they could withstand cold weather.

Leeks have been cultivated in western Europe since the Middle Ages, and remain a popular vegetable in Europe to this day. They are especially associated with Wales. In 640 CE, Welsh soldiers wore pieces of leek on their helmets to distinguish themselves from their Saxon foes in battle. The leek appears on the national emblem of Wales, and is that country's national vegetable.

The cultivation of leeks spread to North America with the arrival of the first European settlers during the 1600s. Although the leek isn't as popular in North America as it is in Europe, it has enhanced a wide variety of dishes with its unique flavor and aroma. In addition to their popularity in Europe (especially France), leeks are an important part of Indonesian and Turkish cuisines. In Indonesia, leeks are a major ingredient in *bamo goring*, the Indonesian version of lo mein. In Türkiye, leeks are a common ingredient in many dishes, and recipes focusing on braised leeks (*zeytinyağlı pırasa*) are enjoyed as a comforting winter favorite.

The part of the leek that is commonly consumed is the white, lower stem. The upper green portions are edible but not normally consumed because of their toughness, but can be added to soup or finely chopped in a food processor or blender. Considered both a table vegetable and a condiment, perhaps the most popular way to use leeks is to make them into soup, both as a featured vegetable (such as in cream of leek soup or leek and potato soup) and as a flavorful addition to other soups, like minestrone. They are also delicious when marinated, and can be added raw to salads. Leeks can be an ingredient in quiche, or savory pies and cakes, and also make a good addition to casseroles, pasta dishes, and stir-fries. They also work well as an ingredient in dips or as a tasty pizza topping.

Leeks are very healthy. They are low in calories and high in fiber and vitamin K. In addition, they contain folate, which plays a part in cell development. Like their cousins, onions and garlic, leeks are known for their high antioxidant activity and the ability to accumulate significant amounts of potassium and iron. Leeks show antibacterial, cardioprotective, cholesterol-reducing, antiviral, hypoglycemic, and anticancer activities. Leek consumption is known to improve liver and gastrointestinal tract functioning, quicken metabolic processes, promote blood circulation, and has been found to be useful in rheumatism treatment and to decrease blood pressure. Leeks also help protect against anemia, enhance brain activity, inhibit blood platelet aggregation, and lower fat and blood sugar levels. Finally, eating leeks on a regular basis reportedly decreases the risk of prostate, colon, stomach, and breast cancers. Antimicrobial and antifungal effects of leek have been recorded in laboratory analyses.

The world's top leek-producing country is Indonesia, followed by Türkiye, France, South Korea, and Belgium. Although leeks are grown in many regions of the United States, they are not considered a major crop. Most of the leeks consumed in the U.S. are imported from Mexico.

Resources

Golubkina, Nadezhda A., Timofey M. Seredin, Marina S. Antoshkina et al. "Yield, Quality, Antioxidants and Elemental Composition of New Leek Cultivars under Organic or Conventional Systems in a Greenhouse." *Horticulturae* 4, no. 4 (2018): 39.

Lang, Kristine. "Leeks: Harvest and Storage." South Dakota State University Extension website. March 30, 2023.

Mahr, Susan. "Leeks." Wisconsin Horticulture, Division of Extension. University of Wisconsin-Madison. Accessed January 4, 2024.

Swamy, K. R. M., and R. Veere Gawda. "Leek and Shallot," in *Handbook of Herbs and Spices* Vol. 3. Sawston, UK: Woodhead Publishing Series in Food Science, Technology and Nutrition, 2006, 365–389.

"Which Country Produces the Most Leeks?" Helgi Library website. December 3, 2023.

Xie, T., Q. Wu, H. Lu et al. "Functional Perspective of Leeks: Active Components, Health Benefits and Action Mechanisms." *Foods* 12, 17 (2023):3225.

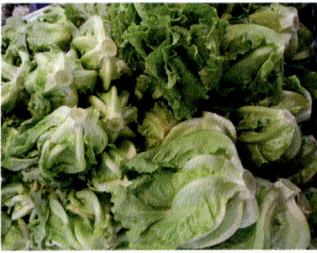

Lettuce

Lettuce (*Lactuca sativa*) is a leafy green that is among our most popular vegetables. Grown around the world, lettuce is mostly eaten raw in salads, sandwiches, and on top of burgers. There are three major types of lettuce: "head" lettuce (of which the iceberg variety is the best known); "leaf" lettuce, which includes red leaf; butterhead (with varieties such as Boston and bibb); and "cos" lettuce, such as romaine.

It was believed that lettuce is indigenous to Egypt, but recent comparisons of genetic material show that the first cultivated lettuce grew in the Caucasus mountains about six thousand years ago. The main lettuce varieties found today were developed later, through breeding and selection in the Middle East, then in Egypt; cultivation later spread through ancient Greece and Rome, as well as central Europe. Lettuce was reported to have been introduced to China by traders via the Silk Road between 600–900 CE, and to North America by explorer Christopher Columbus in the late fifteenth century.

Like other ancient foods, lettuce has been the subject of myth and legend. Among the ancient Egyptians, lettuce was considered a sacred plant of *Min*, the god of reproduction, and was thought to help the deity "perform the sexual act untiringly. (Smith, 2013)"

In contrast, in Greek mythology, Aphrodite's lover, Adonis, was killed in a bed of lettuce by a boar sent by Artemis, who was envious of his hunting prowess. The boar may have also been sent by Persephone, who was envious of his affection for Aphrodite, or by Ares, who was jealous of Aphrodite. In this complex myth, lettuce was associated with male impotence and death rather than male potency and life.

With further breeding and selection, farmers in other parts of the world were able to make improvements to lettuce cultivation over the centuries. According to Nienke Beintem of Wageningen University in the Netherlands (Beintem 2021, 21), "Prickles on the leaves disappeared somewhere on the way to Egypt. The big, soft leaves of the butterhead lettuce emerged in Europe. And only in America did the crunchy iceberg lettuce appear on the scene."

Lettuce is among the healthiest of vegetables, although deep-green, leafy lettuces like Romaine and Boston provide more nutrients than the popular pale green iceberg variety. Lettuce is a good source of vitamin A, which promotes eye health and helps prevent macular degeneration. It is also rich in both vitamin C, an antioxidant, and vitamin K, which helps strengthen bones. Lettuce is also composed of 95 percent water, so eating lettuce (especially with other vegetables) helps increase hydration. Leafy lettuce varieties also contain folate, iron, and beta-carotene.

Lettuce has a long history of medicinal uses, with its appearance in several writings as early as 2680 BCE, as a healing herb. It has been used by both folk healers and modern physicians to help relieve pain, stomach problems, and inflammation, as well as to treat urinary tract infections. Recent studies have provided scientific evidence of lettuce's pharmacological potential, including its antimicrobial, antioxidant, neuroprotective, and hypnotic (sleep-inducing) effects. The chemical composition of lettuce also reveals the presence of different classes of terpenoids, flavonoids, and phenols, which also promote good health.

A comprehensive review of the phytochemicals, nutrition, metabolism, bioavailability, and health benefits in lettuce was published in the June 2022 issue of *Antioxidants* (*Basel*), where the authors (Shi et al. 2022, 1158) discuss the numerous medicinal properties of lettuce:

> Especially due to its antioxidant compounds, lettuce can provide some potential health benefits in cardio-protective, anti-cancer, anti-diabetic, and anti-aging. Furthermore, several researchers found that hydroponic *Lactuca sativa* can heal diseases such as oxidative damage, cancer, Alzheimer's disease, and diabetes.

The article also stated that regular consumption of lettuce supported liver health and the nervous system, and could help reduce bone loss and osteoporosis among older women, due in part to the presence of vitamins K and K_2.

Lettuce is grown around the world, and is a favorite addition to home gardens during the summer months. When it comes to commercial production, China is the world's leading lettuce grower, followed by the United States, India, Spain, and Italy. In the United States, most lettuce is produced on farms in California and Arizona.

Resources

Beintem, Nienke. "Tracing the Origin of Lettuce." *Wageningen World*. Wageningen University & Research. February 2021, 20–21.

de Candolle, Alphonse. *Origin of Cultivated Plants*. New York: D. Appleton and Company, 1908, 95.

Fisher, Nan. "The History of Lettuce." Mother Earth Gardener website. February 21, 2018.

"Health Benefits of Lettuce." WebMD. September 9, 2022.

Kuete, Victor, ed. *Medicinal Spices and Vegetables from Africa*. New York: Academic Press, 2017.

Shi, M., J. Gu, H. Wu et al. "Phytochemicals, Nutrition, Metabolism, Bioavailability, and Health Benefits in Lettuce - A Comprehensive Review." *Antioxidants (Basel)* 11, 6 (2022): 1158.

Smith, K. Annabelle. "When Lettuce was a Sacred Sex Symbol," *Smithsonian Magazine*, July 16, 2013.

Wikipedia. "Lettuce," Accessed February 9, 2025.

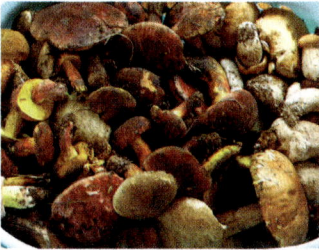

Mushroom

Americans love mushrooms. Although eaten as a vegetable, mushrooms are actually the spore-bearing fruiting body of a fungus, with cultivated varieties of the *Agaricus bisporus* family being the most popular. Mushroom growers in the United States produced over 700 million pounds of both white and brown mushrooms in a recent year. Another seventy-six tons of mushrooms were imported, mostly from Canada, Mexico, and South Korea.

But mushrooms aren't appreciated by everyone. Although more than 38,000 varieties of mushroom are considered edible, "edible" is not the same as "tasty." Many wild mushrooms are poisonous, some even deadly. For most people—including this writer—it's difficult to know which wild mushrooms are safe to eat. For this reason, mushroom lovers tend to stick to the dozen or so tried-and-true commercial mushroom varieties available at supermarkets, greengrocers, and farmers markets.

Mushrooms have been around since time immemorial. For the ancient Egyptians, mushrooms were considered the "food of the gods." They believed that eating mushrooms could help them live longer— or even make them immortal. Wild mushrooms, cultivated in Greece around 200 BCE, were first written about in the works of the Greek playwright Euripides (480–406 BCE). Early Greeks consumed a drink made from the ergot fungus during religious ceremonies, which allowed them to experience expanded levels of consciousness.

According to the *Mixtec Vienna Codex* (13–15 centuries CE), mind-altering mushrooms were used in religious ceremonies by Mayans, Aztecs, and other Indigenous peoples of ancient Mexico. Montezuma II, the last ruler of the Aztecs, is said to have eaten a mushroom called *teonanacatl* (flesh of the gods) at his coronation ceremony.

Although country folk in Europe have been collecting mushrooms for food since prehistoric times, many medieval Europeans distrusted mushrooms, which they associated with witchcraft, evil, and death. Being neither a plant nor an animal, mushrooms were connected with mystery, magic, and aspects of nature that humans cannot control. Attitudes began to change when the French introduced mushrooms into their haute cuisine in the 1600s. It is said that King Louis XIV loved white "button" mushrooms, and had them growing in his garden at the Château de Versailles. By the 1800s, more than three hundred mushroom farmers were cultivating white button mushrooms (then called "les champignons de Paris") in Parisian catacombs and abandoned underground quarries. By the late nineteenth century, Americans were growing mushrooms in their cellars and cooking them in their kitchens.

As mentioned earlier, the mushroom most familiar to consumers in the United States is the "agaricus" family of mushroom, which is composed of a stipe (stem), a pileus (cap), and lamellae (gills). The most popular mushroom of this genus is the white button mushroom mentioned earlier, which was first described by the French botanist Joseph Pitton de Tournefort in 1707. Some 80 percent of the mushrooms consumed in the United States are of the white button type. Other agaricus varieties originated in Italy, including the brown crimini and portabella. Seasonal species like morels, oysters, and chanterelles are often gathered from forests and offered for sale at farmers markets.

Mushroom cultivation in Asia extends back more than 1,100 years. In contrast to Europeans, Asians embraced mushrooms early on as both food and medicine. Mushrooms have been part of Traditional Chinese Medicine for centuries, and today many mushroom species are being studied by Western science to verify their nutritional and medicinal properties. Mushrooms have also played an important role in Ayurveda, the ancient healing system practiced extensively in India and Nepal.

The best-known Asian mushrooms for eating include the shiitake, enoki, lion's mane, white beech, oyster, king oyster, maitake, matsutake, and paddy straw. Reishi mushrooms are used primarily in medicine, while shiitake, lion's mane, and matsutake mushrooms are used as both food and medicine. Shiitake mushrooms have been found to reduce inflammation, boost immunity, and lower cholesterol. They also contain lentinan, which promotes brain function and enhances certain immune system functions that may aid in the fight against cancer. Lion's mane (known as "monkey head" in China and Taiwan) have powerful anti-inflammatory and antioxidant properties; they are often prescribed to reduce stress and anxiety, and may even help patients suffering from dementia. Many Chinese, Japanese, and Korean mushroom varieties are now being grown in North America, and are widely available at specialty greengrocers and Asian supermarkets, the latter which often sell dried mushrooms as well. Mushroom-based nutritional supplements are available online and at pharmacies and health food stores.

Mushrooms are commonly consumed in dried, raw, and cooked forms, and play an important role in cuisines around the world. They can be served alone or as a welcome addition to Chinese, Japanese, French, Indian, Mexican, Italian, or Korean dishes. The versatile mushroom can be used to make or enhance the flavor of sauces and gravies, soups, pizzas, casseroles, omelets, stir-fried dishes, hot pots, dumplings, vegetable pies, enchiladas, and pasta, rice, and noodle dishes. Some varieties can be added to salads. Portabella mushrooms are often used in place of meat, especially standing in for burgers or steak.

Mushrooms are low in calories and fat, and are highly nutritious, with each variety having its own unique nutritional profile. One serving of five medium button mushrooms is an excellent source of the B vitamins riboflavin (28 percent Daily Value, or DV), niacin (20 percent DV), pantothenic acid (27 percent DV), and copper (32 percent DV). Button mushrooms also contain 4 milligrams of *ergothioneine* per 100 gram serving. Researchers are investigating this amino acid to determine whether it can reduce inflammation in the lungs and damage to the liver, kidneys, and brain.

One whole portabella cap is an excellent source of copper (27 percent DV), selenium (28 percent DV) and niacin (24 percent DV), and contains 2 mg of ergothioneine per 100 gram serving. Portabellas also contain polysaccharides, polyphenols, and carotenoids, which have been found to have anti-inflammatory, antioxidant, and anticancer properties. Eating portabella mushrooms on a regular basis promotes digestive health, and may also improve mental cognition.

The study of mushrooms and other fungi—known as *mycology*—has recently been embraced by Western science. Mycology is believed to have tremendous potential regarding the use of mushrooms and fungi in environmental preservation, sustainable agriculture, nutrition, and health. Although more research into these fungi needs to be done, a 2023 article appearing in *Food Reviews International* summarized the many documented nutritional and health benefits of mushrooms:

> In the aspect of nutritional value, mushrooms are high in protein and insoluble fiber, while low in fat and sodium, making them a low-energy, healthy food. Mushrooms contain a large amount of beneficial bioactive substances for health, including phenolic compounds, as well as tocopherols, terpenoids, and phytosterols. Mushroom polyphenols have antioxidant, anti-inflammatory, anti-cancer, anti-tyrosine [retards browning of foods], anti-hyperglycemic, and other

biological activities beneficial to human health and medical applications, especially in the various degenerative disease and cancer treatments. (Zhou et al. 2024, 924)

With the exception of Antarctica, mushrooms are grown throughout the world. China is by far the largest producer, followed by Japan, Poland, and the United States. Most of the mushrooms grown in the U.S. are from Pennsylvania, where farmers have been cultivating mushrooms for over 150 years. Most mushroom farms in Pennsylvania can be found in the borough of Kennett Square, located in the Delaware Valley between Philadelphia and Wilmington, Delaware. Kennett Square calls itself "The Mushroom Capital of the World," and is home to an annual mushroom festival, usually held in early September.

Resources

André, Annie. "Button Mushrooms and Their Forgotten Paris Catacombs Origin." *Annie André Blog.* Updated January 10, 2024.

Avey, Tori. "Magical Mushrooms: The Allure of Edible Fungi." Food. PBS. org. April 1, 2014.

"A brief cultural history of the mushroom." Deutsche Welle. October 17, 2022.

Grucza, Ariel. "What are the Health Benefits of Portabella Mushrooms?" WebMD. June 7, 2022.

"Leading Producers of Mushrooms and Truffles Worldwide . . ." Statista website. 2021.

"Shiitake Mushrooms: Health Benefits, Nutrition and Uses." WebMD. September 19, 2022.

U.S. Department of Agriculture. "Mushrooms." National Agricultural Statistics Service. August 26, 2022.

Venkat, S. R. "What are the Health Benefits of Lion's Mane Mushrooms?" WebMD. May 20, 2022.

Zhou, Ying, Minghang Chu, Farhad Ahmadi et al. "A Comprehensive Review on Phytochemical Profiling in Mushrooms: Occurrence, Biological Activities, Applications and Future Prospective." *Food Reviews International* 40, no. 3 (2024): 924–951.

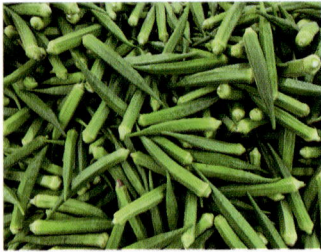

Okra

Okra (*Hibiscus esculentus*), a vegetable with edible seed pods, is a member of the hibiscus–mallow family, along with cotton, hibiscus, and cacao. It has been a quintessential food in the southern United States for centuries, but the origins of this tropical vegetable have been traced to the White Nile in what is now Sudan, which drains into the southwestern highlands of Ethiopia. Cultivated by the ancient Egyptians, okra seems to have spread out of Africa to the Middle East and the Indian subcontinent some two thousand years ago. It was first reported in Brazil in 1658, probably brought from Africa during the early years of the slave trade. It is also likely that okra was also introduced to the United States when slaves were brought to its shores from western Africa, beginning in 1619.

It appears that African women bound for the United States used to braid okra seeds into their hair before being forced to board transatlantic slave ships, hoping they would somehow—and someday—be free to plant their own crops. The name "okra" is believed to be a corruption of *nkru-ma*, a name used by the Asante (Ashanti) people who lived in what is now Ghana.

Some food historians have given credit to the French-speaking Creoles for popularizing the vegetable, known to them as *gumbo*. The name gumbo—still commonly used for okra in parts of the Gulf Coast of the U.S.—is taken from the Bantu word *ki ngombo*, or *quingombo*, which seems to verify its introduction to America during the slave trade, which lasted from the seventeenth to the nineteenth centuries.

Okra also traveled east to what are now India and Pakistan, and quickly became a highly sought after and popular food. More than a dozen varieties of okra are grown today in India alone.

When cut open, okra pods produce a slimy mucus, which led white slave owners to use okra as a thickening agent for soup. Gumbo, a hearty stew developed by Creoles in Louisiana, consists primarily of a strongly flavored stock along with celery, bell peppers, and onions, with okra as a thickener. Okra can also be fried, with the crisp exterior balancing out the interior sliminess.

Known variously as Lady's Finger, or as *bhindi* in Hindi, okra is used extensively in southern Asian cuisines today. Some of the most popular okra dishes include bhindi masala, bhindi ka aalan (okra curry), and dahi bhindi (tangy Indian okra in yogurt). Okra is also popular in regional African cuisines, and is an important vegetable in both Brazil and the Dominican Republic.

While not a nutritional powerhouse, making okra part of one's daily diet is good for health. In addition to protein and dietary fiber, okra is especially rich in vitamins C and K, and is a good source of vitamin B_3 (thiamin) and vitamin B_6 (pyridoxine). It is also a good source of calcium, manganese, and magnesium.

Okra is also a rich source of phytochemicals such as tannins, alkaloids, carbohydrates, terpenoids, steroids, flavonoids, and polyphenols, which have been variously shown to have antioxidant, antimicrobial, and anticancer activities. Polyphenols in particular have been linked to lowering blood pressure, cholesterol, and inflammation which can cause heart disease. Okra can also help regulate blood sugar. The pectin found in okra supports the growth of friendly bacteria in the intestines and promotes bowel movement regularity.

Okra is grown in the United States, but it is not a major crop. Most of the okra that is produced in the world is grown in India, followed by Nigeria, Mali, Sudan, and Pakistan.

Resources

Cleveland Clinic. "5 Health Benefits of Okra." healthessentials. September 27, 2023.

Deen, G. R., F. A. Hannan, F. Henari, S. Akhtar. "Effects of Different Parts of the Okra Plant (*Abelmoschus esculentus*) on the Phytosynthesis of Silver Nanoparticles: Evaluation of Synthesis Conditions, Nonlinear Optical and Antibacterial Properties." *Nanomaterials (Basel)* 12, 23 (2022): 4174.

Kate and Isabel. "Okra: How it Got to the United States, How to Grow It and How to Eat It." *Farm Blog.* Pomona College. Accessed February 2, 2024.

Klingaman, Gerald. "The History of Okra: Where Does Okra Come From?" University of Arkansas System Division of Agriculture. September 2, 2005.

"Okra." Apni Kheti website. Accessed April 10, 2025.

Wikipedia. "Okra." Accessed February 2, 2024.

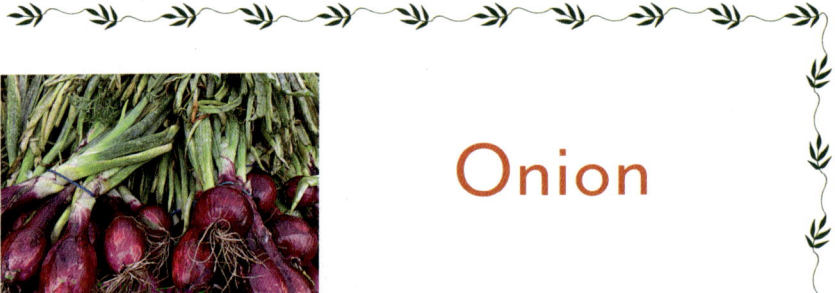

Onion

Onions are the fourth most popular vegetable in the United States after potatoes, tomatoes, and sweet corn. Americans eat some 21.9 pounds of onions a year per person. The most common onion is the "bulb" onion (*Allium cepa*), which is grown in practically every country on the planet.

Many archaeologists, botanists, and food historians believe that onions originated in Central Asia. Other research suggests that onions were first grown in what are now Iran and Pakistan, and still others believe it is probably native to northwestern India, Baluchistan, and Afghanistan. However, most researchers agree the onion has been cultivated for five thousand years or more. Since onions grew wild in various regions, they were probably consumed for thousands of years before being domesticated simultaneously in different parts of the world. Onions may be one of the earliest cultivated crops because they were less perishable than other foods of the time, making them transportable. They were also easy to grow in a variety of soils and climates.

Ancient Vedic writings from India mentioned that onions grew in Chinese gardens as early as five thousand years ago, while in Egypt onions can be traced back to 3500 BCE. There is evidence that the Sumerians of Mesopotamia were growing onions as early as 2500 BCE: a Sumerian text from that era mentions a farmer plowing over the city governor's onion patch.

In ancient Egypt, onions were considered sacred. The onion symbolized eternity to the Egyptians, who buried onions along with their Pharaohs. The Egyptians saw eternal life in the anatomy of the onion because of its circle-within-a-circle structure. Paintings of onions appear on the inner walls of pyramids and tombs. Onions were also widely grown in ancient Greece and Rome, where they were treasured as both a food and as medicine.

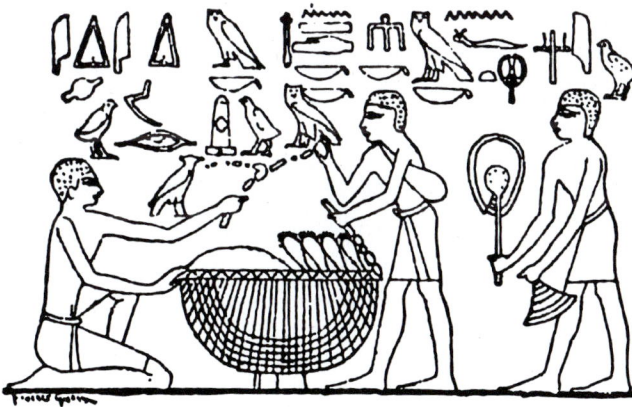

Onions being sold in an Egyptian market.
Maspero (Gaston), Life in Ancient Egypt and Assyria, *New York, 1882.*

The Romans are said to have introduced the onion to the rest of Europe, including what are now Germany and Great Britain. During the Dark and Middle Ages, onions and cabbages were Europe's two most important foods.

In 1620, the first pilgrims brought onions with them to the New World from England on the Mayflower, and it soon became an important staple crop. According to diaries of early colonists, bulb onions were planted as soon as the pilgrim farmers could clear the land. However, they soon found that strains of wild onions already grew throughout North America. Native Americans used wild onions in a variety of ways, eating them raw or cooked, as both a seasoning and a vegetable.

Onions are extremely versatile. They can be baked, boiled, braised, grilled, fried, roasted, sautéed, or eaten raw in salads. They are commonly chopped and used as an ingredient in a wide variety of cooked dishes, and may also be used as a main ingredient in their own right, as in onion soup, creamed onions, or onion chutney. Their layered structure makes them easy to hollow out once cooked, and to then stuff, as with *Soğan dolması*, a popular Bosnian dish.

There are more than twenty onion cultivars in cultivation today, although three are the most common. Most of the onions (an estimated 87 percent) consumed in the United States are *yellow* or *brown* onions. These categories include several varieties including the Vidalia, Walla Walla, and Bermuda. They turn a rich, dark brown when caramelized, and are used in a wide variety of soups, sauces, stews, and stir-fried dishes. *Red* or *purple* onions have a sharper, more pungent flavor than yellow onions, and are often eaten grilled or raw in salads and sandwiches. *White* onions are mild in flavor and have a golden color when cooked. They are commonly used in sautéed dishes and sauces, and are often added raw to potato and pasta salads.

Onions have long been considered a medicinal food. The ancient Greeks used onion to fortify athletes before participating in the Olympic games. Before competition, athletes would consume literally pounds of onions, drink onion juice, and would even rub onions on their bodies. The Roman author and naturalist Pliny the Elder catalogued Roman beliefs about the efficacy of the onion for curing vision and inducing sleep. He also wrote about its ability to treat mouth sores, dog bites, toothaches, dysentery, and lumbago. Native Americans used wild onions to treat colds, coughs, asthma, and other breathing problems. In China, traditional physicians believe that onions, as well as garlic, stimulate sexual appetite and increase the production of semen. For this reason, Buddhist monks are not allowed to consume foods made with onions, garlic, or their relatives.

Modern scientific research has shown that the onion is one of the healthiest of foods. In addition to providing dietary fiber, vitamin C, potassium, calcium, and iron, onion consumption has been associated with a reduced risk of cancer, heart disease, and diabetes because of its high level of phenolic and flavonoid compounds that possess high antioxidant activity. Overall, onions are rich in diverse phytochemicals including organosulfur compounds, phenolic compounds, polysaccharides, and saponins.

A recent article published in the peer-reviewed journal *Frontiers in Nutrition* highlighted the numerous ways that eating onions are good for health:

> Accumulated studies have revealed that onion and its bioactive compounds possess various health functions, such as antioxidant, antimicrobial, anti-inflammatory, anti-obesity, anti-diabetic, anticancer, cardiovascular protective, neuroprotective, hepatorenal [liver and kidney] protective, respiratory protective, digestive system protective, reproductive protective, and immunomodulatory properties. (Zhao et al. 2021, 1)

China and India are the world's two largest onion producers, followed by the United States, Egypt, Iran, and Pakistan. The largest onion-producing states in the U.S. are Washington, Idaho, Oregon, California, and Georgia, while Québec and Ontario are the two largest onion producers in Canada.

Resources

Iowa State University. "Onions." Agricultural Marketing Research Center website. October 2021.

Mehta, Indu. "Origin and History of Onions." *IOSR Journal of Humanities and Social Science*, 22, no. 9 (2017): 7–10.

New Mexico State University. "[Onion] History," Onion Breeding Program website. 2023.

"Onion History." National Onion Association website. Accessed February 5, 2024.

Trinklein, David. "Onion: A Brief History." Integrated Pest Management website. University of Missouri. March 1, 2011.

"World Onion Production by Country." AtlasBig.com. Accessed February 5, 2024

Zhao, X. X., F. J. Lin, H. Li et al. "Recent Advances in Bioactive Compounds, Health Functions, and Safety Concerns of Onion (*Allium cepa* L.)." *Frontiers in Nutrition* 8 (2021): 1–23.

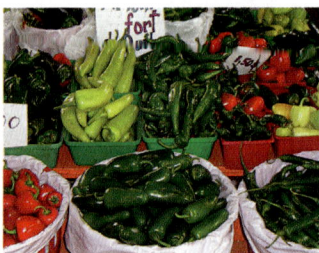

Pepper

Both bell (sweet) peppers and chili peppers are members of the nightshade family, meaning they are related to tomatoes, potatoes, and eggplants. While there are several types of bell peppers (green, yellow, purple, brown, and red varieties), there are literally hundreds of types of chili peppers, all with varying degrees of hotness.

Both sweet peppers and chili peppers (both are of the genus *Capsicum*) are said to have originated in the northern Amazon basin, and later spread north through South and Central America, Mexico, the West Indies, and what are now the southern United States. Fossilized remains of a relative of modern chili peppers discovered in ancient ruins in southwestern Ecuador show that peppers have been cultivated for at least six thousand years.

Chili peppers have a long history of medicinal use by Indigenous peoples of the Americas. For example, the Mayans used chili pepper to treat asthma, coughs, and sore throats. Both Aztecs and Mayans mixed pepper with maize flour to produce *chillatolli*, which was traditionally used to cure the common cold. It has been reported that in Colombia, the Tukano people use chili peppers to relieve a hangover. In Mexico, chili peppers have long been associated with male potency, probably due in part to their often-elongated forms and the fact that they contain *capsaicin*, a phytochemical that increases blood flow throughout the body.

Wild chilies were used as a spice in tropical America (the region nearest the equator including the top half of South America, all of Central America, and all but the northernmost parts of Mexico), which led to their domestication in pre-Colonial times. There are five primary cultivated species, all of which originated in different places. The oldest is believed to be *Capsicum annuum*, which originated either in what is now Mexico or the northern part of Central America. It found its way to Europe earlier than other pepper varieties, and is considered the most important pepper cultivar today. Today, chili peppers are most closely identified with Mexico, India, China, Korea, and Thailand, where they are grown extensively in all five countries, and play a major role in their regional cuisines. In China, for example, chili peppers are used extensively in the cuisines of Szechuan, Hubei, Hunan, and Yunnan, while cuisines from around India (especially the south) use chili peppers in a wide variety of curries, soups, and vindaloo dishes.

There are more than 150 different varieties of peppers, and their pungency, or "heat," is measured using the "Scoville heat unit" scale (SHU). *Mild* peppers, like bell, pimento, and Padrón, rate between 0–1,000 SHU; *medium* peppers, including the serrano, poblano, cayenne, jalapeño, and chipotle, have SHU ratings between 5,000–50,000; *extra hot* habaneros, Thai and Tien Tsin, range from 100,000–400,000 SHU; while some *super-hot* peppers, like the Bhut Jolokia (ghost), Guntur Sanaam, and Carolina Reaper, have SHU ratings that soar into the millions.

Like cherries, scientists believe that the seeds of wild chili peppers were primarily spread by birds. It appears that, because birds lack the taste receptors to feel the "sting" of hot peppers, they had no problem eating them; their digestive systems also left the seeds intact. After the seeds were excreted, many grew into plants.

Christopher Columbus is said to have been the first to bring chili peppers to Europe, although most chili pepper distribution to Europe and Asia has been attributed to Portuguese and Spanish traders. Chili peppers are believed to have been introduced to China in the late 1400s by Spanish traders, and the Portuguese explorer Vasco da Gama introduced fresh chili peppers to India (probably through Goa, then a Portuguese colony) in the 1500s.

Sweet peppers are widely used in raw salads, but can also be baked, roasted, steamed, or pan fried. They can be eaten alone or combined

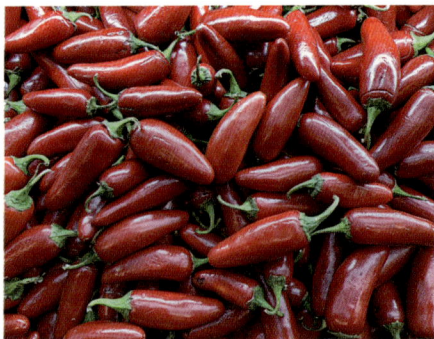

Jalapeno peppers

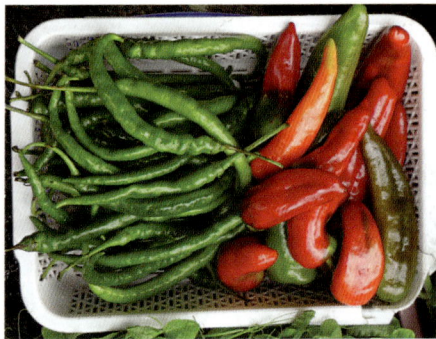

Hot peppers in China

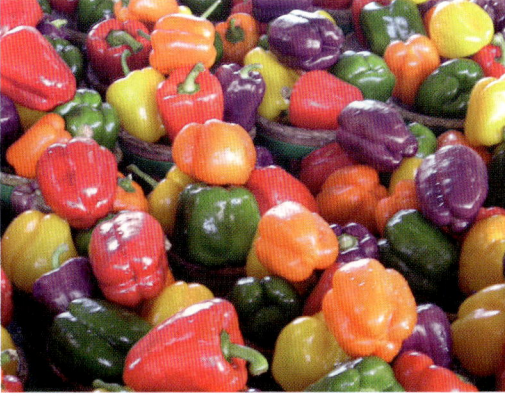

Bell peppers

with other foods in soups, stir-fried dishes, casseroles, and curries. They are often enjoyed baked and stuffed. As mentioned earlier, chili peppers "spice up" countless Mexican, Chinese, Indian, Thai, and Tex-Mex dishes. They can be chopped and added to soups, eggs, and sandwiches; they can also be used in making salsa, sauces, and jams. Powdered chili peppers can be added to sauces, or as an ingredient in tacos and fajitas; they can also be sprinkled over cooked vegetables. Koreans are the highest per-capita consumers of red pepper, a primary ingredient in *kimchi*, a fermented cabbage dish that is eaten at literally every meal.

Chili peppers are nutritious, providing dietary fiber, vitamins A and C, and iron. They are also a rich source of phytochemicals with antioxidant and anti-diabetic activities. Capsaicin is a compound found in hot varieties of chili peppers which provides their characteristic flavor and pungency. Scientists have studied capsaicin extensively in recent years, and have found that it helps prevent and even treat a wide variety of health problems including obesity, diabetes, cardiovascular conditions, respiratory diseases, itch, gastric and urological disorders, pain-related conditions, and cancer.

Research presented at the 2020 American Heart Association's Scientific Sessions meeting analyzed data from 570,000 adults in the United States, Italy, China, and Iran, comparing those who regularly consumed chili peppers with those who rarely or never did. The study—which was led by Bo Xu, MD, a leading cardiologist at the Cleveland Clinic's Heart, Vascular, and Thoracic Institute—found that consumption of chili pepper may reduce the relative risk of cardiovascular disease mortality by 26 percent. Chili pepper consumption was also associated with a 25 percent reduction in death from any cause and 23 percent fewer cancer deaths compared to people who never or only rarely consumed chili pepper.

The most important growers of bell (sweet) peppers in the United States are California, Florida, Georgia, and New Jersey, while the principal growers of chili peppers are Arizona, California, New Mexico, and Texas. China is by far the largest producer of chili peppers in the world (over 16 million tons a year), followed by Mexico, Türkiye, Indonesia, India, Spain, and the United States.

Resources

Azlan, Azuna, Sharmin Sultana, Chan Suk Huei, and Muhammad Rizal Razman. "Antioxidant, Anti-Obesity, Nutritional and Other Beneficial Effects of Different Chili Pepper: A Review." *Molecules* 27, no. 3 (2022): 898.

Bray, Matt. "Chili Pepper History: Where do Peppers Come From?" PepperScale website. March 11, 2022.

Fattori, V., Miriam S. N. Hohmann, Ana C. Rossaneis, et al. "Capsaicin: Current Understanding of Its Mechanisms and Therapy of Pain and Other Pre-Clinical and Clinical Uses." *Molecules* 21, 7 (2016): 844.

"China Explained: How the Chili Pepper Took Over Chinese Cuisine." RADII website. Accessed January 8, 2024.

Iowa State University. "Bell and Chili Peppers." Agricultural Marketing Resource Center website. October 2021.

"People who eat chili pepper may live longer?" American Heart Association website. American Heart Association Scientific Sessions Report, Presentation P1036. November 9, 2020.

Vanbuskirk, Sarah, and Kristin Mitchell. "Health Benefits of Chile, Chile Peppers, and Chili Powder." Nourish by WebMD website. November 10, 2022.

Vegetables 2020 Summary. National Agricultural Statistics Service website. United States Department of Agriculture. February 2021.

"The World's Top Chili Pepper Producing Countries," *WorldAtlas* website. Accessed January 15, 2024.

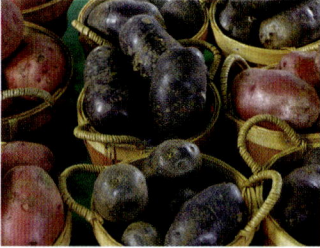

Potato

The potato (*Solanum tuberosum*) is the most popular vegetable in the United States. Coming from a family of eastern European Jews, potatoes have been a three-meal staple for as long as I can remember. They were enjoyed baked, as hash browns, mashed, or as potato pancakes, potato knishes, and potato latkes. Like most people, I always assumed that potatoes originated in Ukraine or Russia, two of the world's major potato producers and consumers, but they are actually indigenous to South America.

Potatoes are believed to have originated in the Central Andes mountain range, and were first cultivated by the Aymara and the Incas thousands of years ago, in an area known today as the Titicaca Plateau, which encompasses parts of what are now Peru and Bolivia. The Aymara are said to have developed more than two hundred potato varieties before the arrival of the Spanish in 1532. However, recent genomic evidence shows that the potato more likely originated in what is now northern Chile. In any event, Peruvian white potatoes are the genetic "parents" of 99 percent of the potatoes grown in North America and Europe. More than three thousand varieties of potato are grown in the Andes, which stretches from Colombia to Chile. Being used to eating only white potatoes since childhood, I was surprised to discover literally dozens of potato varieties of different colors and sizes at local markets when I first visited Bolivia and Peru during the 1970s.

The potato first made its appearance in Europe around 1570, having been brought from South America by the Spanish conquistadores. From Spain, potato cultivation spread slowly to Italy and other European countries. A popular urban myth claims that potatoes were introduced to the British Isles (which then included Ireland) from the state of Virginia by either Sir Walter Raleigh or his travel companion, the astronomer and ethnographer Thomas Herriot, in either 1585 or 1586. But a more likely theory is that they came to the British Isles from Spain. The English author William Coles wrote, in 1657 about "the potatoes which we call Spanish because they were first brought up to us out of Spain, grew originally in the Indies [. . .]" In any case, by 1600, the potato had entered Spain, Italy, Austria, Belgium, Holland, France, Switzerland, Germany, Portugal, England, and Ireland.

Potato cultivation also expanded to Asia, and was introduced in China toward the end of the Ming Dynasty, which ended in 1644. As the population increased in China during the middle period of the Qing Dynasty (1735–96), potato cultivation became more widespread. Potatoes were introduced to India (probably Goa) by Portuguese traders in the early seventeenth century, followed by British traders who introduced potatoes to Bengal. By the end of the eighteenth century, potatoes (known in India and Pakistan as *aloo*) had been cultivated across northern India's hill regions.

In the early 1700s, a colony of Irish Presbyterians who settled in colonial New Hampshire introduced the potato to North America, and they were first planted in what is now Washington state by the Spanish explorer Salvador Fidalgo in 1792. However, potatoes didn't become an important crop in North America until the mid-1800s. Like peppers, tomatoes, and eggplants, potatoes are part of the nightshade family, which includes several poisonous plants. As a result, many people associated the potato with the Devil, and farmers refused to grow them, let alone eat them for lunch or dinner.

Potatoes didn't become popular in the United States until Thomas

Jefferson served them to guests at the White House during his presidency in the early 1800s. The potato's appeal in the U.S. was strengthened by more than one million Irish immigrants who arrived in the 1840s due to the potato famine (known simply as "The Great Famine") that destroyed much of Ireland's potato crop and caused widespread starvation.

The renowned American horticulturist Luther Burbank is credited with developing more than eight hundred new varieties of flowers, fruits, and vegetables, including a potato. In 1872, he created a large, brown-skinned, white-fleshed potato—the Russet Burbank—which has become one of the world's most predominant varieties.

Potatoes are incredibly versatile, and are enjoyed throughout the world. They can be eaten boiled, baked, steamed, roasted, scalloped, diced, stuffed, fried, or grated, and are a primary ingredient in dumplings, knishes, and potato pancakes. They are also eaten cold in potato salad, and as potato chips. Most of the potatoes (some 63 percent) grown in the United States are processed and sold as French fries, dehydrated potatoes, and other refined potato products. Some of the fresh potatoes sold in North America include the Russet, Yukon Gold, Kennebec, Adirondack Blue, Red Bliss, German Butterball, and Red Thumb. Lesser known—but no less delicious—varieties can be found in farmers markets and specialty greengrocers. Potatoes are also used as animal feed.

With the exceptions of French fries and potato chips, potatoes are considered by nutritionists to be a healthy food. In addition to starch, potatoes provide protein, vitamins (especially vitamins B and C), and minerals like magnesium, iron, copper, zinc, and especially potassium, which aids in the workings of the heart, muscles, and nervous system. Potatoes have also been found to contain a variety of healthy phytochemicals including polyphenols, anthocyanins, and carotenoids. Potato skin also contains dietary fiber, which is important for digestive health.

Potatoes that have a vivid color (such as bright yellow, orange, or purple varieties) are more nutritious than white potatoes: purple potatoes, for example, are richer in anthocyanins and other antioxidants that may prevent heart disease and cancer and also support brain health. Colorful potatoes also have lower glycemic index (GI) levels than white varieties, which means they help regulate blood sugar levels better than white potatoes do.

It may be surprising to know that most of the world's potatoes are grown in China and India, two Asian countries where rice is "king." They are followed by the United States, Ukraine, and Russia. Alberta, Manitoba, and Prince Edward Island are the three major potato growing provinces in Canada; Idaho is the biggest producer of potatoes in the United States, followed by Washington, North Dakota, Wisconsin, and Colorado. By the late 1940s, New York's Long Island was one of the top five largest potato-producing areas in the United States, but the island's estimated one thousand potato farms were largely replaced by housing developments and wineries by the 1970s.

Resources

"A Brief History of the Potato." National Gardening Association website. Accessed January 18, 2024.

"Canadian potatoes, from farm to fork." Statistics Canada website. December 20, 2022.

Chapman, Jeff. "The Impact of the Potato," *History Magazine*. Accessed January 18, 2024.

de Candolle, Alphonse. *Origin of Cultivated Plants*. New York: D. Appleton and Company, 1908, 46.

de Haan, Stef, and Flor Rodriguez. "Potato Origin and Production." in Jaspreet Singh and Lovedeep Kaur, eds., *Advances in Potato Chemistry and Technology*. New York: Academic Press, 2016: 1–32.

Good Food Is Good Medicine. "Potato Health Benefits and Why You Should Eat More Spuds." Health Tips. UC Davis website. May 18, 2022.

Iowa State University. "Potatoes." Agricultural Marketing Resource Center website. November 2021.

Lettice, Eoin. "The Potato and Sir Walter Raleigh: Never let the facts spoil a good story." *Communicate Science* blog. June 29, 2011.

McWilliams, Brendan. "A Short History of the Potato." *Irish Times* website. September 18, 1997.

"Potato History." Washington State Potato Commission website. Accessed January 18, 2024.

Wikipedia. "History of the Potato," Accessed January 18, 2024.

Wikipedia. "Potato." Accessed January 18, 2024.

Radish

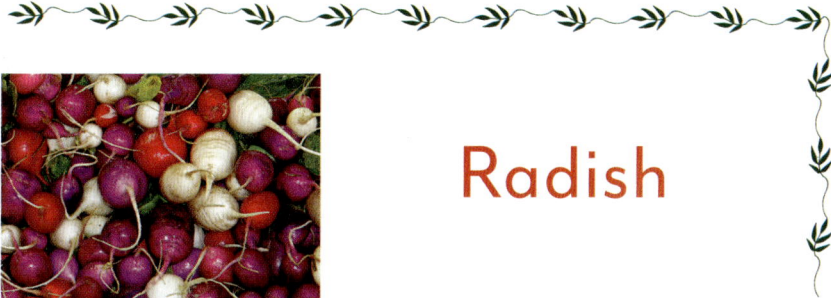

The main edible part of the radish plant (*Raphanus sativus*) is its swollen taproot. The enlarged roots are available in a wide range of sizes, shapes, and colors depending on the cultivated variety. Early-maturing European "salad" types—the variety most available in supermarkets— can be round, oval-shaped, or cylindrical. They are usually red, white, or red with a white tip, and have crisp white flesh with a spicy flavor. Chinese (also called Japanese or Oriental) radishes are often white, large, feature a conical shape and white flesh, and tend to have a mild, slightly peppery flavor.

The radish is a fast-maturing root plant, and wild varieties likely originated in central and western China into India. Evidence of indigenous radishes have also been found in areas ranging from the Mediterranean to the Caspian Sea. Radishes have been cultivated for thousands of years, and were grown by both the ancient Egyptians and Greeks. According to the Greek historian Herodotus (c. 484–424 BCE), the radish was an important crop in ancient Egypt, and images of radishes were painted on the walls of the Pyramids about four thousand years ago. The first written records that mention radishes come from the third century BCE. Ancient Greek and Roman texts noted the characteristics of radishes, and described them variously as small, large, round, long, mild, and sharp.

Radishes were first grown in western Europe in the mid-sixteenth century. After the Americas were "discovered" by European explorers during the late 1400s, the radish was one of the earliest vegetables to be brought over from Europe. European radishes are mostly eaten raw as a stand-alone snack food or added to salads. Although they are often discarded, the leaves of the radish plant are also edible, and can be enjoyed as a salad green or added to soup or blended vegetable juices.

The Chinese, or Oriental, radish, known as *daikon* in Japan, was first cultivated in China nearly two thousand years ago, and was known in Japan at least one thousand years ago. The Chinese radish is an important ingredient in Korean, Chinese, Japanese, Vietnamese, and Indian cuisines where it is served raw, pickled, or cooked. Daikon is often used in soups, stews, and stir-fried dishes.

Both radish varieties are rich in dietary fiber and also contain vitamin C, small amounts of vitamin B, and a healthy balance of minerals including potassium, magnesium, calcium, and iron. Radishes also contain mustard oils (specifically mustard oil glycosides), which is what gives the vegetable its spicy flavor. Mustard oils have been found to have antibacterial and antifungal properties, and also support good digestion.

The Oriental radish has been an integral part of Traditional Chinese Medicine for centuries, and has been widely used for its ability to stimulate the flow of *qi* (circulating life force) in the body. It has a long history of treating lung problems and urinary tract infections, and is still prescribed by traditional Chinese doctors today.

Recent scientific studies have found that Western radishes help regulate blood sugar levels, enhance liver function, and reduce blood pressure. They are also a good source of natural nitrates that improve blood flow. Pickled radishes have been shown to have greater antioxidant activity due to fermentation, while radish sprouts have been found to have higher concentrations of beneficial phytochemicals than radish taproots. Radish leaves also contain high concentrations of vitamins and minerals, especially beta-carotene, vitamin C, calcium, and potassium. Other laboratory studies have found that Chinese radishes contain no fewer than 609 plant compounds. Some of them have been shown to have strong antioxidant activity, possessing anticancer, antimicrobial, anti-inflammatory, and antibacterial properties.

The world's major radish producing countries include China, Japan, and South Korea. Radishes are grown throughout North America, led by California and Florida.

Resources

Gamba, Magda, Eralda Asllanaj, Peter Francis Raguindin et al. "Nutritional and phytochemical characterization of radish (Raphanus sativus): A systematic review." *Trends in Food Science & Technology*113 (2021): 205–218,

Hadley, H., and R. Fordham. "Vegetables of Temperate Climates" in *Encyclopedia of Food Sciences and Nutrition*, Second edition. New York: Academic Press, 2003, 5946–48.

Hanlon, P. R., and D. M. Barnes. "Phytochemical composition and biological activity of 8 varieties of radish (Raphanus sativus L.) sprouts and mature taproots." *Journal of Food Science*76, 1 (2011): C185–92.

Pennsylvania State University. "Radish." Plant Village website. Accessed January 17, 2024.

"Radish History: Varieties of Radishes." Vegetable History. Vegetable Facts website. Accessed January 17, 2024.

Tan, Sharlene. "What Are the Health Benefits of Daikon Radishes?" Nourish by WebMD. May 19, 2022.

Whitbourne, Kathryn. "Radish: Health Benefits, Nutrition and Uses." Nourish by WebMD. September 19, 2022.

Yang, Qiu, et al. "Radish Genetic Resources." Crop Genebank Knowledge Base website. Accessed January 17, 2024.

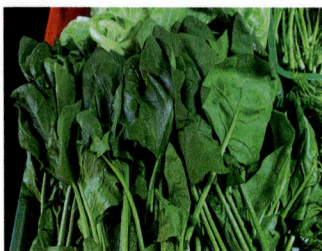

Spinach

Despite enjoying "Popeye" cartoons on television and in comics as a child growing up in the 1950s, I wasn't a fan of spinach. Like several other green vegetables, it was introduced to me at our elementary school cafeteria, taken from a can and cooked until it was a greenish-brown mush. It wasn't until my mother bought fresh spinach at a farm stand one summer and sautéed it in garlic that I grew to love spinach. Sixty years later, I eat it often, both raw in salads or lightly sautéed.

Spinach (*Spinacia oleracea*) is native to southwestern Asia. It was first cultivated in Persia (now Iran) over two thousand years ago, and was also found growing in gardens in Nineveh and Babylon. It eventually spread to the Mediterranean countries, and was successfully cultivated by Arab farmers as early as the eighth century. The first references to spinach are from the text *Sasanian Persia*, written around 226–640 CE. In 647 CE, spinach was taken from Nepal to China where it became known as "Persian green." Arab traders brought spinach seeds to Spain during the eleventh century, and spinach cultivation spread to the rest of Europe by the fourteenth. Spinach was especially popular in France, and was first introduced to the French court by the Florentine noblewoman Catherine de' Medici when she married King Henri II in 1533. Spinach is believed to have been brought to North America with early European colonists, but did not became widely cultivated until the 1920s. In 1930, spinach became the first vegetable in the United States to be frozen and sold commercially.

There are three basic types of spinach, which should all be carefully washed before use. *Savoy* has dark green, crinkly, curly leaves and is sold in bunches in most supermarkets. *Flat-* or *smooth-leaf spinach* has broad, smooth leaves. It is often grown for canned and frozen spinach, as well as baby foods and other processed foods. *Semi-savoy* has slightly crinkled leaves. It has a similar texture to the savoy, but is easier to clean. It is grown for both fresh market and processing.

Spinach is popular cooked (steamed or sautéed) as a side dish or added to stir-fried dishes, pasta recipes, casseroles, stews, and soups, and is the main ingredient in spinach pie (spanakopita), a popular Greek delicacy that's also enjoyed throughout southern Europe and the Middle East. Spinach is also highly valued in traditional Indian cuisine—where it is called *saag*—and is used to make various curries (*bhaji*) and much-loved mushroom saag and saag paneer. Fresh, raw spinach has become an increasingly popular component of dips and a major ingredient in vegetable salads. It is also a nutritious ingredient in fresh vegetable juices and both fruit and vegetable shakes.

Spinach is one of the most nutrient-dense of all plant foods. High in fiber and low in calories, spinach is an excellent source of vitamins C, K, A, E, riboflavin (vitamin B_2), and pyridoxine (vitamin B_6); it is also a good source of folate, iron, calcium, magnesium, and potassium. Cooking has been known to degrade folate and vitamin C content, although cooked spinach provides higher levels of vitamin A and iron as opposed to raw. Spinach contains oxalic acid that can negatively impact the amount of iron and calcium that is actually available for absorption by the body.

Spinach is rich in beneficial phytochemicals. An article about spinach appearing in the peer-reviewed journal *Food & Function* documents many of its health-enhancing attributes:

> Spinach-derived phytochemicals and bioactives are able to (i) scavenge reactive oxygen species and prevent macromolecular oxidative damage, (ii) modulate expression and activity of genes involved in metabolism, proliferation, inflammation, and antioxidant defense, and (iii) curb

food intake by inducing secretion of satiety hormones. These biological activities contribute to the anti-cancer, anti-obesity, hypoglycemic [reduce blood sugar levels], and hypolipidemic [reduce harmful cholesterol levels] properties of spinach. (Roberts and Moreau 2016, 3337)

Most of the spinach grown in the United States is from California, followed by Texas, Arizona, and New Jersey. China is by far the world's largest producer of spinach worldwide, followed by the United States, Kenya, and Türkiye.

Resources

de Candolle, Alphonse. *Origin of Cultivated Plants*. New York: D. Appleton and Company, 1908, 98–99.

Iowa State University. "Spinach." Agricultural Marketing Resource Center website. August 2021.

Mahr, Susan. "Spinach. *Spinacia oleracea*." Wisconsin Horticulture Division of Extension website. University of Madison–Wisconsin. 2023.

"The Origin and History of Spinach." CliffordAWright.com. Accessed November 18, 2023.

Roberts , J. L., and R. Moreau. "Functional properties of spinach (Spinacia oleracea L.) phytochemicals and bioactives." *Food & Function* 7, 8 (2016): 3337–53.

"Spinach." *New World Encyclopedia* website. Accessed November 18, 2023.

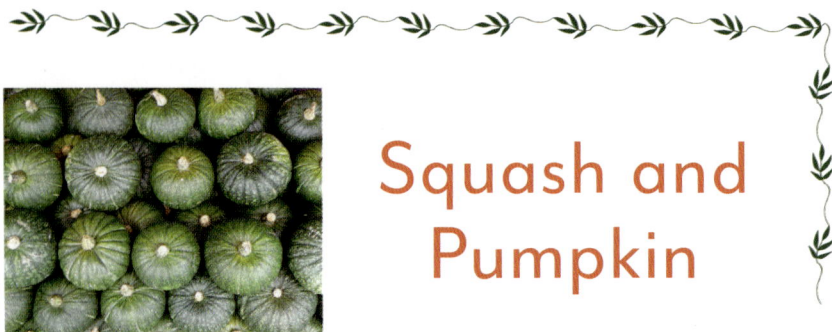

Squash and Pumpkin

Squashes, indigenous to North and Central America, were first cultivated by native peoples over ten thousand years ago. Mexico is presently the center of species diversity: of fifteen types of squash found in the Americas, thirteen are cultivated in Mexico today. Mexican cooks treasure squash and squash blossoms as a major ingredient in traditional dishes like *cemitas* and *tlayudas*, as well as a wide variety of soups and casseroles.

Squashes belong to the genus *Cucurbita*, which includes melons (originally from the Mediterranean), peppers (South America), watermelon (Africa), and pumpkins (North America). Squash originated from wild plants in Mexico and Central America. Domestication began some eight thousand years ago and spread from southern Canada all the way south to Argentina and Chile. Centers of domestication stretched from the Mississippi River watershed and Texas, through Mexico and Central America, to both northern and western South America.

Squash was a major source of food for Native Americans, and is considered the oldest cultivated food on the continent. Squash was the first of the "three sisters" crops planted by Native Americans, which later included corn and beans. According to an article published by the University of California:

> Corn served as the trellis upon which the beans could climb; beans were nourished by the sunlight and kept the corn stalks stable on windy days, while also nourishing their soil; and pumpkins sheltered the corn's shallow roots and prevented weeds from taking hold. (Oliveira, University of California website)

Squash was grown by the Pueblo tribes in what is now the southwestern United States. It was also cultivated and eaten by many other Indigenous peoples in North America, including the Apache, Iroquois, Hopi, Navajo, Papago, Zuni, and Yuman.

Like cucumbers, tomatoes, and eggplant, squashes are technically a fruit, since they contain seeds and come from the flowering part of the plants. Because they are cooked (and eaten) as a vegetable, you'll find them in the "vegetable" section of your local supermarket.

Botanists have classified twenty-seven major types of squash, which are generally divided into "summer" and "winter" varieties. *Winter squashes* have thick skins and can keep unrefrigerated for months after harvesting. The most common varieties of winter squash include spaghetti, acorn, kabocha, banana, buttercup, and "sugar pumpkin" squash, which is mainly used for pumpkin pie and can be a major (and nutritious) ingredient in muffins, cakes, and soups. Cultivation of the Connecticut field pumpkin goes back to Colonial times and is the most popular variety for jack-o'-lanterns for Halloween.

Summer squash is harvested earlier in the year than winter squash, and tends to have a soft and tender skin. They should be eaten within two weeks after purchase. The most popular varieties include yellow squash, zucchini squash, and chayote squash.

Originally, wild squash was round and bitter in flavor. Over many centuries of domestication, the flesh gradually became sweeter. Squash is mostly eaten cooked, and can be enjoyed on its own as a side dish (roasted, sautéed, steamed, or baked) or as an ingredient in a wide range of casseroles, stir-fried dishes, pasta, and soups. Squashes are also used in baking—two of the most famous baked squash creations being zucchini bread and pumpkin pie. Pumpkin pie was developed by early American colonists who experimented with foods indigenous to North America. Pumpkin pie wasn't considered a "holiday" food until 1827, when author Sarah Josepha Hale dedicated a chapter of her book, *Northwood: A Tale of New England*, to describing a traditional Thanksgiving dinner, which included pumpkin pie. Pumpkin seeds will be discussed in a later section.

Squashes (especially varieties with deep yellow or orange flesh) are excellent sources of vitamin A (beta-carotene), vitamin B complex, vitamin C, and vitamin E, along with essential minerals like calcium, magnesium, potassium, and iron. They also contain phenolic compounds, such as flavonoids, phenolic acids, proteins, and carbohydrates.

An article published in a recent issue of *South African Journal of Botany* summarizes some of the many health benefits of eating squash:

> It could reduce the risk of coronary heart disease, the blood glucose levels, and the serum cholesterol level. Moreover, it prevents oxidative stress and improves immunity due to its antioxidant activities. [. . .] They are also a good source of dietary fiber and essential micronutrients including antioxidants that support heart health, healthy skin, and protect against cell damage due to free radicals. (Enneb et al. 2020, 166)

Remember that nutritional content of squash will vary according to each type. For example, a 100 gram serving of *acorn* squash contains 1200 International Units (IU) of vitamin A, while the same serving of *butternut* squash will provide 6400 IU.

The six largest squash-producing countries are China, India, Ukraine, Russia, Spain, and Mexico. California is the largest grower of squash in the United States, followed by Florida, Georgia, and Michigan. The United States is among the largest importers of squash in the world, with more than 90 percent imported from Mexico.

Resources

Cleveland Clinic. "Everything You Should Know About the Benefits of Squash." healthessentials website. March 31, 2023.

Composition of Foods, Agricultural Handbook No. 8. Washington, D.C.: United States Department of Agriculture, 1963.

Davis, Chad. "Pumpkin or Sweet Potato Pie? There's a Rich History Behind Both." Harvest Public Media. NPR website. November 22, 2023.

Enneb, S., S. Drine, M. Bagues et al. "Phytochemical profiles and nutritional composition of squash (Cucurbita moschata D.) from Tunisia." *South African Journal of Botany* 130 (2020): 165–171.

Murphy, Hugh. "Foods Indigenous to the Western Hemisphere," American Indian Health and Diet Project website. University of Kansas. Accessed November 30, 2023.

Oliveira, Rosane. "10 Things You Probably Didn't Know about Pumpkins." University of California website. October 28, 2018.

"Squash, Gourds and Pumpkin Production." NationMaster website. Accessed November 30, 2023.

Wikipedia. "*Cucurbita*." Accessed November 30, 2023.

Yadav, M., S. Jain, R. Tomar et al. "Medicinal and biological potential of pumpkin: an updated review." *Nutrition Research Reviews*. 23, 2 (2010):184–190.

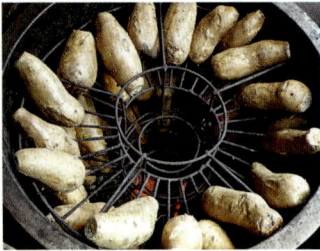

Sweet Potato

The sweet potato (*Ipomoea batatas*) is believed to have originated in the West Indies, near the coast of Mexico's Yucatan Peninsula, Belize, and Honduras. Despite its name, the sweet potato is not related to the potato. Sweet potatoes are members of the morning glory family (Convolvulaceae), while white potatoes are part of the nightshade family (Solonaceae). Strangely, sweet potatoes and yams (discussed later) are not related either, although both tuberous root vegetables are often marketed as the same food.

It is believed that Christopher Columbus first brought sweet potatoes (called *batatas* in the Island Carib and Kari'nja languages) to Europe. They were cultivated in Virginia as early as 1648, and George Washington grew sweet potatoes on his farm at Mount Vernon. Portuguese traders soon introduced sweet potatoes to Africa, and from there to Java (now part of Indonesia) and India. The acclaimed American botanist George Washington Carver was fascinated by sweet potatoes, and eventually developed over one hundred different products—including twenty-six different foods—from the plant during his tenure at the Tuskegee Institute (now Tuskegee University) from 1896 to 1943. During World War I, the sweet potato flour that he developed was used to extend wheat flour in baked goods.

There are literally hundreds of sweet potato varieties, though they can be divided into five basic types: orange skin with orange flesh, red skin with orange flesh, yellow skin with white flesh, purple skin with white flesh, and purple skin with purple flesh. As can be imagined, each variety has its own special flavor and texture.

In the United States, sweet potatoes are usually eaten as a traditional holiday vegetable at Thanksgiving, Christmas, and Easter. Sweet potato pie is a Thanksgiving favorite, and was likely introduced by enslaved Africans during the seventeenth century.

However, sweet potatoes are as versatile as white potatoes, and have a much higher nutritional value. They can be enjoyed baked, boiled, broiled, fried, grilled, and microwaved, or used in soups, stir-fried dishes, casseroles, stews, pies, and salads. Sweet potato leaves are both tasty and nutritious, and can be prepared like spinach or other leafy greens. Originally fed to pigs, they are now considered a delicacy in China and Taiwan, and can be found on the menu in many fine Chinese restaurants. They are sometimes available at Asian markets in North America, offered for sale at premium prices.

Between 2000 and 2016, the popularity of sweet potatoes in the United States increased by 42 percent, and reached a modest per capita consumption of 5.7 pounds by 2022.

In parts of Asia and Africa, sweet potatoes are considered vital to survival, as opposed to an occasional holiday treat. They are an essential breakfast staple in many African countries, and are also considered the ultimate comfort food. In rural Zimbabwe, they are the subject of a popular song; translated from Shona to English, it says, "That sweet potato in the pot: who should I eat it with?" Sweet potatoes are a versatile food, and are enjoyed in many different ways according to national tastes. Nigerians, for example, prefer their sweet potatoes in porridge, fermented drinks, or just plain boiled, while in Indonesia sweet potatoes are enjoyed in sweets, cakes, desserts, and potato puffs.

Nutritionists have begun to refer to the sweet potato as a "low-cost superfood" due to its relatively low price and strong nutritional profile. Sweet potatoes furnish us with protein and low glycemic carbohydrates, which provide long-term energy without sharply increasing blood sugar levels. They also contain dietary fiber, which supports the growth of healthy gut bacteria and promotes bowel regularity. Sweet potatoes also contain an extensive range of micronutrients including minerals (manganese, copper, potassium, and iron), vitamins (mainly B complex, C, E, and provitamin A [as carotenoids]), anthocyanins (found primarily in purple sweet potatoes), and flavonoids. Their high concentrations of beta-carotene and vitamin A have especially been found to support eye health and help prevent macular degeneration—the most common cause of vision loss. Just one sweet potato provides 102 percent of the vitamin A that a normal adult needs each day.

Recent laboratory and clinical studies have shown that the sweet potato is one of the healthiest foods one can eat, as it provides a spectrum of nutritional and medicinal benefits at low cost. According to a scientific review of sweet potatoes published in the journal *Antioxidants* (*Basel*):

> Sweet potato is considered an excellent source of dietary carotenoids and polysaccharides, whose health benefits include antioxidant, anti-inflammatory and hepato-protective activity, cardiovascular protection, anticancer properties, improvement in neurological and memory capacity, metabolic disorders, and intestinal barrier function. Moreover, the purple sweet potato, due to its high anthocyanin content, represents a unique food option for consumers, as well as a potential source of functional ingredients for healthy food products. (Laveriano-Santos et al. 2022, 1648)

The world's largest producer and consumer of sweet potatoes is China, followed by India and Indonesia in Asia, and Malawi, Nigeria, Tanzania, Mozambique, and Ethiopia in Africa. The United States is the world's eighth largest sweet potato grower, with North Carolina being the most important sweet potato growing state.

Resources

Booth, Stephanie. "Health Benefits of Sweet Potatoes." WebMD. July 17, 2023.

"Carver Sweet Potato Products." Tuskegee University website. Accessed October 28, 2023.

Davis, Chad. "Pumpkin or Sweet Potato Pie? There's a Rich History Behind Both." Harvest Public Media. NPR website. November 22, 2023.

Harper, Douglas. "Potato." Online Etymology Dictionary. Accessed October 28, 2023.

Iowa State University. "Sweet potatoes." Agricultural Marketing Resource Center website. November 2021.

Laveriano-Santos, E. P., A. López-Yerena, C. Jaime-Rodríguez et al. "Sweet Potato Is Not Simply an Abundant Food Crop: A Comprehensive Review of Its Phytochemical Constituents, Biological Activities, and the Effects of Processing." *Antioxidants (Basel)* 11, 9 (2022): 1648.

"Sweet Potato Basics." National Gardening Association website. Accessed October 28, 2023.

"Sweet Potato Facts and Figures." International Potato Center (CIP) website. Accessed October 28, 2023.

"Sweet potato memories: love 'em, rely on 'em . . . hate 'em," *Goats and Soda*. National Public Radio website. November 23, 2023.

"Sweet Potato Production FAQ." Our World in Data website. Food and Agricultural Organization of the United Nations. 2023.

"Top Sweet Potato Growing Countries." *WorldAtlas* website. Accessed October 28, 2023.

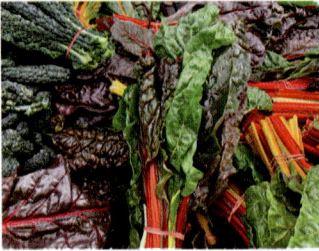

Swiss Chard

Swiss chard (*Beta vulgaris* var. *cicle*) is a colorful, leafy green that is a descendant of the sea beet. Chard was highly valued by early Arabs, as well as the Greeks and Romans; it was likely the plant referred to by Aristotle as a "red-stalked leafy green plant" around 350 BCE.

Chard has been under cultivation in the coastal areas of Europe since at least the third century CE, and has been growing in Britain since at least 1597, when the English botanist John Gerard recorded growing it in his famous book *The Herball or Generall Historie of Plantes*. The name *chard* is derived from the Latin word for "thistle" (*carduus*), but the vegetable was also called silver beet, beet spinach, seakale beet, and leaf beet.

Except for its name, Swiss chard has nothing to do with Switzerland; chard is believed to have originated in Sicily, and was given its name by Dutch seed merchants during the nineteenth century to distinguish it from French leafy green varieties. Although chard is a close relative of spinach, it is often compared to kale.

Until the 1850s, Swiss chard was categorized as a specialty plant, and was cultivated primarily in Europe. It has long been cultivated in central Croatia, and was referred to as "the queen of the Dalmatian garden." Chard is believed to have been introduced to the American colonies by European immigrants, and was originally grown for its beet-like bulb rather than to be eaten as a leafy green. Chard became increasing popular in the United States after the Civil War, and was grown as both an ornamental plant and as food. Because the red or yellow middle rib of each green leaf is bitter in flavor, nineteenth-century Americans separated the leaves from the middle rib for cooking. It was also used raw in salads.

Swiss chard can be enjoyed raw or cooked. It can be steamed or sautéed, and can also be used in soups and stews, casseroles, omelets, and frittatas. Young uncooked leaves can be enjoyed in salads and sandwiches. Swiss chard has traditionally been a part of Mediterranean cuisine, although it has also played an important role in the culinary traditions of Egypt, Croatia, and Türkiye.

Like other leafy greens, Swiss chard is packed with antioxidants, and contains high levels of vitamins A, C, and K, along with magnesium, manganese, potassium, copper, iron, and dietary fiber. The leaves have the highest amount of fiber, sodium, magnesium, and vitamin C, while the stems are high in potassium. Once used as a cure for a variety of ailments including dandruff, anemia, jaundice, and toothache, modern pharmacology has found that a diet rich in chard can lower the risk of obesity, diabetes, and heart disease—it can even inhibit cancer growth. Eating chard can help maintain bone health, improve digestion, regulate blood sugar levels, and contribute to healthy brain function.

Swiss chard contains several antioxidants called flavonoids, including quercetin, kaempferol, rutin, and vitexin. As mentioned earlier, kaempferol is a powerful anti-inflammatory compound that may have anticancer properties. Research shows that vitexin may help prevent heart disease by lowering blood pressure, reducing inflammation, and blocking the formation of blood clots. The high fiber content of chard can help support both good digestion and elimination, while helping to regulate blood sugar levels.

South Africa and Italy are among the world's leading producers of Swiss chard, followed by the United States, where most of the commercial crop is grown in California.

Resources

Chewy Media. "The Swiss Chard: A Little History and Growing Instructions." Harvesting History website. Accessed October 29, 2023.

"Fascinating Facts: Chard." The Royal Horticultural Society website. 2023.

Jagdish. "Swiss Chard Farming, Planting, Cultivation Practices." AgriFarming website. Accessed October 29, 2023.

Kubala, Jillian. "Swiss Chard: Nutrition, Benefits, and How to Cook It," healthline website. March 29, 2022.

Ninfali, Paulino, and Donato Angelino. "Nutritional and functional potential of Beta vulgaris cicla and rubra," *Fitoterapia* 89 (2013): 188–99.

"Swiss Chard Market Summary," Produce Blue Book Services website. Accessed October 29, 2023.

Westenhiser, Tara. "Swiss Chard." Food Source Information. Colorado State University website. Accessed October 29, 2023.

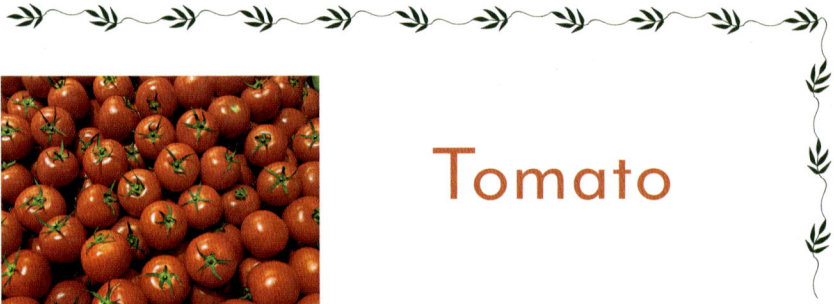

Tomato

When asked, "Where did tomatoes come from?" most would answer, "Italy!" because tomatoes have played a major role in Italian cuisine for hundreds of years. Yet, all cultivated tomatoes can be traced to a single species, *Solanum lycopersicum*, which grew wild in South America. There are sixteen relatives of this species, and they thrived in the narrow coastal region from northern Chile, through Peru, to Ecuador, including the Galapagos Islands, about 80,000 years ago.

Domestication of these wild (blueberry-sized) tomatoes began some seven thousand years ago. As they slowly spread through Mesoamerica—by both bird and human migrations—tomatoes gradually evolved into larger varieties, to the size of the cherry tomatoes we enjoy today. The name "tomato" comes from the Aztecs, from the Nahuatl word *tomatl*. This has led many to believe that tomatoes are native to Mexico, and many cultivated tomato varieties did originate there.

Spanish explorers brought the domesticated tomato to Europe during the sixteenth and seventeenth centuries. Being a member of the nightshade family (which also includes potatoes, peppers, and eggplant), tomatoes were not initially popular in Europe because people believed the brightly colored fruit (eaten as a vegetable) was poisonous. The first mention of the *pomi d'oro* ("golden apple")—Italians' first term for "tomato"—was in Tuscany in 1548, and tomatoes were highlighted in Italian cookbooks soon after. However, tomatoes didn't become popular in Italy until the eighteenth century. They now play an essential role in Italian cuisine, and can be found in a wide variety of Italian dishes, especially pizza and pasta dishes.

Tomatoes are believed to have arrived to the southern United States from the Caribbean during the 1700s, but weren't widely cultivated until the early 1800s. It appears that an article published by Dr. John Bennett in 1834, extolling the health benefits of the tomato, marked the beginning of its acceptance in the United States. Tomatoes are now the second favorite vegetable in the United States, after potatoes. They are also the most popular vegetable grown in America's home gardens. There are dozens of popular tomato varieties grown in North America, and over ten thousand tomato cultivars exist throughout the world.

Tomatoes are incredibly versatile, and are mostly eaten raw in salads. They can also be baked and stuffed. Tomatoes are also enjoyed as juice, and as primary ingredients in a wide variety of soups, sauces, and main dishes in many of the world's cuisines. In addition to the multitude of traditional Italian recipes, tomatoes are also widely used in Mexican cuisine, including in salads, soups, egg dishes, guacamole, bean dishes, rice and noodle dishes, casseroles, and, of course, all kinds of salsa. Tomatoes also form the base of Indian chutneys, curries, and birjanis, plus at least four of India's most famous soups: mulligatawny, rasam, sambar, and shorba. In Türkiye, tomatoes are often paired with eggplant dishes like soslu patlican, along with esogelin corba (a tomato-based soup), kisor (made with bulger), all kinds of kebabs, and yapak dolma, a delicious appetizer made with grape leaves.

Tomatoes are highly nutritious. In addition to providing dietary fiber, tomatoes are a good source of phenolic compounds (phenolic acids and flavonoids), carotenoids (lycopene, and alpha- and beta-carotene), vitamins A and C, and glycoalkaloids (tomatine). Red tomatoes are especially a good source of lycopene, which has been found to lower the risk of heart disease by 14 percent—this percentage can be increased by combining tomatoes with olive oil, which improves the body's utilization of lycopene.

The many benefits of eating tomatoes are highlighted in an appearing in the peer-reviewed *Journal of Food Sciences and Technology*:

> Bioactive constituents present in tomato have antioxidant, anti-mutagenic, anti-proliferative [inhibit tumor cell growth], anti-inflammatory, and anti-atherogenic [against atherosclerosis] activities. [. . .] [The] protective role of tomato (lycopene as a potent antioxidant) in humans against various degenerative diseases are known throughout the world. Intake of tomato is inversely related to the incidence of cancer, cardiovascular diseases, ageing, and many other health problems. (Chaudhary et al. 2018, 2833)

The authors of this article also pointed out that, unlike some fruits and vegetables, the nutritional and antioxidant properties of this "wonder fruit" do not decrease during normal cooking.

China is the largest tomato producer in the world, followed by India, Türkiye, the United States, and Egypt. California, Michigan, Indiana, and Ohio are the major growers of processed tomatoes destined for ketchup, pasta sauce, salsa, juice, and soup in the United States. California and Florida are leading growers of fresh tomatoes.

Canada is a major producer of greenhouse tomatoes, with the highest production in Ontario, British Columbia, and Québec. Fresh tomatoes are also imported into the United States from Mexico and Canada.

Resources

"Canadian tomatoes, from farm to fork." Statistics Canada website. May 18, 2021.

Chaudhary, P., A. Sharma, B. Singh, and A. K. Nagpal. "Bioactivities of phytochemicals present in tomato." *Journal of Food Science and Technology* 55, 8 (2018): 2833–2849.

Cleveland Clinic. "What Are the Health Benefits of Tomatoes?" healthessentials website. July 26, 2023.

"The history of tomatoes: How a tropical became a global crop." *The Garden Scoop* blog. University of Illinois Extension website. July 25, 2020.

Iowa State University. "Tomatoes." Agricultural Marketing Resource Center website. November 2021.

Lehoullier, Craig. "The History of Tomatoes in America." *Grit* website. April 6, 2015.

"World Tomato Production by Country." AtlasBig.com. Accessed November 21, 2023.

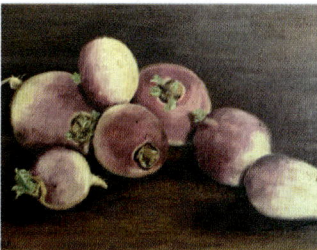

Turnip

Turnips (*Brassica rapa* subsp. *rapa*) are indigenous to Europe, and have been used by humans as both a vegetable and as fodder for livestock since 2500–2000 BCE. In northern and eastern Europe, as well as in Asia, it is common to eat only the turnip tubers, whereas in southern parts of Europe, turnip tops and greens are also consumed.

The turnip is a relative of kale, cauliflower, and cabbage, and, like its cousins, different kinds of turnips have been known since pre-Christian times. Some of those varieties bore Greek place names, indicating early culture and agricultural development by the ancient Greeks. Farmers found turnips easy to grow, and cultivation eventually spread east to China, reaching Japan by 700 CE.

During the first century CE, the Roman author and naturalist Pliny the Elder described long turnips, flat turnips, and round turnips. He wrote of turnips using the names *rapa* and *napus*. In Middle English, *napus* became *naep*; the name "turnip" was derived from this word, along with *turn* ("made round"). The turnip was a popular food in the British Isles. During the reign of Henry VIII, turnip roots were generally boiled or baked. The tops were cooked as "greens," and the young shoots were used in salads.

The European types of turnip are the most common, and were developed in the Mediterranean area. The center of cultivation of the Asiatic varieties of turnip is in middle Asia, west of the Himalayas. There are also two secondary centers in eastern Asia and Asia Minor, today's Türkiye.

The turnip was brought to North America by the French explorer Jacques Cartier, who planted it in Québec in 1541. It was later introduced to Jamestown, Virginia, by British colonists in 1609, and to Massachusetts during the 1620s. Native Americans began growing turnips soon after.

Like other root vegetables, turnips are versatile. They can be boiled and mashed as a tasty alternative to mashed potatoes, or they can be added to soups, stews, stir-fries, and casseroles. Raw turnips can also be chopped and added to salad, or can be used in coleslaw recipes. Turnip greens can be cooked or added to salads. One of my favorite Chinese appetizers is turnip cake, in which shredded turnip is fashioned into a square, which is then pan-fried and served with a thick, soy-based dressing.

Turnips are a good source of vitamins and minerals, including folate, calcium, magnesium, phosphorous, and potassium. Turnip greens (which most people throw into the garbage) are loaded with dietary fiber and vitamins A, C, and K.

The turnip has been used by folk healers since ancient times to treat a wide range of health problems including headaches, chest complaints, rheumatisms, edemas, gonorrhea, syphilis, and even rabies. Contemporary scientific research has found that the turnip is a powerful healing food, primarily due to its wide variety of health-promoting phytochemicals such as *glucosinolates*, which have been found to help prevent cancer, including those of the breast and prostate. Turnips are also rich in lutein, an antioxidant that supports eye health and helps prevent macular degeneration and cataracts. An article appearing in *The Journal of Food Science* in 2018 states:

> Recent pharmacological investigation on turnips have revealed the antitumor, antihypertensive, antidiabetic, antioxidant, anti-inflammatory, hepato-protective [liver protective], and nephron-protective [kidney protective] effects. The anticancer property was found to be the most promising biological activity of turnip. (Paul et al. 2019, 19)

China is the world's largest commercial grower of turnips, followed by Uzbekistan and the United States.

Resources

Bonvissuto, Danny. "Health Benefits of Turnips." WebMD. September 2021.

Paul, S., C. A. Geng, T. H. Yang et al. "Phytochemical and Health-Beneficial Progress of Turnip (*Brassica rapa*)." *Journal of Food Science* 84 (2019): 19–30.

"Production of Turnip," Tridge.com. 2023.

Tacer-Caba, Z. "Different sources of glucosinolates and their derivatives," in *Glucosinolates: Properties, Recovery and Applications*. New York: Academic Press, 2020, 143.

"Turnip and Its Hybrid Offspring." Aggie Horticulture. Texas A&M University. Accessed December 10, 2023.

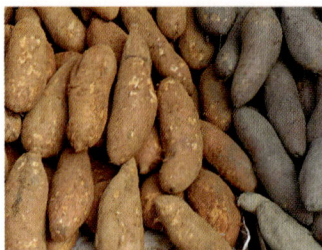

Yam

Yams are often confused with sweet potatoes, but they are not the same. Yams (*Dioscorea* sp.) belong to the Dioscoreaceae family, while sweet potatoes (*Ipomoea batatas*) are members of the Convolvulaceae (morning glory) family. Although they are both starchy tuber vegetables and tend to look alike, yams are generally larger than sweet potatoes, and can grow up to five feet (1.5 meters) long and weigh up to 132 pounds (60 kilograms). Yams are cylindrical in shape, and their skin is usually brown and rough. By contrast, the skin of sweet potatoes is smooth, and ranges in color from yellow, orange, red, brown, and purple. Sweet potatoes also tend to be long and tapered in shape. Yams are more difficult to peel than sweet potatoes when raw, although they are easy to peel when cooked. Yam flesh is usually white or yellow, although mature yams can have flesh that is pink or purple. Yams are drier and starchier, compared to sweet potatoes. They also have a milder flavor.

Unlike sweet potatoes, which are indigenous to and were domesticated in the West Indies, yams were domesticated independently at least three times in three different continents, starting over ten thousand years ago: in mainland Southeast Asia and the Pacific (*Dioscorea alata*), in Latin America (*Dioscorea trifida*), and in Africa (*Dioscorea rotundata*). African yams are mainly produced in the "yam belt," a region including what are now the Republic of Côte d'Ivoire (Ivory Coast), Ghana, Togo, Benin, Nigeria, and Cameroon. Over six hundred varieties of yams are known, and 95 percent of these are grown in Africa. It is believed that African yams eventually found their way to the Caribbean. They are considered an important staple food in many parts of Africa and the Pacific Islands, including Papua New Guinea and Japan.

It is no surprise that yams are considered sacred in many traditional societies, and have long played a role in community festivals and ceremonies. In southeastern Nigeria, a yam-related festival is held in many communities at harvest time. Among the Igbo people, the yam is often depicted as a male totem figure. The most widely grown yams are the yellow and white varieties. Others include Filipino purple, Kush Kush, Indian, Chinese, and Japanese mountain yams.

Yams can be enjoyed much like potatoes and sweet potatoes. In western Africa, yams are eaten boiled, fried, baked, or roasted in combination with tomato stew and a variety of sauces. Kush kush, a popular Caribbean comfort food, features yams that are mashed and sautéed with onions, chili peppers, herbs, and spices. Yams can also be processed into chips, flakes, and flour.

Aside from being a good source of dietary fiber, yams are also rich in manganese and potassium. Unlike yams with white flesh, yellow, orange, and purple-hued yams are high in antioxidants such as vitamins C and A, as well as complex carbohydrates, which help regulate blood sugar. Deep orange varieties of yams contain abundant beta-carotene, which the body converts to vitamin A.

Yams have long been part of traditional medicine traditions. For example, the Chinese yam is used in both Chinese cuisine and is an important part of Traditional Chinese Medicine. It is prescribed to strengthen the stomach, spleen, lungs, and kidneys, and to treat a wide range of health problems including digestive disorders, general weakness, frequent urination, poor appetite, excessive vaginal discharge, premature ejaculation, and chronic wheezing and coughing.

Yams have similar health benefits to sweet potatoes, including antioxidant, anti-inflammatory and hepato-protective activity, cardiovascular protection, anticancer properties, improvement in neurological and memory capacity, and protection from metabolic disorders. In addition, recent studies have found that wild yam root contains *diosgenin*, a plant steroid that has been shown to limit the progression of both osteoporosis arthritis and rheumatoid arthritis. It has also been shown to reduce LDL or "bad" cholesterol levels. Other laboratory and clinical studies have found that yams help protect the cardiovascular system, help prevent diabetes, relieve post-menopausal symptoms, and are antimicrobial and anti-inflammatory.

Today, western Africa produces over 90 percent of the world's yam crop, with Nigeria being the largest grower, followed by Ghana and the Ivory Coast. Tropical countries in South America (primarily Colombia), along with the West Indies, Asia (including China, India, and Vietnam), and the Pacific islands (especially Indonesia, Papua New Guinea, Taiwan, the Philippines, and Okinawa in Japan) also produce yams for local consumption.

Resources

Brown, Mary Jane. "Sweet Potatoes vs Yams: What's the Difference?" healthline.com. September 21, 2017.

Chan, Vicky. "Chinese Yam–Nourishing to Spleen, Lungs & Kidneys." ChineseMedicineLiving.com. November 8, 2013.

"Health Benefits of Yams." WebMD. August 30, 2023.

Kiss, Juniper. "Where Did Greater Yams Come From?" Botany One website. July 2, 2020.

Lebot, Vincent, Floriane Lawac, and Laurent Legendre. "The greater yam (*Dioscorea alata* L.): A review of its phytochemical content and potential for processed products and biofortification." *Journal of Food Composition and Analysis* 115 (2023): 104987.

Obidiegwu, Jude E., Jessica B Lyons, and Cynthia A Chilaka. "The *Dioscorea* Genus (Yam)—An Appraisal of Nutritional and Therapeutic Potentials." *Foods* 9, 9 (2020): 1304.

Scarcelli, Nora, Philippe Cubryl, Roland Akakpo et al. "Yam genomics supports West Africa as a major cradle of crop domestication." *Science Advances* 5, 5 (2019): eaaw1947.

"Yam," *New World Encyclopedia* website. Accessed February 9, 2025.

Photo on p. 227 by Bruno Weltmann

Culinary Herbs and Spices

Culinary herbs are the fresh or dried leaves of special varieties of vegetables, which are used as food flavorings. By contrast, spices come from the root, stem, seed, fruit, flower, or bark of a plant. Both are usually dried and ground. Hundreds of plants are grown for these purposes. Some of the more popular herbs consumed in North America include basil, cilantro, chives, dill, mint, oregano, parsley, pepper, rosemary, sage, and thyme. Common spices include ginger, cinnamon, black pepper, and turmeric. Some plants, like cilantro (coriander), can be both an herb *and* a spice, as both leaves and seeds from the plant are used.

All herbs and spices contain active chemical ingredients that are used for specific purposes:

- *Alkaloids* are organic compounds of plant origin that contain at least one nitrogen atom and have pronounced physiological actions on humans. They provide many drugs (including morphine and quinine) as well as poisons, like atropine and strychnine.
- *Bitters* are phytochemicals (chemicals found in plants) that have a sharp, bitter flavor and stimulate the appetite.
- *Enzymes* are substances produced by plants that act as a catalyst to bring about specific biochemical reactions.
- *Essential oils* are concentrated extracts that retain the natural smell or flavor of the plants from which they came.
- *Glycosides* are compounds formed by a simple sugar that combine with another compound by what is called a "glycosidic bond." Many medications are derived from glycosides. For example, Iridoid glycosides (derived from lavender) lower blood pressure by relaxing the smooth muscles in blood vessels.
- *Tannins* are chemical compounds also known as *polyphenols*. They are found in many plants, including the skin and seeds of grapes, and act as the plant's natural defense mechanism against animals and insects.

- *Vitamins and minerals* are considered essential nutrients for life because, acting together, they perform hundreds of roles in the body including support for the nervous system, promoting wound healing, strengthening bones, and bolstering the immune system. They also convert food into energy and repair cellular damage.

All of the herbs and seasonings included in this section are widely used in foods. In addition to their ability to provide flavor to many dishes, they also contain important phytochemicals that have proven medicinal value. Although many of the health claims for these foods go back thousands of years, modern researchers at leading universities have begun to discover that many of these health-promoting claims can be proven scientifically.

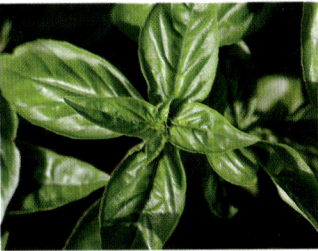

Basil

Photo by Amada44

Basil (*Ocimum basilicum*) is one of the world's most popular herbs. It originated in tropical and subtropical areas of southern and southeastern Asia, including India, Pakistan, and Thailand, and has been cultivated for at least five thousand years. Because of its popularity, basil is often referred to as the "king of herbs." There are now more than 150 basil varieties, the most common being sweet Italian, Genovese, Bush (Greek), purple, and scented basils.

The name "basil" may have been derived from the Greek words

basileus, meaning "king," or *basilikon*, meaning "royal." The Latin word *basiliscus* refers to Basilisk, a mythical fire-breathing dragon. According to Roman legend, basil is the antidote to the venom of this monster. The botanical name *Ocimum* is derived from the Greek term "to be fragrant."

In India, basil was sacred to the Hindu gods Krishna and Vishnu, and it was believed that if a leaf of basil were buried with the dead, the deceased person would go to heaven. Basil has also been used as a medicinal plant in both Traditional Chinese Medicine and Ayurveda, India's traditional medicine system. In ancient Egypt, the plant was associated with conservation and antibacterial properties; basil was used in the mummification process, and has been found inside Egyptian tombs.

Basil gradually spread to both China and the Middle East as the result of the spice trade, and is said to have arrived in Greece and Italy around 350 BCE. During the 1600s, the English used basil as a flavoring in their food, and also as an insecticide. Sprigs of basil were hung in doorways to ward off flies and "evil spirits." Basil has been cultivated in the Americas for over two hundred years.

Both the Italians and the Portuguese have long considered basil to be a symbol of love. In Italy, a courting young man would wear a sprig of basil to signal serious intentions to his prospective bride, while in Portugal basil sprigs are traditionally given to a lover or loved one along with a poem during certain religious holidays.

Basil can be used fresh or dried to flavor a wide variety of foods including vegetables, pasta, rice, poultry, and fish. Although long a favorite ingredient in curries and other savory Thai dishes, basil is probably best known as a flavoring in Italian cuisine, including pasta with tomato and basil, pasta with pesto, and Caprese salad. Basil is commonly preserved in vinegar or olive oil, which adds a delightful flavor to both for use in salad dressings. It is also used in jelly, honey, tea, and liquor. The flowers of basil are also edible, and can be an attractive addition to salads and other dishes.

Basil is highly nutritious. It contains generous amounts omega-3 fatty acids, folate, and vitamins A, C, and K, and it is rich in essential minerals such as manganese, copper, iron, calcium, and magnesium. Basil has been used in Ayurvedic medicine for centuries, to treat a wide variety of health problems including pain relief, diabetes, sinus congestion, and heart disease. Modern science has found that the antioxidants and other phytochemicals in basil have powerful anti-inflammatory and antibacterial properties, and can support skin health, alleviate stress, support liver function, relieve indigestion, help the body maintain optimum blood pressure levels, and protect against age-related macular degeneration and other eye diseases.

Egypt and the United States are the primary countries in which basil is grown and exported.

Resources

"Basil History and Culture." US Basil Consortium, Rutgers University website. Accessed December 5, 2023.

"Basil: The King of Herbs." SPICEography.com. Accessed December 5, 2023.

De Innocentis, Ivana. "History and Origin of Basil." *The Food Hub*. TUMN. Accessed December 5, 2023.

Rindels, Sherry. "Basil." Yard and Garden, Iowa State University. March 21, 1997.

Wikipedia. "Basil." Accessed December 5, 2023.

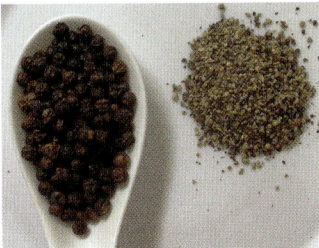

Black Pepper

The black pepper plant (*Piper nigrum*) is a flowering vine that traces its origin to what is now Kerala State in southern India. What we know as "black pepper" is the vine's green berries, which are dried and used as a seasoning. After harvesting, the berries are dried in the sun or by machine for several days, during which the fruit around the seed shrinks and darkens into a thin, wrinkled, black layer. Once dried, the fruits are called peppercorns. White pepper consists of the seed only, with the skin of the fruit removed.

Black pepper, which belongs to the *Piper* genus, is not a relative of chili peppers, which belong to the *Capsicum* genus. However, they are both technically a form of berry produced by their host plants, although chili peppers are larger and come in many shapes and colors.

Like chili peppers, black pepper has been used as a seasoning for more than four thousand years. It is one of the most popular spices in the world, and is used in every type of national cuisine. Black pepper has a sharp, pungent flavor that adds depth and heat to a wide variety of dishes.

The history of black pepper is complex. It has been used as both a spice and medicinal plant in India since prehistoric times. Black pepper has been traded for thousands of years and has often been referred to as "Black Gold." Ancient Egyptians used black pepper as both a seasoning and a preservative. There is evidence that black pepper was placed in the nostrils of Pharaoh Ramesses II after his death in 1213 BCE as part of his mummification. Pepper was known in Greece in the fourth century BCE, and was believed to have been introduced by traders via the Arabian Sea.

Black pepper, commonly known as just "pepper," was a highly valued seasoning in the Roman Empire during the first century CE. After the fall of Rome, pepper began to spread through the Middle East and the rest of Europe, and eventually arrived in the Americas. Black pepper is believed to have been introduced to China during the second century BCE, and was first found in markets in Sichuan. It was generally very expensive in Imperial China until the fifteenth century; Ming treasure voyages to India returned with such large quantities of pepper, it caused prices to drop.

Although we don't consume large amounts black pepper at a time, it is a highly nutritious food that deserves a greater role in our diets. In addition to dietary fiber, black pepper is a rich source of manganese, iron, potassium, vitamin C, and vitamin K. One of the most beneficial effects of black pepper is that it contains *piperine*, a chemical that not only provides pepper's distinctive flavor but enhances the bioavailability of other foods: it helps the body to transport and absorb other healthy foods that we consume—especially those containing iron and beta-carotene—making those nutrients more accessible and available. It is especially useful when combined with turmeric, another healthy spice which is indigenous to India. Black pepper helps the body absorb *curcumin*, a powerful antioxidant and anti-inflammatory compound found in turmeric.

Black pepper has been used in Ayurvedic, Siddha, and Unani medicinal systems in India for centuries. The Syriac *Book of Medicines*, published in Damascus during the thirteenth century CE, prescribed pepper to treat constipation, diarrhea, earache, gangrene, heart disease, hernia, hoarseness, indigestion, insect bites, insomnia, joint pain, liver problems, lung disease, oral abscesses, sunburn, tooth decay, and toothaches.

In addition to its nutritional benefits, recent laboratory findings have shown that black pepper is a good source of antioxidants, and has proven anti-inflammatory properties. It is also considered a good substitute for salt to enhance the flavor of foods. Black pepper is being studied for its ability to stimulate the pathways of the nervous system in the brain, boosting neurological health and reducing cognitive malfunction and memory impairment.

A recent article about black pepper—especially exploring its *piperine* and essential oil—appearing in *Clinical Phytoscience* emphasizes the therapeutic value of this amazing spice:

> [P]iperine is the naturally occurring and principal bioactive alkaloid constituent of black pepper owing to its potential therapeutic properties, including cerebral brain functioning and increased nutrient absorption. The BPEO [black pepper essential oil] has several biological roles, including antioxidant, anti-inflammatory, anticancer, anti-obesity, antidepressant, antidiabetic, antimicrobial, gastroprotective, and insecticidal activities. (Ashokkumar et al. 2021, 7)

Pepper is one of the most popular spices in the world. The country with the highest volume of pepper consumption is Vietnam, followed by India and the United States. The countries with the highest levels of black pepper consumption per capita are Bulgaria, Singapore, and Vietnam. The top five black pepper producing countries are Vietnam, Indonesia, India, Brazil, and China.

Resources

Ashokkumar, K. M. Murugan, M. K. Dhanya et al. "Phytochemistry and therapeutic potential of black pepper [*Piper nigrum* (L.)] essential oil and piperine: a review." *Clinical Phytoscience* 7, 52 (2021): 7–52.

"Black Pepper: History, Flavor, Benefits, Uses." SPICEography.com. Accessed December 6, 2023.

"Black Pepper: Origin, History and Uses." Agriculture in India website. Accessed December 6, 2023.

Cleveland Clinic. "What Are the Health Benefits of Black Pepper?" healthessentials. August 4, 2021.

Wikipedia. "Black pepper." Accessed December 6, 2023.

"World Pepper Market 2020: Historic Review of 2007-2018 with Projections to 2025." GlobeNewswire.com. February 25, 2022.

"The World's Tope Black Pepper Producing Countries." *WorldAtlas* website. Accessed December 6, 2023.

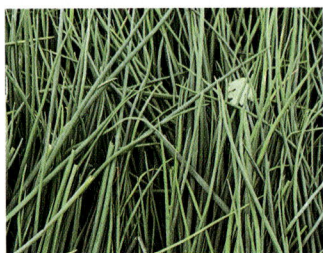

Chive

Chives (*Allium schoenoprasum*) are members of the onion family, which also includes shallots, garlic, scallions, and leeks. This herb grows in dense clumps of slender bulbs, each bulb producing hollow, tubular leaves that are eight to twenty inches (20–51 cm) long. Chives have a mild yet tasty onion flavor, and have been used as a food, a seasoning, and a medicine for thousands of years.

Although there has been some disagreement about their place of origin, archaeological evidence suggests that chives have been cultivated in China for at least four thousand years, and were possibly introduced to Europe by the explorer Marco Polo in the late 1200s CE. There is also some evidence that chives are also indigenous to Siberia and Greece. Some historians believe that chives are native to parts of North America (especially near the Great Lakes Huron and Superior), while others maintain that it was first introduced to America by European colonists during the seventeenth century.

Because chives tend to thrive in the wild, they were not actively culti-vated in Europe until the Middle Ages, which lasted from 476–1453 CE. In medieval Europe, chives were used to discourage insects, and were also grown as a decorative plant. Chives produce a dense yet delicate purple flower that attracts pollinators. Early Chinese doctors prescribed chives to treat digestive disorders and kidney problems. Lore surrounding chives includes the tale that they were given to Alexander the Great in Siberia. And the recommendation in ancient Rome was that those who wanted to be kissed should avoid eating chives. Like onions and garlic, chives were considered to be an aphrodisiac in China, and were prescribed by tradi-tional doctors to treat erectile dysfunction; chives even carried the old nickname "get-it-up grass." In order to reduce sexual desire and maintain chaste thoughts, Buddhist monks have long been prohibited from eating them. Chives, garlic, and onions are still not allowed in Buddhist vegetar-ian cuisine today.

Chives have been a popular seasoning and garnish in many parts of the world. Ancient Greeks and Romans used chives to season soups, stews, and salads. During the Middle Ages in Europe, chives were used to flavor breads and other baked goods. In France, chives are one of the *fines herbes*, a term to describe the core set of herbs used in French cuisine. In his 1806 book *Attempt at a Flora* (*Försök til en flora*), the Swedish botanist Anders Jahan Retzius describes how chives are used to add flavor to pancakes, soups, fish, and sandwiches. In China, chives are known as *jiu cai*, and are used more as a vegetable than as a seasoning or garnish; chives are often stir-fried and served as a side dish to other foods, and are also cooked with eggs. Due to their high demand by Asians living abroad, fresh chives are easily found in Asian markets in North America and Europe.

Like its relatives in the onion family, chives are nutritious. They provide a modest amount of dietary fiber, and contain a generous amount of Vitamin K, which helps strengthen bones and has been found to limit damage to neurons, a major feature of Alzheimer's disease. Chives also contain organosulfur compounds, which may help prevent cancers of the prostate and esophagus. In addition, chives provide choline, a phytochemical that promotes sleep and improves memory.

Recent scientific evaluation of chives by pharmacologists at Punjabi University in India has identified its potential medicinal use as an anti-inflammatory, anticancer, antioxidant, anthelmintic (expels intestinal worms), or antihypertensive agent. Investigations of their medicinal uses in contemporary medicine are still in the early stages, and more research is necessary.

Chives are easy to grow and have long been a welcome addition to home gardens all over the world. Both China and the United States are major commercial producers of chives. They are also grown extensively in Mexico, Canada, India, and parts of South America.

Resources

"Chives." Roots of Medicine. University of Iowa. Accessed December 8, 2023.

"Chives: An Ancient Herb with a Delicate Flavor." SPICEography.com. Accessed December 8, 2023.

de Candolle, Alphonse. *Origin of Cultivated Plants*. New York: D. Appleton and Company, 1908, 72.

Singh, Varinder, Gargi Chauhan, Pawan Krishan, and Richa Shri. "*Allium* schoenoprasum L.: a review of phytochemistry, pharmacology and future directions." *Natural Product Research* 32, 18 (2018): 2202–2216. Wikipedia. "Chives." Accessed December 8, 2023.

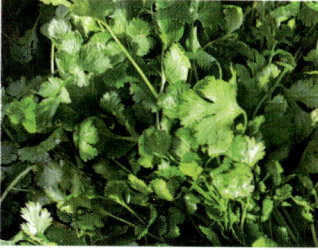

Coriander and Cilantro

Coriander (*Coriandrum sativum*) is a much-loved culinary herb and a member of the Apiaceae family, which also includes carrots, fennel, parsley, celery, anise, and cumin. It is commonly used in Latin American and Asian cuisines, and is sometimes referred to as "Mexican parsley" or "Chinese parsley."

Many are confused about the differences between coriander and cilantro, because these names are often used interchangeably. "Coriander" usually refers to the whole plant or only the seeds, which are usually ground and used as a spice. "Cilantro" typically refers to the leaves and stalk of the plant, which are used fresh or dried.

Like the other herbs and spices in this book, coriander's history as both an herb and a spice is a long one. Coriander is native to the eastern Mediterranean. Coriander seeds that date back eight thousand years have been found in caves in Israel, and it appears to have been cultivated in Greece since at least 6000 BCE. The *Ebers Papyrus*, an Egyptian text that dates from around 1550 BCE, mentioned uses of coriander, and its seeds were found in the tomb of King Tutankhamen, who died in 1323 BCE. Coriander seeds are referred to as one of the bitter herbs in the Bible, and were eaten at the first Passover.

The early Romans used coriander to flavor their bread, as an aromatic, and medicinally to relieve flatulence. The herb was intro-duced to the Americas in the 1600s. Since that time, it has played an important role in spicing up dishes from the American Southwest, Mexico, and throughout Latin America. Coriander is considered one of the three most important culinary herbs in India, and is used exten-sively to flavor curries, masalas, and chutneys. It is also an important ingredient in *berbere*, an essential spice mixture from Ethiopia.

Cilantro has become one of the most popular culinary herbs in the United States, and chefs use a lot of it. The leaves and tender stems are used in curries, sauces, salsas, soups, and salads. Cooking deepens its characteristic sharp flavor.

Cilantro's nutritional profile is impressive. The plant contains high amounts of vitamins A, B$_2$ (riboflavin), folate, vitamin C, and especially vitamin K. Coriander seeds contain essential oils that have been shown to have antibacterial effects. The seeds also contain phy-tochemicals that may lower blood pressure by causing blood vessels to dilate. Several studies have shown that consuming cilantro on a regular basis may reduce symptoms of neurological diseases like Alzheimer's and Parkinson's. Coriander and cilantro also have exten-sive histories in folk medicine. They have been an essential part of the Indian Ayurvedic tradition of medicine for centuries, and have been used to treat eye problems, constipation, digestive problems, headache, and skin problems.

Resources

Ortega, Ynes. "Cilantro." Food Source Information, Colorado State University website. Accessed December 8, 2023.

"Cilantro: A Healthy and Versatile Herb." SPICEography.com. Accessed December 8, 2023.

"Coriander." *Encyclopaedia Britannica*. Updated January 17, 2025.

"Coriander–Uses, Side Effects and More." WebMD. Accessed December 8, 2023.

"Health benefits of Cilantro." WebMD. September 19, 2022.

Jaiswal, Shalini. "Top 15 Health Benefits of Coriander Herb." TheAyurveda.
    org. July 22, 2020.
Wikipedia. "Coriander." Accessed December 8, 2023.

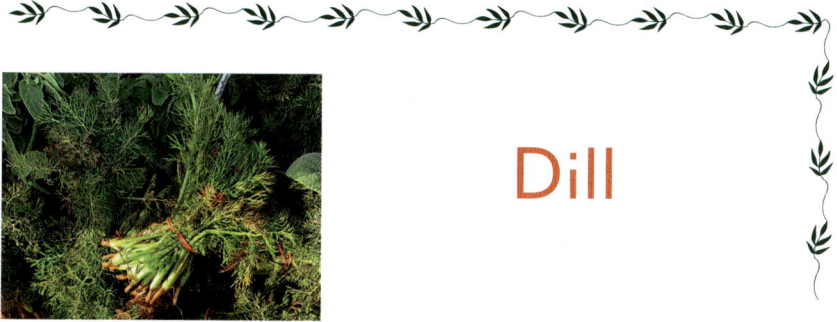

Dill

Dill (*Anethum graveolens*) is an ancient seasoning for both Scandinavian and eastern European dishes, although the seeds are best known for giving character to dill pickles, vinegar, and potato salad.

Dill is believed to have originated in the Mediterranean region, although the name "dill" is derived from an Old Norse word meaning "to soothe." Dill was cultivated in Babylonian gardens in what is now parts of Iraq and Syria as far back as 3000 BCE, and was also used as a medicinal herb in Egypt at about the same time. In 1550 BCE, the *Ebers Papyrus*, which included descriptions of over nine hundred medical prescriptions based mostly on plants, included dill as one of the components of a medicine to relieve pain. Oil scented with dill was burned in Greek homes to freshen the atmosphere, and the plant's essential oil was used to make wine.

Dioscorides, the Greek physician and pharmacologist (40–90 CE) wrote that scorched dill seeds had the ability to heal the wounds of soldiers, a practice which was also shared by the Romans. Roman gladiators were fed meals seasoned with dill because it was believed that consuming the herb would give them courage. In Medieval Europe, sprigs of dill were used to protect homes (and people) from witchcraft, and were hung on doorways and worn as charms. Dill was also added to love potions and aphrodisiacs to make them more effective.

By the seventeenth century, dill could be found growing in many English kitchen gardens. It was most likely introduced to America by English settlers. John Winthrop, who led a group of Puritans to form the Massachusetts Bay Colony in 1630, was known to have grown dill.

Along with chives and parsley, dill is considered a staple culinary herb in northern, central, and eastern Europe. Most of the dill used in the United States is in the form of seeds used to make pickles. The slightly bitter seeds are also used by home cooks as a condiment to flavor vegetable and meat dishes, soups, stews, casseroles, sauces, and vinegar. The dill weed itself has a stronger flavor than its seeds, and can be added chopped or whole to soups, stews, casseroles, pasta, and egg dishes. It can also enhance the flavor of many types of sauces.

Since people generally use dill in small quantities, the herb doesn't add many nutrients to one's daily diet. However, dill is a good source of B vitamins (especially riboflavin, pyridoxine, and folate) as well as vitamin C. It also contains generous amounts of essential minerals including manganese, iron, calcium, potassium, and magnesium. Dill is packed with flavonoids, which have been linked with reducing "bad" cholesterol and supporting heart health in general. The phenolic acids found in dill exhibit antioxidant, antimicrobial, and antitumor activities. Dill has also been found to manage type 2 diabetes, gastrointestinal problems, urinary infections, and insomnia.

Although dill is grown in the United States and Canada, most of the dill North Americans use, whether commercially in pickle manufacturing or in the home kitchen, is imported from India, Egypt, and Canada.

Resources

Bremness, Lesley. *Herbs*. New York: Dorling Kindersley, 2002, 229.
"Dill: Not Just for Pickles." SPICEography.com. Accessed December 12, 2023.
"Health Benefits of Dill." WebMD. September 19, 2022.

Ozliman, S., G. Yaldiz, M. Camlica et al. "Chemical components of essential oils and biological activities of the aqueous extract of *Anethum graveolens* L. grown under inorganic and organic conditions." *Chemical and Biological Technologies in Agriculture* 8, 20 (2021).

"The Herb Society of America's Essential Guide to Dill." HerbSociety.org. Accessed February 9, 2025.

Wikipedia. "Dill." Accessed December 12, 2023.

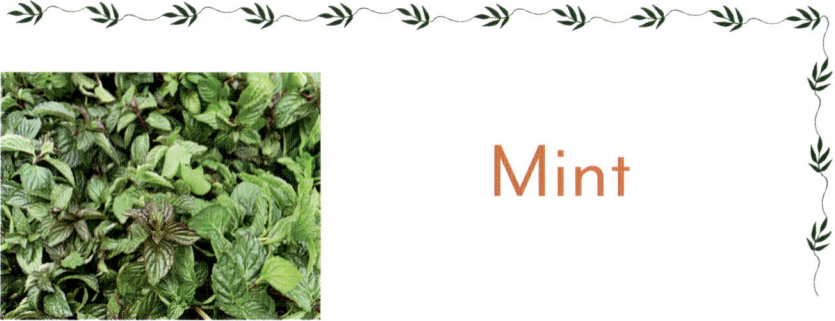

Mint

Mint (*Mentha*) is one of the world's most popular herbs. Spearmint (*Mentha spicata*) and peppermint (*Mentha* x *piperita*) are the most frequently cultivated varietals. Peppermint is a cross between spearmint and watermint, *Mentha aquatica*. When first discovered, peppermint was classified as its own species, but is now most commonly thought of as a hybrid.

Mint can trace its ancestral roots to the eastern Mediterranean region thousands of years ago. Mint was highly regarded by the ancient Egyptians, and archaeologists have found dried mint leaves in Egyptian tombs. The *Ebers Papyrus*, a medical text that dates from 1550 BCE, mentions mint as a digestive medicine, also used to reduce flatulence.

The ancient Greeks and Romans valued mint for its refreshing smell; they used mint in funerary rites, and living people rubbed mint on their skin to scent their bodies. The origin of mint has been highlighted in Greek mythology. A nymph named Minthe attracted the attention of Hades, the god of the underworld. Persephone, Hades's jealous wife, attacked Minthe and attempted to trample her to death. In order to save her life, Hades turned Minthe into an herb.

In the mythological story of Baucus and Philemon, the Roman poet Ovid notes that the two lovers placed mint on eating surfaces underneath food offerings for the gods because of its attractive smell. Both the Greeks and Romans commonly used peppermint to flavor sauces, and as perfume infused in wine. The Greeks believed that mint was a symbol of hospitality, and used it to decorate their tables.

The Romans eventually brought mint and mint sauce to Britain; they strewed mints in feasts and banquets as a token of welcome to their guests. The poet Geoffrey Chaucer referred to the use of mint growing wild in English rural pathways. Mint was also mentioned in other European literary works as well as in plant catalogues, including John Gardiner's *Feate of Gardening* in 1440. Mint was introduced to Thailand and Japan in the 1800s; the Japanese began distilling peppermint oil to produce menthol centuries ago.

When the pilgrims landed in America on the Mayflower, mint was one of the plants they brought with them, and so it has been cultivated in American gardens for hundreds of years. It is also found growing wild in many parts of the world.

Mint is probably the world's most popular herb. The Greeks used it in a traditional drink made with fermented barley. Ancient Romans used the herb as a flavoring in wines and sauces. As a seasoning, mint can be chopped and added to salads, sprinkled over fruit, or combined with basil to make mint pesto. Peppermint tea can be enjoyed hot or cold, and is often used as a digestive aid. Mint is used in a wide variety of soaps, toothpaste, mouthwashes, chewing gum, candies, and breath fresheners.

As far back as the early 1620s, European physicians suggested rinsing the mouth with mint boiled in white wine and vinegar. They also recommended rubbing the gums with dry mint powder, as "a good lotion for the teeth and mouth[,] and rottennesse of the gummes. (Pickering, 2023)" Mint tea has been used as a digestive aid and to promote restful sleep for thousands of years.

Peppermint has antiseptic, anti-parasitic, antiviral, and sweat-inducing properties. Peppermint oil relieves body aches and pains with its anti-spasmodic properties. There is growing interest in the medicinal value of mint, especially its antibacterial properties, stress reducing capabilities, and its ability to fight cancerous tumor cells. Modern physicians have noted that drinking peppermint tea has been found to reduce stomach pain, bloating, and gas, and to help regulate bowel movements in people suffering from irritable bowel syndrome (IBS). However, they've also found that consuming mint can worsen symptoms of patients diagnosed with gastroesophageal reflux disease, or GERD.

A growing number of food scientists and medical professionals believe that mint is one of the healthiest of herbs. The authors of a recent scientific paper published in the peer-reviewed journal *Molecules* even used the unscientific term "wonderful" in the article's title: "The Wonderful Activities of the Genus *Mentha*: Not Only Antioxidant Properties." The authors summarized:

> Among medicinal plants, mint (*Mentha* species) exhibits multiple health beneficial properties, such as prevention from cancer development and anti-obesity, antimicrobial, anti-inflammatory, anti-diabetic, and cardioprotective effects, as a result of its antioxidant potential, combined with low toxicity and high efficacy. (Tafrihi et al. 2021, 1118)

About 70 percent of the world's peppermint and spearmint are grown in the United States. Oregon, Washington, Idaho, Indiana, California, and Wisconsin are the top peppermint-producing states, while Washington, Oregon, Indiana, Idaho, and Michigan are the top spearmint-growing states. Other major mint growers worldwide are Europe and Japan.

Resources

Boyles, Margaret. "12 Uses of Mint Leaves, From Health to Home." *The Old Farmer's Almanac*. September 11, 2023.

Bremness, Lesley. *Herbs*. New York: Dorling Kindersley, 2002, 190-91.

"Health Benefits of Mint." WebMD. Accessed December 12, 2023.

"Mint," Hamilton College Academics website. Accessed December 12, 2023.

"Mint: A Healing Burst of Cool Flavor," SPICEography.com. Accessed December 12, 2023.

"Peppermint: Uses, Side Effects and More." WebMD. Accessed December 12, 2023.

Pickering, Victoria. "Plant of the Month: Mint." JSTOR Daily website. Accessed December 12, 2023.

Tafrihi, M., M. Imran, T. Tufail et al. "The Wonderful Activities of the Genus *Mentha*: Not Only Antioxidant Properties." *Molecules*. 26, 4 (2021): 1118–1140.

"The U.S. Produces Over 70% of the World's Mint," *AgHires* blog. Accessed February 9, 2025.

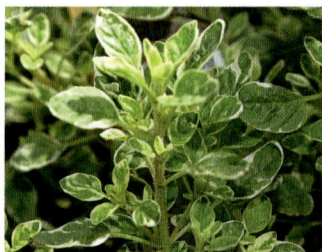

Oregano

Photo by David J. Stang

Oregano is an herb that appears to have originated in two separate parts of the world: the Mediterranean variety (*Origanum vulgare*) and the Mexican variety (*Lippia Graveolens*). Both varieties have traditionally been harvested in the wild. The name *Origanum* is derived from the Greek, meaning "joy of the mountain" since oregano thrives in high-elevation climates. Mexican oregano comes from a different botanical family. It has a stronger flavor than Mediterranean oregano yet shares similar nutritional and medicinal profiles.

As one can tell from its name, Mediterranean oregano is indigenous to the Mediterranean region and western and southwestern Eurasia, which encompasses an area that spans today's Egypt, Türkiye, Italy, and Spain. Oregano has been a popular seasoning since ancient Egyptian, Greek, and Roman times, and is used to add flavor to vegetables, wine, meat, and fish.

According to Greek mythology, Aphrodite, the goddess of love and beauty, created oregano as a symbol of happiness. This led early Greeks to use oregano in marriage ceremonies to celebrate happiness and in funeral services to bring peace to both the departed and their grieving relatives and friends.

The Greek physician Hippocrates (460–370 BCE) used oregano as an antiseptic, and to prevent lung ailments and gastrointestinal distress. Oregano leaves were also used in ancient Greece and Rome to treat skin sores, muscle aches, stomach distress, and colds. Medieval Europeans chewed oregano leaves for relief of rheumatism, toothache, indigestion, and cough. Dr. Robert Eglesfeld Griffith's *Medical Botany*, published in Philadelphia in 1847, includes historical information on the use of oregano oil to increase menstrual flow, induce perspiration, and as a liniment to relieve body aches and pains.

Along with basil, oregano has traditionally been a popular seasoning in many Italian dishes, including pizza, pasta, tomato-based sauces, vegetable dishes, and salads. In Greece, oregano has been added in dried form to pickled olives and used to flavor cheese, and is added fresh to almost every Greek dish, including meat dishes, vegetable dishes, and salads. In Türkiye, oregano is known as *Guvey Out*, and is used to flavor soups, legumes, and cabbage dishes, as well as the famous döner kebab.

Although oregano is the most popular imported seasoning sold in the United States today, it was largely unknown until American troops returned from Italy after World War II. Soldiers had discovered what they called "the pizza herb" in southern Italy, and loved its fragrance and pungent flavor. Oregano has since become an American staple, and

Americans consume more than 14 million pounds of oregano a year. In addition to pizza and pasta dishes, oregano is often used to season soups, stews, casseroles, legume-based dishes, and breads.

Along with red pepper and cumin, Mexican oregano is a staple ingredient in chili powder. Mexican oregano adds flavor to a wide variety of traditional Mexican recipes, along with ingredients found in Tex-Mex dishes, like shredded cheese, beans, meat, chili peppers, and tortillas. It is best known for adding flavor to various types of chili.

Although oregano contains a variety of vitamins and minerals (including vitamins A, C, and K and potassium, iron, and calcium), we use oregano in such small amounts, its nutritional impact is small.

Like many of the other herbs included in this book, oregano has been used as a medicinal plant for thousands of years. And it has recently become a subject of scientific study due to its newly discovered antioxidant, anti-inflammatory, antimicrobial, and neuroprotective properties. A recent study has shown that taking oregano as a dietary supplement for three months can reduce LDL ("bad") cholesterol while increasing levels of HDL ("good") cholesterol. Another study showed that taking oil of oregano for six weeks killed intestinal parasites, including *Blastocystis hominis*, *Entamoeba hartmanni*, and *Endolimax nana*. Scientists are also exploring oregano's role in cancer prevention and for treating diseases like diabetes and depression. At a time when there is concern about drug-resistant diseases, researchers have found that oregano oil can kill eleven types of microbes that are resistant to antibiotics, offering great promise for future medical treatment.

Resources

Brazier, Yvette. "What Are the Health Benefits of Oregano?" Medical News Today website. April 4, 2023.

Bremness, Lesley. *Herbs*. New York: Dorling Kindersley, 2002, 196.

Egelsfeld Griffiths, R. *Medical Botany: or, Descriptions of the more important plants used in medicine: with their history, properties, and mode of administration*. Philadelphia: Lea & Blanchard, 1847, 511.

Martyris, Nina. "GIs Helped Bring Freedom to Europe, and a Taste for Oregano to America." *The Salt*. National Public Radio website. May 9, 2015.

"Oregano." McCormick Science Institute website. Accessed December 19, 2023.

"Oregano," Roots of Medicine. University of Iowa. Accessed December 19, 2023.

"Oregano: A Staple Herb That Packs a Punch." SPICEography.com. Accessed December 19, 2023.

"Oregano—Uses Side Effects and More." WebMD. Accessed December 19, 2023.

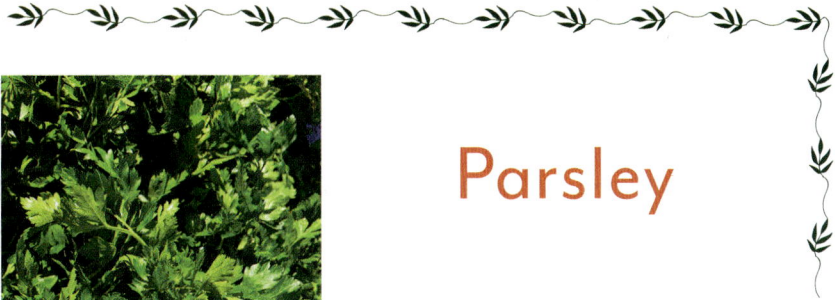

Parsley

Parsley's name (*Petroselinum crispum*) comes from the Greek word *petro*, meaning "stone." This was due to the fact that parsley was first discovered growing on Greece's rocky hillsides thousands of years ago. Greek legend tells us that the herb grew up from the place where the blood of young Opheltes was spilled when he was bitten by a serpent. While some early Greeks viewed parsley as a symbol of death, it was also symbolic of victory and dedicated to Zeus, the Greek god of sky and thunder. Parsley was woven into crowns and worn at dinner by ancient Greeks to increase gaiety and increase appetite. The ancient Romans used parsley as a digestive aid; they also sprinkled it on dead bodies to cover the smell of decay. Charlemagne (748–814 CE), the King of the Franks, King of the Lombards, and Holy Roman Emperor ordered that parsley be planted in his gardens.

Although parsley was considered a medicinal herb, many Europeans associated parsley with death during the Dark Ages, which began in the 1330s CE and lasted approximately two hundred years. Christians were forbidden to transplant parsley in the belief that doing so invited death and crop failure. After the Dark Ages, Europeans began to view parsley in a more positive light, and it became a popular food and seasoning—especially in Italy and France. Parsley was reported to be growing in English gardens by 1548, and a domesticated form of parsley was introduced to Peru from Spain at about the same time. Parsley arrived at American settlements in Virginia by 1612.

Parsley leaves have been eaten in the Middle East for thousands of years, and (along with bulger) are a main ingredient in tabouleh salad, perhaps one of the tastiest and most nutrient-rich salads ever invented. Parsley leaves are a popular ingredient in other salads, and are also used as a garnish. Ground parsley root is used to add flavor to soups, casseroles, stir-fried dishes, and stews.

Parsley has a strong nutritional profile, and also contains many phytochemicals that are good for health. It is a rich source of vitamins A, C, K, and folate, and is a good source of calcium, potassium, and magnesium. Parsley leaves also yield fatty acids, and an essential oil from the seeds is used in condiments and seasonings, as well as in fragrances for perfumes, soaps, and creams.

Parsley leaves, roots, and seeds have a long history in medicine. They contain diuretic properties and are able to reduce the release of histamine, which often manifests as seasonal allergies. Parsley has also been used medicinally to improve digestion, relieve rheumatism, and tone uterine muscles after birth. Parsley leaf infusions are used as a tonic for hair, eyes, and skin. The antioxidant properties in parsley are believed to prevent skin damage due to free radicals and help prevent heart disease, diabetes, and cancer. The flavone *apigenin* in parsley is being studied for its anti cancer effects. The apigenin content of fresh parsley is reportedly 215.5 milligrams per 100 grams—the highest of any plant.

Results of a modern study by researchers at the Tehran University of Medical Science in Iran summarized the exceptional medicinal benefits of parsley:

> [A] wide range of pharmacological activity including antioxidant, hepatoprotective [protects liver function], brain protective, anti-diabetic, analgesic, spasmolytic [relieves spasms or convulsions], immunosuppressant, anti-platelet, gastroprotective, cytoprotective [reduces stomach acid], laxative, estrogenic [enhances fertility], diuretic, hypotensive [reduces blood pressure], antibacterial, and antifungal activities have been exhibited for this plant in modern medicine. (Farzaei et al. 2013, 815)

Such findings have inspired physicians and nutritionists alike to recommend that parsley become a more important part of our daily diets.

Resources

Bremness, Lesley. *Herbs*. New York: Dorling Kindersley, 2002, 264.

de Candolle. Alphonse. *Origin of Cultivated Plants*. New York: D. Appleton and Company, 1908, 91.

Farzaei, M. H., Z. Abbasabadi, M. R. Shams et al. "Parsley: a review of ethnopharmacology, phytochemistry and biological activities." *Journal of Traditional Chinese Medicine* 33, no. 6 (2013): 815–26.

Grivetti, Louis E. "Parsley." *Nutritional Geography*. University of California, Davis. Accessed December 19, 2023.

"Health benefits of Parsley." WebMD. November 27, 2022.

"Parsley: An Understated Herb." SPICEography.com. Accessed December 19, 2023.

Simon, James E., Jack Rabin, and Laura Clavio. "Parsley: A Production Guide." Cooperative Extension Service. Purdue University. Accessed December 19, 2023.

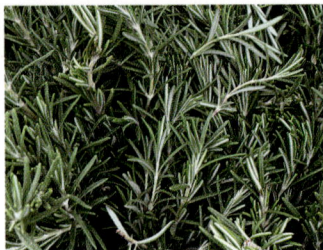

Rosemary

Rosemary comes from the leaves of the evergreen shrub *Rosmarinus officinalis*. The plant's botanical name is derived from the Latin words *ros* (dew) and *marinus* (belonging to the sea). It was called "Rose of Mary" to honor the Virgin Mary. This herb is believed to be native to the hills along the western Mediterranean, including Portugal and Spain.

Recorded use of rosemary dates back to ancient Egypt, with the first mention of the herb found on cuneiform stone tablets dating back to 5000 BCE. Egyptians used it for embalming corpses starting in 3500 BCE. There is also record of King Ramesses III—who reigned from 1186–1155 BCE—offering 125 measures of rosemary to the Egyptian god Amun at Thebes. In ancient Greece, rosemary was valued for its alleged ability to strengthen the brain and improve memory: students took rosemary to improve their memory and wore rosemary garlands when studying for examinations. In Shakespeare's *Hamlet*, Ophelia says, "There's rosemary, that's for remembrance. Pray you, love, remember."

Rosemary has long been a plant of European myth and legend. In Portugal, the plant was associated with elves and was called *alecrirn*, meaning "elfin-plant." Sicilian tales mentioned that baby fairies slept in beds of rosemary flowers. In Spain, rosemary was called *romero*, or "pilgrim's flower," referring to the story about the Virgin Mary resting under a rosemary bush during the Israelites flight from Egypt, known as The Exodus. Some devout Christians today plant a "Mary Garden," which almost always includes rosemary.

Like the Egyptians, the French used rosemary during Medieval times to embalm the dead. It was also carried by visitors to English prisons as a precaution against typhus. During times of plague, sprigs of rosemary leaves were inserted into the hollow heads of canes carried by physicians. Like in ancient Greece, rosemary continues to be used as a symbol for remembrance. During war commemorations and funerals, rosemary is planted around graves throughout much of Europe.

Rosemary is an important part of the culinary traditions in many Western countries, especially in Italy and southern France. Rosemary is found in the French herb blends *bouquet garni* and *herbes de Provence*. In Italy, it is commonly used to top Focaccia bread, and chopped rosemary is infused into olive oil as a dip for bread in many Italian restaurants. Rosemary is used to season a wide variety of meat and fish dishes, as well as soups, stews, casseroles, stir-fried vegetables, and salads. It also works well with grains, mushrooms, potatoes, onions, and peas.

Although rosemary is mainly used as a seasoning, it contains generous amounts of B vitamins including pantothenic acid, niacin, riboflavin, thiamin, and folate. In addition, the antioxidants and other phytochemicals found in rosemary have been linked to immune system support, stress reduction, and—yes—improved memory. Rosemary has traditionally been used as an anti-inflammatory and analgesic agent, and is currently being studied for anti cancer and liver-protecting properties.

A recent study by researchers at the College of Pharmacy at the University of Illinois mentioned that rosemary contains several classes of phytochemical compounds including diterpenes, polyphenols, and flavonoids. Carnosol and carnosic acid are two of the most abundant phytochemicals found in rosemary, and these compounds contribute up to 90 percent of its antioxidant potential. In their peer-reviewed article, published in the *International Journal of Nutrition*, the researchers added that several *in vivo* studies have showed that rosemary has a positive impact on gastrointestinal (GI) health through decreased oxidative stress and inflammation in the GI tract.

Rosemary is primarily grown commercially in Spain. It is also widely grown in Portugal, France, and the United States.

Resources

Datiles, M. J., and P. Acevedo-Rodriguez. "Rosmarinus officinalis (rosemary)." CABI Compendium. CABI Digital Library website. December 4, 2014.

"Health Benefits of Rosemary." WebMD. September 16, 2022.

Mahr, Susan. "Rosemary, *Rosemarinus officinalis*." Wisconsin Horticulture. University of Wisconsin. Accessed December 17, 2023.

"Rosemary." McCormick Science Institute website. Accessed December 17, 2023.

"Rosemary: The Herb of Remembrance." SPICEography.com. Accessed December 17, 2023.

Veenstra, J. P., and J. J. Johnson. "Rosemary (*Salvia rosmarinus*): Health-promoting benefits and food preservative properties." *International Journal of Nutrition*6, 4 (2021): 1–10.

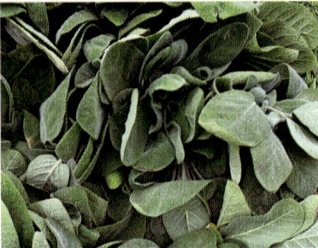

Sage

Sage (*Salvia officinalis*) is an important culinary herb and medicinal plant that traces its origins back thousands of years to what are now Albania and Bosnia. There are more than nine hundred species of sage, yet only a handful are used as food. Although sage is widely cultivated, a large proportion of it is still collected in the wild. The name *Salvia* is derived from the Latin word *salvere*, meaning "to save," and is an acknowledgement of the plant's medicinal properties, which are found primarily in its leaves.

Ancient Egyptians used sage as a remedy for infertility more than four thousand years ago; physicians prescribed it to treat serious diseases and epidemics, like the plague. Sage was also used as one of the main ingredients in the mixture of herbs used in embalming rituals to allow the deceased to move on to the afterlife.

In ancient Greece, the physicians Dioscorides and Galen recommend sage to increase urination, promote wound healing, increase fertility, and to promote regularity in the menstrual cycle. In medieval Europe, sage was regarded as a sacred plant believed to protect against black magic, fire, and hail, and was given to women to ease both conception and childbirth.

Charlemagne (747–814 CE) required that all of the monasteries under his control plant sage in their gardens. In addition to being used an incense during religious services, sage was also prescribed during the Middle Ages to treat a wide range of health problems including fevers, liver disease, and epilepsy. It was also used to improve memory: the English herbalist John Gerard (1545–1607) claimed that sage (usually as a tea made from the leaves) was beneficial for the brain and would improve memory, an opinion that was later supported by the physician and herbalist Nicholas Culpeper (1616–1654). In India, Ayurvedic physicians used sage leaves to treat intestinal gas, upset stomach, and infections of the mouth, nose, and throat. In China, a variety of sage (*Salvia miltiorrhiza*) has been used in Traditional Chinese Medicine to strengthen the liver and kidneys, and to treat cardiovascular and cerebrovascular diseases, typhoid fever, colds, and joint pain.

White sage (*Salvia apiana*) is a variety of sage indigenous to North America. It has a long and rich history of ceremonial and religious use by Native Americans. Smudge sticks are bundles of dried sage that are lit on fire; the smoke is then used to cleanse the atmosphere of negative energy.

In addition to widespread medicinal and ceremonial use, sage has been highly regarded as a culinary herb for centuries. The main flavor of sage comes from several aromatic compounds which gives it a strong flavor similar to rosemary. Dried sage leaves are widely used in Balkan, Greek, Italian, and European cuisines in general, and to season sausage, poultry, and fish in particular. Fresh sage leaves can be fried to a crispy texture and added to pasta and gnocchi dishes. Fresh sage flowers are tossed in salads and, like the leaves, can be made into a satisfying herbal tea. In the United States, sage is the classic herb added to stuffing served at Thanksgiving. Sage is also a main component in many commercial poultry and Italian seasoning blends.

Although it contains a variety of vitamins and minerals (including vitamins A, C, K, and folate, and magnesium and potassium), the herb is consumed in such small amounts, its nutritional impact is small. However, sage has been found to be rich in antioxidants and other phytochemicals, and there is now much scientific interest in its medicinal properties. Research has been conducted regarding sage's ability to lower blood glucose and cholesterol, reduce inflammation, and even to treat Alzheimer's disease. Several double-blind scientific studies have evaluated sage's ability to improve mood and cognitive ability among human subjects—including those suffering from Alzheimer's disease— with positive results.

More than half of the world's sage supply is harvested from Albania, Croatia, and Montenegro. It is also cultivated in Bosnia, Serbia, and the United States.

Resources

Bremness, Lesley. *Herbs*. New York: Dorling Kindersley, 2002, 127.

Dubey, Divyanjali. and Neha Mishra. "Pharmacology and Medicinal Properties of Sage Plant." 35–47.

Engels, Gayle. "Sage." *Herbalgram* #89, 1–4. Accessed December 17, 2023.

Hamidpour, M., R. Hamidpour, S. Hamidpour, and M. Shahlari. "Chemistry, Pharmacology, and Medicinal Property of Sage (Salvia) to Prevent and Cure Illnesses such as Obesity, Diabetes, Depression, Dementia,

Lupus, Autism, Heart Disease, and Cancer." *Journal of Traditional and Complementary Medicine* 4, 2 (2014): 82–88.

"History of Sage." Salvia website. Accessed December 17, 2023.

Outlaw, Sara. "Sage Throughout the Ages." The Herbal Academy website. September 26, 2016.

"Sage." McCormick Science Institute website. Accessed December 17, 2023.

"Sage: The Essential Old World Herb." SPICEography.com. Accessed December 17, 2023.

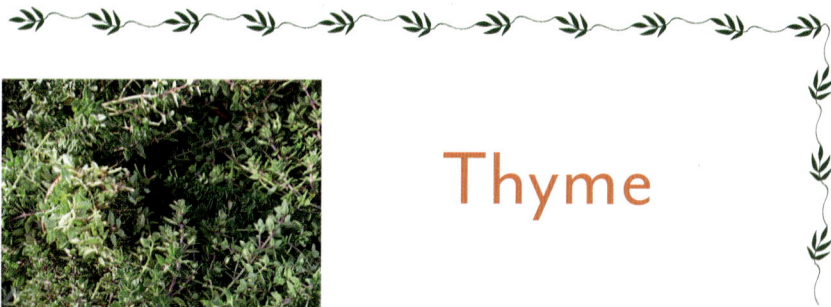

Thyme

Thyme (*Thymus vulgaris*) is a woody, broadleaf evergreen perennial native to southwestern Europe and southeastern Italy, which quickly spread throughout the Mediterranean basin. There are hundreds of thyme cultivars, yet only a few are commonly used in kitchens today. These include "garden" or English thyme, lemon, French, German, caraway, and orangelo varieties. The origin of the word "thyme" comes from the Greek word *thýmon*, which means "courage." The word may also be derived from the Greek word *thymos*, meaning "perfume" or "fumigate," since thyme was often burned in Greek temples to purify the atmosphere. The species name, *vulgaris*, means "common" or "widespread" in Latin.

Like other herbs highlighted in this book, thyme has been valued as both a culinary herb and medicinal plant for thousands of years. Along with rosemary and sage, the ancient Egyptians used thyme for embalming; the Romans also used thyme to keep food supplies from spoiling.

As mentioned earlier, the early Greeks considered thyme a symbol of courage, and Greek soldiers rubbed their chests with thyme leaves to receive strength and vigor; they also bathed with thyme water before going into battle.

The belief that thyme was a symbol of courage continued in Europe through the Middle Ages. Thyme became an ornament on tunics and scarves which women would embroider for their knights; sprigs of thyme were also given to soldiers upon leaving for battle. In medieval Europe, wild thyme was thought to attract fairies, especially on midsummer's eve. It was also believed that placing branches of thyme under one's pillow could keep nightmares away.

The first recorded evidence for the medical uses of thyme dates back to the first century CE in Dioscorides's *De materia medica* and Pliny's *Natural History*. Before that time, the herb had long been prized by both the ancient Greeks and Romans for its antiseptic properties. It has been reported that the Greeks treasured a type of honey that was obtained from a species of thyme, and recognized its ability to treat diseases of the breast. Galen, the Greek physician and philosopher (129–216 CE), considered thyme a powerful antiseptic and prescribed it in powdered form to patients suffering from joint pain. Traditional folk healers have prescribed thyme to treat bronchitis and coughs, and, during the nineteenth century, constituents of thyme oil were used by dentists as an oral antiseptic to treat abscesses and gum inflammation. Thymol, an antiseptic, is still used as an active ingredient in various commercially produced mouthwashes, and before the advent of modern antibiotics, thyme oil was used to medicate bandages.

The use of thyme as a culinary herb dates back to 2700 BCE, when it was mentioned in a cuneiform tablet with instructions on preparing dough made with pulverized thyme, figs, and pears. The Etruscans and Romans also used thyme in the kitchen, as well as to perfume wines and flavor cheeses. Thyme remains an important herb in many of Europe's cuisines, especially in southern parts of Europe. In France, *bouquet garni* is made up of fresh branches of thyme tied together with other fresh herbs (such as rosemary, parsley, and bay), which is added to soups, sauces, and stews (the bundle is removed before serving). Dried thyme is also part of *herbs de Provence*, a spice blend from southern France. In the Middle East, thyme is an important component of the seasonings *zahtar* (a combination of sumac, sesame, salt, and herbs) and *dukka*, an Egyptian blend of nuts, seeds, and spices.

Europeans traditionally use thyme to add flavor to fish dishes, and the herb is considered an ideal ingredient to flavor vegetable salads; thyme also pairs well with legumes, cooked grains, and summer vegetables (such as tomatoes, zucchini, eggplant, and peppers), as well as carrots, onions, mushrooms, potatoes, and squash. Thyme is also used in soups, omelets, marinades, and sauces, and is even suitable for flavoring fresh fruit salads. Louisiana's Creole cuisine is known for its extensive use of thyme. It is also a key component of Jamaican jerk seasoning, which can also contain allspice, peppers, cloves, cinnamon, nutmeg, garlic, brown sugar, ginger, and salt.

Like most of the other herbs presented in this book, thyme is a good source of dietary fiber and vitamins A, B$_6$, and C. It is also a good source of minerals, especially potassium, calcium, iron, manganese, magnesium, and selenium.

Thyme is beginning to be studied for the medicinal value of its leaves and their essential oil, which consists of thymol (30–70 percent), carvacrol (3–15 percent), p-cymene, terpinene, and a number of secondary components. Thyme leaves also contains antioxidants and phytochemicals such as glycosides, saponins, and tannins. Carvacrol, for example, has been found to exert antibiotic-like effects like streptomycin, penicillin, and vancomycin.

The antimicrobial activity of thyme has been shown to kill fungi and bacteria including *Staphylococci*, *Streptococci*, *Pneumococci*, *Enterococci*, *Candida albicans*, and *Corynebacterium*. One study revealed that thyme oil was able to decontaminate lettuce infected with the bacterium *Shigella*. Its natural antimicrobial and anti-inflammatory properties, together with the herb's antispasmodic and expectorant action, make thyme an excellent remedy for diseases of the upper airways including flu, bronchitis, sore throat, cough, and cold.

Studies have shown that thyme promotes the death of cancer cells and thus may be helpful to fight certain types of cancer, including of the breast and colon. The authors of a detailed review of the phytochemicals in and therapeutic uses of thyme, which appeared in the May 2022 issue of *Nutrients* (Hammoudi Halat et al. 2022, 2104), wrote: "The current status of knowledge regarding thyme depicts a wide plethora of nutritional and therapeutic benefits and provides powerful recommendations for future research directions."

The herb is cultivated primarily in eastern and southern Europe and northern Africa, but also in the United States.

Resources

Bissanti, Guido. "Thyme," Un mondo esosostenible. January 27, 2023.

Hammoudi Halat, D., M. Krayem, S. Khaled, and S. Younes. "A Focused Insight into Thyme: Biological, Chemical, and Therapeutic Properties of an Indigenous Mediterranean Herb." *Nutrients*14, 10 (2022): 2104.

"Thyme." McCormick Science Institute website. Accessed December 17, 2023.

"*Thymus vulgaris*." North Carolina Extension Gardener. North Carolina State University Extension. Accessed December 17, 2023.

Grains

A *grain* is a small, hard, dry fruit (known as *caryopsis*)—with or without an attached hull layer—that is harvested for human or animal consumption. Whole grains (or foods made from them) contain all the essential parts and naturally-occurring nutrients of the entire grain seed in their original proportions. Grains have been a staple food for humans for thousands of years, including wheat, rye, corn (maize), oats, barley, and rice. Corn is both a vegetable and a grain—however, since most eat corn as a vegetable in the United States and Canada, we have included it in the "vegetables" section of this book.

Amaranth

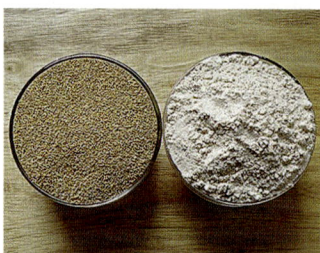

Photo by Diejun Chen, USDA ARS

Amaranth (*Amaranthus hypochondriacus*) is one of the world's oldest grains. Amaranth seeds have been found in archaeological sites in northern Argentina that date back seven to eight thousand years, and it was likely domesticated six thousand years ago. An early form of amaranth was found near the city of Tehuacán in Mexico dating from 4000 BCE.

Along with corn and beans, amaranth was a major crop among the early Aztecs, and was considered a food of immortality. It was often used in religious ceremonies, including one honoring Huitzilopochtli, the god of war: An image of the god was created from amaranth grains and honey. After the celebration—which included human sacrifice—the image was broken into pieces and distributed to the surviving attendees to eat. Snacks made from popped amaranth mixed with honey are popular in Central and South America today.

Amaranth has been found in Ozark rock shelters dating from 1100 CE, and colonial explorers wrote about obtaining amaranth seeds from Indigenous peoples living along the Colorado River in present-day Arizona and Utah. The history of amaranth has also been traced to Southeast Asia and China. Amaranth seeds found in the Indian state of Utter Pradesh date back three thousand years, leading some food historians to believe that it may have also originated in Asia. However, genomic research has led to the belief that amaranth more likely originated in the New World and made its way to India and China via ancient transoceanic trading routes that predated European exploration.

After the Spanish conquest of Central and South America during the sixteenth century, amaranth cultivation spread to the Caribbean, Africa, and Asia, where it is primarily consumed as a leafy green vegetable. Due to its high nutritional content, amaranth has been increasing in popularity in both Europe and North America, where it is basically consumed as a grain. Amaranth's nutrient content, drought tolerance, and overall resilience to disease has inspired food scientists to develop more advanced techniques for both breeding and cultivation of what is generally considered an underutilized plant.

Amaranth's use in food products is varied. While on a visit to Oaxaca in Mexico, I first tried amaranth as a cooked breakfast cereal and found its subtle flavor delicious. Amaranth is widely used in its intact form, like rice or polenta, and is said to pair well with squash and corn. It may also be processed into flour, and is a puffed or popped component of commercial cereals and granola bars. In Africa and Asia, amaranth leaves are usually picked fresh and eaten raw in salads, or cooked as a side dish.

Amaranth's nutritional profile is impressive. It is one of the few grains that is a complete protein because it contains all nine of the essential amino acids. Amaranth is gluten free and provides both vitamins C and B_6 (pyridoxine), as well as essential minerals including iron, calcium, magnesium, manganese, phosphorus, and selenium. Food scientists believe that amaranth may play a key role in underdeveloped countries, and may someday be recognized as one of the promising nutritional, healthy crops with the potential to feed the global population.

Amaranth contains *lunasin*, a peptide believed to have both anti-inflammatory and cancer-fighting benefits. It is also the best plant source of *squalene,* a powerful antioxidant used as a dietary supplement for diabetics and those suffering from hypertension or metabolic disorders. Amaranth oil has antibacterial and anti-tumor properties, and has been used to treat burns and wounds. Research has also shown that amaranth may also help reduce serum cholesterol levels.

A recent review of the nutritional and therapeutic properties of amaranth was published in the journal *Foods*:

> There are reports in the scientific literature regarding the beneficial activity of amaranth on the cardiovascular and nervous systems, hypoglycemic effect, antimicrobial activity, and antioxidant activity. Amaranth is widely used in the pharmaceutical industry to produce medicinal products against atherosclerosis, stomach ulcers, tuberculosis, as well as antiseptic, antifungal, and anti-inflammatory preparations. (Barniak and Kania-Dobrowolska 2022, 623)

Relatively small amounts of amaranth are being grown in the United States, and the grain is finally reemerging as a commercial crop in Mexico. Amaranth is grown primarily in China, but also in Africa, Russia, South America, and parts of eastern Europe.

Resources

"Amaranth." Agricultural Utilization Research Institute website. July 1, 2003.

"Amaranth: May Grain of the Month," Oldways Whole Grains Council website. Accessed February 1, 2024.

Baraniak, J., and M. Kania-Dobrowolska. "The Dual Nature of Amaranth-Functional Food and Potential Medicine." *Foods* 11, 4 (2022): 618–30.

"Health Benefits of Amaranth." WebMD. August 22, 2022.

Joshi, D. C. S. Sood, R. Hosahatti et al. "From zero to hero: the past, present and future of grain amaranth breeding." *Theoretical and Applied Genetics* 131 (2018): 1807–1823.

Myers, Robert L. "Grain Amaranth: A Lost Crop of the Americas." The Jefferson Institute website. October 2002.

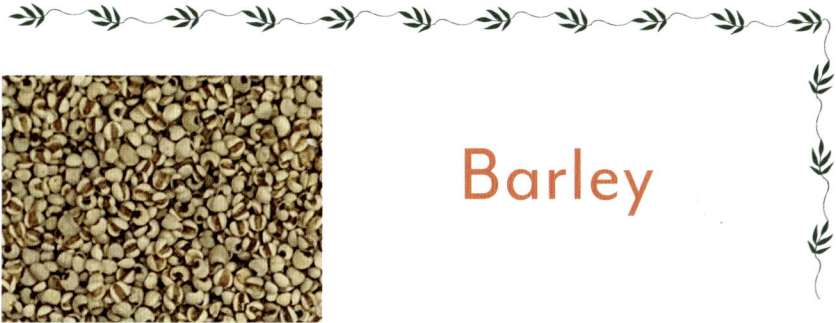

Barley

Barley (*Hordeum vulgare*) is one of the most ancient human foods. Archeological evidence suggests the existence of barley in Egypt along the River Nile around 17,000 years ago, while evidence from sites in the Fertile Crescent (including from present-day Israel and Jordan to southern Türkiye, Iraqi Kurdistan, and southwestern Iran) indicate that barley was first domesticated almost ten thousand years ago. It is believed to have descended from a wild relative known as *Hordeum spontaneum*. Today, there are well over fifty different cultivars of barley that are used as either human food or animal feed.

Barley domestication eventually spread east to the Indus Valley, the Himalayas, and China, and west to Europe and northern Africa, including present-day Ethiopia and Morocco. There is evidence that barley was cultivated in 5000 BCE in Egypt and 1500 BCE in China. It has long been an important part of Traditional Chinese Medicine, where it has been used to strengthen the spleen and pancreas, relieve stomach and digestive problems, and support the nervous system.

The ancient Egyptians used barley to produce beer and bread, and the Greeks would roast it to use for porridge; roasting the barley grain produced malt, which would ferment and become slightly alcoholic. It was also used as a staple in the diet of the legendary gladiators of ancient Rome, and was also referenced in the Bible, in John 6:9–10: "It was with five barley loaves and two fishes that our Lord fed the five thousand."

In modern times, barley is most often eaten as porridge or added to soups and salads. It makes a good filling for stuffed peppers and tomatoes, and is also used as an extender for vegetable proteins. As mentioned earlier, barley has been milled into flour since early Egyptian times, and is still used today for making breads, muffins, and pancake batter. Pearl (de-hulled) barley is the most popular variety sold in the United States, although whole barley can be found in Asian supermarkets in major cities across North America and Europe.

While oats and oatmeal have become famous for their nutritional and health benefits, the nutritional and medicinal profiles of barley are even greater. Like other grains, barley is rich in dietary fiber, which benefits digestion and elimination; it also helps us to control both our body weight and blood sugar levels. Barley is especially high in beta-glucan, a type of dietary fiber that has been linked to facilitating weight reduction as well as improving insulin sensitivity, lowering blood pressure, and increasing a feeling of satiation between meals.

Barley is an excellent source of niacin and a good source of vitamin B_6; it also provides minerals such as manganese, selenium, phosphorous, and iron. In addition, barley is rich in phytochemicals like *flavonoids* that may help reduce LDL "bad" cholesterol and protect against heart disease and stroke. Scientists believe that the *lignons* in barley have antioxidant, anti-tumor, antiviral, and antibacterial properties. Other health-promoting phytochemicals include phenolic acids, tocopherols, phytosterols, and folates.

A peer-reviewed article published the *Journal of Food and Drug*

Analysis in 2017 summarizes the nutritional and therapeutic benefits of this ancient grain:

> Epidemiological studies have associated the regular consumption of barley with its potential to reduce the risk of certain diseases, such as chronic heart disease, colonic cancer, high blood pressure, and gallstones. Reports of barley's role in maintaining a healthy colon, inducing immunostimulation, and generally boosting the immune system, among others, have been established. These therapeutic potentials are attributed to the presence of the bioactive components of vitamins, minerals, fiber, and other phytochemicals. Interestingly, among the myriads of bioactive substances present in barley, fiber component, especially beta-glucan fiber, is mainly credited for barley's health benefits. (Idehen et al. 2017, 148)

Today, barley is the world's fourth largest grain crop behind wheat, rice, and corn. The ten major barley producing countries include Russia, Germany, Canada, Ukraine, France, Australia, the United Kingdom, Türkiye, the United States, and Denmark. Idaho, North Dakota, and Montana are the major producers of barley in the United States, while Alberta, Saskatchewan, and Manitoba are the major growers in Canada. Some three-quarters of the barley grown in the United States is currently used for malt production. The remainder is used for livestock and human food, which makes up only around four percent of total barley production.

Resources

Badr, A., et al., "On the Origin and Domestication History of Barley (*Hordeum vulgare*)," *Molecular Biology and Evolution* 17, no. 4 (2000): 499–510.

Bain, Lisa. "7 Impressive Health Benefits of Barley That Might Surprise You." *Good Housekeeping.* August 21, 2020.

"Barley." Encyclopedia.com. May 17, 2018.

"Barley in TCM." Chinese Nutrition website. Accessed February 1, 2024.

"Brief History of Barley." ThinkBarley.com. April 2022.

Ducleff, Michaeleen. "Less snacking, more satisfaction: Some foods boost levels of an Ozempic-like hormone." *Shots: Health News from NPR*. National Public Radio website. October 30, 2023.

Fuller, D. Q., and A. Weisskopf. "Barley: Origins and Development" in Claire Smith, ed., *Encyclopedia of Global Archaeology*. New York: Springer New York, 2020.

Idehen, E., Y. Tang, and S. Sang. "Bioactive phytochemicals in barley." *Journal of Food and Drug Analysis* 25, 1 (2017): 148–161.

Iowa State University. "Barley Profile." Agricultural Marketing Resource Center website. February 2022.

"Major Crop Production, Canada and Provinces," Government of Canada website. Accessed February 1, 2024.

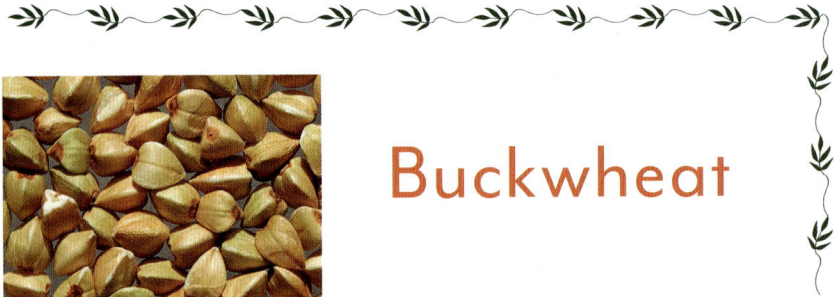

Buckwheat

Photo by B. Boldychev

My grandmother used to serve *kasha* (buckwheat groats, the hulled seeds of the buckwheat plant) when I was a child, and it was one of my favorite foods. It is often prepared with fried onions, mushrooms, and egg noodles in the form of a bowtie, which Eastern European Jews call *varnishkes*.

Buckwheat (*Fagopyrum esculentum*) is considered a "pseudocereal" because it is used as a cereal like wheat and barley, but is not a member of the grass family. Archaeologists have dated the cultivation of buckwheat as early as 2600 BCE in northern China, specifically in Manchuria. It eventually was introduced to Russia from Mongolia, probably in the fourteenth century CE. Buckwheat cultivation then gradually spread throughout Europe during the Middle Ages, from the north to the south.

The first mention of its cultivation in Germany was in a Mecklenburg register in 1436. After Poland, Belgium, and France, buckwheat became established in Spain in the seventeenth century. Buckwheat may also have reached Europe via Anatolia, a region located in modern-day Türkiye.

Buckwheat has been grown in North America since colonial times, and was once commonly found on farms in the northeastern and north-central regions of the United States. Production reached a peak in 1866, at which time buckwheat was primarily used either as a livestock feed or for making flour.

By the mid-1960s, acreage devoted to buckwheat cultivation in the United States had declined. Yet, buckwheat soon enjoyed a resurgence of popularity in the mid-1970s, brought on by the increased demand for commercially prepared breakfast cereals, the popularity of buckwheat flour for pancakes, and by the demand for exports to Japan for making buckwheat noodles (soba), one of Japan's favorite comfort foods.

Buckwheat is a gluten-free food and therefore cannot be used to make bread unless it is added to other flour types. Buckwheat is highly

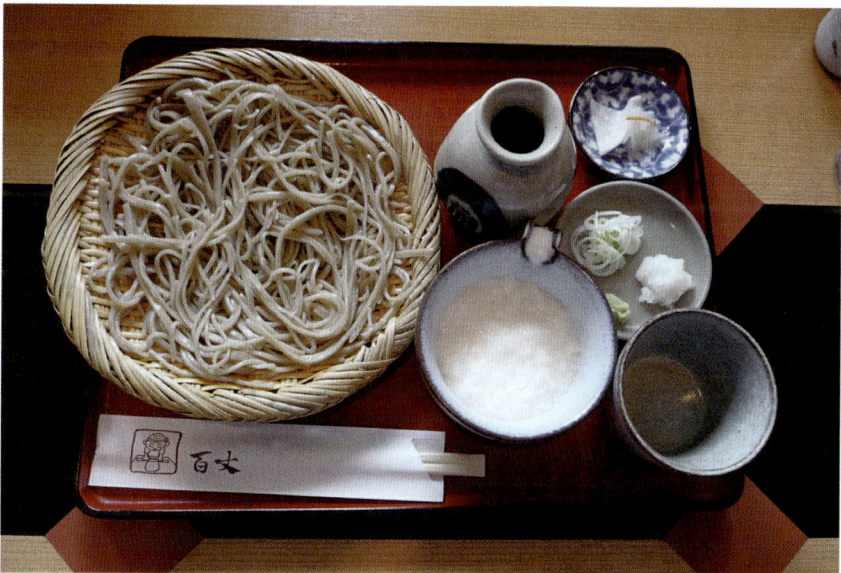

Soba noodles made of buckwheat.

nutritious. In addition to dietary fiber, it has an amino acid composition that is nutritionally superior to all other cereals, including oats. Buckwheat protein is particularly rich in the amino acid lysine; it is also a good source of iron and potassium. An article appearing in *The Journal of Agricultural Science* (Ahmed et al. 2014, 349) summarizes the nutritional, phytochemical, and therapeutic value of buckwheat:

> The vital functional substances in buckwheat are flavonoids, phytosterols, fagopyrins, fagopyritols, phenolic compounds, resistant starch, dietary fibre, lignans, vitamins, minerals, and antioxidants, which make it a highly active biological pseudocereal. Cholesterol-lowering effects that lessen the problems of constipation and obesity are important health benefits that can be achieved through the functional substances of buckwheat.

Eating buckwheat on a regular basis has also been found to offer protective effects against several chronic diseases including hypertension, obesity, cardiovascular diseases, and gallstone formation.

Russia, China, and Ukraine are the world's major producers of buckwheat. Although considered a minor crop in the United States, leading growers include North Dakota, Washington, Minnesota, and New York. The provinces of Manitoba, Ontario, and Québec, traditional growers of buckwheat in Canada, experienced a decline in production not unlike in the United States.

Future trends point to increased production in western Canada. Marta Izydorczyk (Milligan, Grainews website, Glacier FarMedia), a research scientist and program manager for barley and other grains with the Canadian Grain Commission, is one of Canada's most ardent supporters of buckwheat: "It is such a good crop. Everything is there. It has bioactive components such as rutin, proteins that are more nutritious than cereal grains, and it's gluten free, which, at this time, is buckwheat's best 'hook' (Milligan, Grainews website, Glacier FarMedia)."

Resources

Ahmed, A., N. Khalid, A. Ahmad et. al. "Phytochemicals and biofunctional properties of buckwheat: a review." *The Journal of Agricultural Science* 152, 3 (2014): 349–369.

"Buckwheat." Alimentarium.org. Accessed February 1, 2024.

de Candolle, Alphonse. *Origin of Cultivated Plants*. New York: D. Appleton and Company, 1908, 349.

Iowa State University. "Buckwheat." Agricultural Marketing Research Center website. February 2022.

Luthar, Z., A. Golob, M. Germ et al. "Tartary Buckwheat in Human Nutrition." *Plants* (*Basel*) 10, no. 4 (2021): 700.

Milligan, Patty. "Rebuilding Buckwheat Production," Grainews website. Glacier FarMedia. January 22, 2015.

Oplinger, E. S., E. A. Oelke, M. A. Brinkman et al. "Buckwheat." Corn Agronomy. University of Wisconsin. Accessed February 1, 2024.

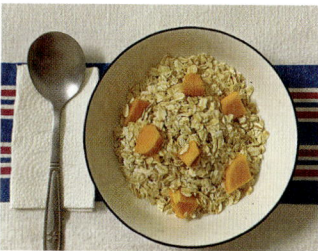

Oats

Oats (*Avena sativa*) were first used as a pasturage or forage crop in southern Europe and northern Africa long before they were grown for grain. Oats date back about 32,000 years, when wild oats were hand ground by paleolithic hunter gatherers. There are many wild oat species, but only four have been cultivated for today's use. *Avena sativa* is primarily sold on grocery store shelves, and is the type of oats we enjoy as oatmeal. Two others—*Avena byzantina* and *Avena strigosa*—are grown for animal feed. The fourth—*Avena abyssinica*—is exclusive to Ethiopia and is rarely exported. Approximately 70 percent of the oats grown in North America are fed to livestock.

Both the ancient Greeks and Romans were acquainted with oats, and called it *bromos* and *avena*, respectively. These names likely referred to wild oat varieties. Oat cultivation was believed to have begun in Greece and northern Italy, and gradually spread to southern areas of the Roman Empire. The earliest mention of oat cultivation in China dates from a historical work on the period from 618 to 907 CE, although oats probably grew wild in China well before that time. Oats are believed to have been brought to North America from southern and northern Europe. They were introduced by the Spanish to what is now Florida in 1513, and to California in 1720. They were brought to the northeastern part of the United States by English and Dutch settlers beginning in 1702. Hybridization of various oat varieties in both the United States and England began in the early 1870s.

Oats are one of the few common grains that are almost always sold whole. *Old-fashioned*, or rolled, oats are steamed and flattened, while *steel-cut* oats consist of the entire grain kernel, and are often sold cracked for faster cooking. *Instant* oats, the most processed form available, are made by cutting oat groats into small pieces, steaming them, and rolling them into thin flakes. Although they can be free of additives, instant oats are often packaged with added sugar, artificial flavors, and milk powder. They are easy to prepare, but tend to have a mushy consistency.

As a gluten-free grain with proven nutritional and health benefits, oats have become a very popular food. They are primarily consumed cooked, as oatmeal, to which fresh or dried fruit, nuts, and seeds can be added to boost flavor, texture, and nutritional value. In addition to cooked oatmeal, oats are a primary ingredient in granola and muesli cereals. Oats are also added to breads, cookies, and energy bars. Oat milk and oat creamer are being marketed as plant-based alternatives to cow's milk and cream. In the United States, oat milk is now ranked second to almond milk in popularity.

Oats are a good source of protein, dietary fiber, calcium, iron, thiamin (vitamin B_1), and niacin (vitamin B_3). Like barley, oats contain a type of fiber called beta-glucan. They also contain a wide variety of phytochemicals including phenolic compounds, which act as a defense mechanism against various pathogens. The consumption of oats is associated with the prevention of diseases like cancer, stroke, and coronary heart diseases. An article published in the *British Journal of Nutrition* says:

> Whether the potential health benefits of oats are linked to their high dietary fiber content (33 percent) compared with other grains, their contribution of beta-glucan that may lower cholesterol concentrations, or their myriad novel phytoconstituents, the preponderance of evidence supports oats' value to human health. (Roger, van Klinken, *British Journal of Nutrition*)

A comprehensive review of the health benefits of oats by researchers at South Dakota State University was published in the November 2021 issue of the journal *Foods*. The article highlighted numerous laboratory and clinical studies that have found that oats are one of the best whole grains for lowering blood cholesterol levels. Oats have also been found to help strengthen the immune system, reduce inflammation, and maintain healthy blood sugar levels, thus reducing the risk of type 2 diabetes. In addition, oats have been found to improve blood pressure, weight management, and bowel movement regularity. Studies reported that oats improve gut health by increasing the presence of friendly bacteria. And, they have been found to help patients suffering from celiac disease, atherosclerosis, or skin problems. Studies are ongoing to investigate the effects of oat consumption on cancer, especially colon cancer.

Oats are grown primarily in the European Union, Russia, Canada, Australia, and the United States. The major oat-producing states are Minnesota, North Dakota, South Dakota, Wisconsin, Michigan, Ohio, and Nebraska. Saskatchewan, Manitoba, and Alberta are the three primary growers of oats in Canada.

Resources

Blakeslee, Karen. "History of Oats." You Asked It! Kansas State University Research and Extension. December 17, 2020.

Clemens, Roger, and B. Jan-Willem van Klinken. "Oats, more than just a whole grain: an introduction." *British Journal of Nutrition* 112, no. S2 (2014): S1–S3.

Coffman, Franklin A. *Oat History, Identification and Classification.* Technical Bulletin No. 1516. Washington: United States Department of Agriculture, 1977.

de Candolle, Alphonse. *Origin of Cultivated Plants.* New York: D. Appleton and Company, 1908, 373.

Heuzé, V., G. Tran, P. Nozière et al. "Oats." Feedipedia.org. Updated April 15, 2016.

"Major Crop Production, Canada and Provinces." Government of Canada website. Modified July 24, 2024.

"Oats." The Nutrition Source. Harvard T.H. Chan School of Public Health. 2023.

Paudel, D., B. Dhungana, M. Caffe, and P. Krishnan. "A Review of Health-Beneficial Properties of Oats." *Foods* 10, 11 (2021): 2591.

Perkins, John. "2022 Oat Production Up Sharply from 2021." Brownfield Ag News website. September 30, 2022.

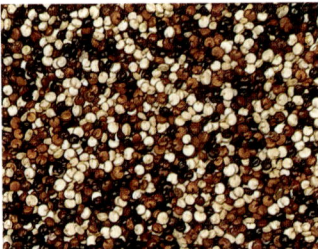

Photo by Fumikas Sagisavas

Quinoa

Quinoa (*Chenopodium quinoa*) is a plant that originated in the Andes Mountains, specifically in the area surrounding Lake Titicaca in Peru and Bolivia. Like amaranth, quinoa is one of the oldest human foods.

It was cultivated by both the Aymara (Aimara) and Inca peoples beginning five to seven thousand years ago. Quinoa is unique in that it is a seed eaten in a manner similar to a grain. The Incas considered quinoa to be sacred, and referred to it as *chisiya mama*, translated variously as "mother grain" or "mother of all seeds."

At the time of Spanish conquest, quinoa cultivation was widely distributed within and beyond the Peruvian and Bolivian Andes. It was grown from Lake Titicaca, southwest to what is now Chile and Argentina, and as far north as Quito (Ecuador) and the Colombian department (state) of Cundinamarca, which includes Bogotá, the nation's capital. In his royal commentaries, the Peruvian-born chronicler Garcilaso de la Vega, "El Inca," (1539–1616) described quinoa as one of the second grains cultivated on earth, somewhat resembling millet or short-grain rice. He also mentioned that the first shipment of quinoa seeds to Europe were dead on arrival and unable to germinate, perhaps because of the high humidity of the sea voyage.

Like other foods eaten as grain, quinoa can be enjoyed as a side dish like rice or buckwheat groats (kasha). It can be flaked and used as a breakfast cereal, and is also made into pasta and various kinds of snack foods. Quinoa can be added to soups or milled into flour to be used in bread, shakes, or breakfast porridges.

Quinoa is one of the rare grains to have reached "superfood" status. It is comparable in energy to beans, maize, rice, and wheat. It is also a good source of high-quality protein, dietary fiber, and polyunsaturated fats. It is rich in B vitamins—especially thiamin, riboflavin, niacin, and folic acid—and minerals, especially calcium, iron, magnesium, phosphorus, potassium, and zinc. Quinoa is a gluten-free grain.

The high amounts of dietary fiber in quinoa have been linked to digestive health and the prevention of both colorectal cancer and diabetes; a randomized controlled medical study revealed that eating quinoa on a regular basis helped lower the risk of diabetes in older adults who had been diagnosed with prediabetes. A comprehensive review published in the journal *Plants* (Basel) in 2021 summarizes the nutritional, phytochemical, and health benefits of this ancient grain:

> Quinoa is a rich source of protein, fibers, minerals, vitamins, and lipids. Quinoa grains contain essential amino acids and polyphenols. The composition of essential amino acids in quinoa is similar to the amino acid requirement pattern and is higher than that in whole grain and refined wheat. Additionally, quinoa contains a significant amount of minerals. A significant quantity of polyphenols is also present in quinoa seeds. The polyphenols show different pharmacological properties such as anti-allergic, antiviral, anti-inflammatory, cardiovascular protective, and anticarcinogenic activity. (Hussain et al. 2021, 2261)[1]

Largely unknown in North America until perhaps forty years ago, commercial demand has been increasing for this highly nutritious and tasty ancient grain. While quinoa continues be a major food source among the Aymara and Inca peoples in Peru and Bolivia today, it has been gaining in importance as an export crop.

Quinoa has been cultivated and commercially produced in the United States since the early 1980s. It has been planted in California, Oregon, New Mexico, Colorado, and Washington, but has only been somewhat successful in the Colorado Rockies. Due to high production costs, almost all of the quinoa North Americans eat today is imported from Peru, Bolivia, and Ecuador, the world's three major producers. While the growth of quinoa consumption outside of its indigenous region has increased the income of Andean farmers, it has also raised concerns over the food security of the original consumers who can no longer afford it.

Resources

Abellán Ruiz, M. S., M. D., Barnuevo Espinosa, C. García Santamaría et al. "Efecto del consumo de quinua (*Chenopodium quinoa*) como coadyuvante en la intervención nutricional en sujetos prediabéticos"

[Effect of quinoa (*Chenopodium quinoa*) consumption as a coadjuvant in nutritional intervention in prediabetic subjects]. *Nutricion Hospitalaria* 34, 5 (2017): 1163–1169.

Cleveland Clinic. "The Health Benefits of Quinoa," healthessentials. June 30, 2023.

Hussain, M. I., M. Farooq, Q. A. Syed et al. "Botany, Nutritional Value, Phytochemical Composition and Biological Activities of Quinoa." *Plants (Basel)*10, 11 (2021): 2258–2276.

Iowa State University. "Quinoa." Agricultural Marketing and Resource Center website. April 2022.

"Quinoa Origin and History." United Nations Food and Agriculture Organization. 2013.

Wikipedia. "Quinoa." Accessed February 6, 2024.

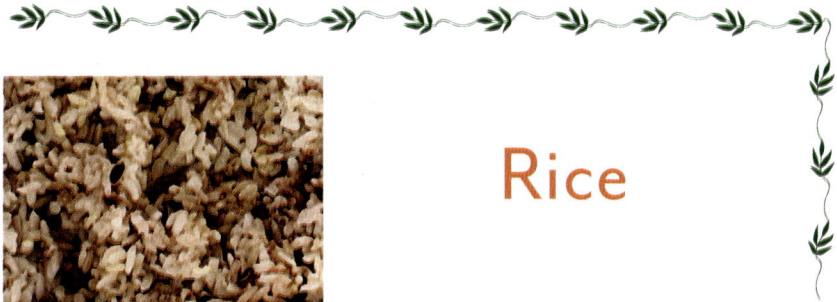

Rice

Among anthropologists, archeologists, and food historians, the genealogy of rice is controversial. There is evidence that rice was first grown in south-central China, in the Yangtze River basin, as early as 6000 BCE. Cultivation gradually spread from there to what are now Korea and Japan. Yet other archaeological evidence suggests that rice was also cultivated in the Ganges River valley in what is now northern India, by people unconnected to those of the Yangtze as far back as 6500 BCE. And there is also evidence that rice was grown in Africa's Inner Niger Delta as far back at 1000 BCE, and had no connection to rice originally grown in China and India. Rice of Asian origin is generally classified as *Oryza sativa*, while African rice—which differs in size, shape, color, and flavor—is classified as *Oryza glaberrima*.

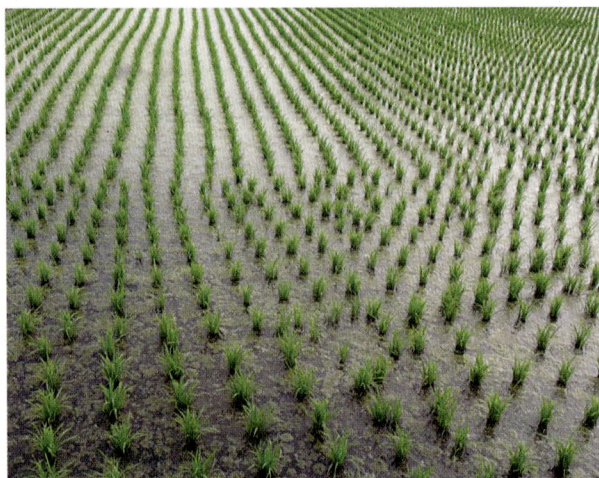

Rice Paddy, Taichung County, Taiwan.

Rice cultivation eventually spread throughout southern Europe and to parts of North Africa. From Europe, rice was brought to the New World in the seventeenth century. It was also brought from Portugal to Brazil and from Spain to Central and South America. Due to its versatility, rice can grow in many parts of the world. It is able to grow in the desert conditions of Saudi Arabia and in the wetland deltas of Southeast Asia. The first time I visited Taiwan in 1995, I found the dark green rice plants growing in clear water to be exceptionally beautiful.

Rice has played an important role in the folklore of many world cultures, especially in Asia. In Alphonse de Candolle's *Origin of Cultivated Plants*, the author wrote about an ancient Chinese ceremony, featuring one of five indigenous species of rice, which involves the Yan Emperor Chin-nong (神農), a mythological Chinese ruler. He was known variously as "Divine Farmer" and "Divine Husbandman," and was credited to have taught early Chinese the basics of agriculture, including the use of the plow. According to de Candolle, "In the ceremony instituted by the Chinese Emperor Chin-nong in 2800 BC, rice plays the principal part. The reigning emperor must himself sow it, whereas the four other species are or may be sown by the princes of his family."

Rice also played an important role in the ancient cultures of Myanmar. According to Dr. Thomas L. Rost, Professor Emeritus of Plant Biology at the University of California, Davis:

> In Myanmar, the Kachins [a people indigenous to northern Myanmar] were sent forth from the center of the Earth with rice seeds and were directed to a country where life would be perfect and rice would grow well. In Bali, Lord Vishnu caused the Earth to give birth to rice and the God Indra taught people how to raise it. And in China rice is the gift of animals. Legend says after a disastrous flooding all plants had been destroyed and no food was available. One day a dog ran through the fields to the people with rice seeds hanging from his tail. The people planted the seeds, rice grew, and hunger disappeared. (Rost, University of California, Davis)

Early Spanish explorers introduced Asian rice to the Caribbean and South America; rice first arrived in Mexico in the 1520s at Veracruz, which was selected for its warm, wet climate. Portuguese colonizers and their African slaves introduced Asian rice at about the same time to Brazil. Rice was likely introduced to what is now South Carolina in 1685, and it became an important crop in the American South, especially in South Carolina and Georgia. Many plantation owners amassed great wealth from the planting of Asian rice, due to an abundance of slave labor. Many slaves from the Senegambia area of western Africa and from coastal Sierra Leone also brought with them knowledge about rice cultivation, of which their masters made good use. Early rice cultivation in the southern states was often dangerous and often lethal. One eighteenth-century writer highlighted their plight:

> If a work could be imagined peculiarly unwholesome and even fatal to health, it must be that of standing like the negroes, ankle and mid-leg deep in water which floats an ouzy mud, and exposed all the

while to a burning sun which makes the air they breathe hotter than the human blood; these poor wretches are then in a furness [*sic*] of stinking putrid effluvia. (West, Slavery in America website)

Rice is one of the world's most important human foods. World rice consumption averages approximately 78.3 kilograms per person per year. Laos has the highest per capita consumption of rice at 254 kilograms a year, followed by Bangladesh (263 kg.), Cambodia (241 kg.), Vietnam (220 kg.), and Indonesia (211 kg.). Per capita yearly consumption in China is 126 kg, while that of India is 97.2 kg. Rice consumption in North America is far smaller: people living in Canada eat just 13 kg. of rice per year, while those living in the United States consume 10.8 kg. In top rice-consuming countries in Asia—such as Bangladesh, Bhutan, Cambodia, Indonesia, Thailand, and Sri Lanka—the share of rice consumption in total calorie intake per day ranges from 40 to 67 percent.

More than *eight thousand* varieties of rice are grown and consumed today, although four main groups are traded globally. Slender, long-grain *Indica* rice comprises the bulk of commercial rice, while the rest is made up of fragrant or aromatic rice, like basmati and Jasmine; the short-grained *Japonica* variety that is used for sushi and risottos; and glutinous, or "sticky" rice, which is used for making sweets. Rice can be found in a variety of colors, including white, brown, red and black (also known as *purple*) rice. Black rice or red rice are sometimes mixed with white to add color to rice dishes in East Asia.

Rice is among the most versatile of human foods. It can be eaten alone or used in a wide variety of soups, side dishes, and main dishes in Asian, Middle Eastern, Latin American, and many other world cuisines. Rice is also used to make breakfast cereals, noodles, and beverages like rice milk, amazake, horchata, rice wine, and stronger alcoholic drinks like Japanese sake and Korean soju.

Rice is a gluten-free food. Although it is generally considered healthy to eat, brown rice—as well as red and black varieties—retains both its germ and bran layer, which are the most nutritious parts of the grain, including protein, vitamins, minerals, and antioxidants. In addition to B vitamins, phytochemicals found in brown rice include dietary fiber, functional lipids, essential amino acids, phytosterols, phenolic acids, flavonoids, anthocyanins, proanthocyanins, tocopherols, tocotrienols, minerals, gamma aminobutyric acid (GABA), and gamma-oryzanol. Brown rice also contains high levels of phytic acid. According to a peer-reviewed article appearing in a recent issue of *Antioxidants* (Basel), the nutrients and phytochemicals found in brown rice are associated with a wide range of pharmacological properties, such as antioxidant, anti-diabetic, anti-cholesterol, and cardio-protective.

Because brown rice contains dietary fiber, it provides an earlier sensation of "fullness" than white rice. In addition, brown rice has a "low" glycemic index (GI) of fifty, while white rice has a GI of seventy, classified as "high." The combination of fiber and a low GI in brown rice helps stabilize blood glucose levels and prevents food cravings, and may therefore help with weight management. The dietary fiber found in brown rice also supports the digestive system and the development of friendly intestinal bacteria. By contrast, eating substantial servings of white rice on a regular basis can lead to elevated blood sugar levels, which over time may increase the risk of weight gain.

More than 90 percent of the world's rice production takes place in Asia, with China, India, Bangladesh, Indonesia, Vietnam, and Thailand the top rice growers. The United States ranks fourteenth in world rice production, with most grown in Arkansas, Louisiana, Mississippi, Missouri, and Texas.

Resources

Biswas, Soutik. "Why India's rice ban can trigger a global food crisis." BBC News website. August 2, 2023.

"Debating the origins of rice." University College London. 2015.

de Candolle, Alphonse. *Origin of Cultivated Plants*. New York: D. Appleton and Company, 1908, 385.

"Glycemic Index of Grains." Glycemic Index Guide website. Accessed February 16, 2024.

Ravichanthiran, K., Z. F. Ma, H. Zhang et al. "Phytochemical Profile of Brown Rice and Its Nutrigenomic Implications." *Antioxidants (Basel)* 7, 6 (2018): 71.

"Rice Consumption Per Capita." Helgi Library website. March 10, 2023.

"Rice Production." Helgi Library website. July 23, 2023.

Rost, Thomas L. "Rice Anatomy: Introduction." University of California, Davis. 1997.

Torrens, Kerry. "Top 5 health benefits of rice." BBC Goodfood website. June 20, 2023.

Veltman, Margaretha A., Jonathan M. Flowers, Tinde R. van Andel et al. "Origins and geographic diversification of African rice *Oryza glaberrima). PLoS ONE* 14 3 (2019).

West, Jean. M. "Rice and Slavery: A Fatal Gold Seed." Slavery in America website. Accessed February 16, 2024.

Wikipedia. "Rice Production in the United States." Accessed February 16, 2024.

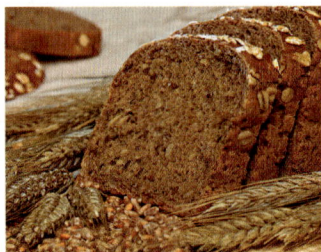

Rye

Photo by Vitalik Radko

Rye (*Secale cereale*) is one of the world's most ancient grains. Rye was descended from weeds, and was first grown in the Euphrates river valley in what is now Syria possibly as far back as 12,000 years ago. Multiple *querns* (grain mortars) placed in food processing stations at several ancient archeological sites—including Abu Hureyra (c. 10,000 BCE), Tell'Abr (9500–9200 BCE), and Jerf el Ahmar

(9500–9000 BCE)—include the presence of charred wild rye, barley, and einkorn wheat grains.

Rye had advantages over wheat and barley in ancient times: it was easier to harvest than wheat, and could be more easily prepared as food, mostly by roasting, grinding, boiling, and mashing. Rye cultivation spread from Syria to Anatolia about 8,600 years ago. Recent genomic studies have found that domesticated rye reached Central Europe (Poland and Romania) about 6,500 years ago. Cultivated rye in Central Europe evolved from weeds that were growing outside their region of origin. Rye cultivation spread from Europe to North America during the sixteenth and seventeenth centuries, and the cold-resistant grain was also introduced to Russia during this time. Today, Russia is one of the world's largest rye producers. Rye was the world's most predominant grain until the nineteenth century, when it was largely replaced by wheat.

Europeans have been grinding rye into flour to make traditional, dense, dark, and delicious rye and pumpernickel breads for centuries. However, most "rye bread" and "pumpernickel" bread sold in North America today is made primarily refined of wheat flour with added colorings to make the bread appear darker. However, both eastern European and artisanal bakeries in North America continue to bake these breads the traditional way, with rye flour. Rye has also been a primary component in the production of alcoholic beverages like beer, rye whiskey, and vodka. Rye has also been used as animal feed and forage.

The nutritional profile of rye bread is strong. Rye flour contains protein and dietary fiber, including beta-glucan, described earlier in this section, which has been linked to facilitating weight reduction, improving insulin sensitivity, lowering blood pressure, and increasing satiation between meals. The carbohydrates found in rye are considered to be in the low to moderate glycemic index (GI) range. In digestion, rye starch is hydrolyzed to sugars more slowly and produces a lower insulin response than wheat, and is therefore a good alternative to refined wheat flour, especially for diabetics.

Rye provides generous amounts of folate, along with vitamins B_1 (thiamin), B_2 (riboflavin), and B_3 (niacin). Rye is also rich in essential minerals, including selenium, manganese, copper, and iron. The dietary fiber and variety of phytochemicals in rye flour may offer health benefits relating to digestive health, heart health, blood sugar control, and weight loss. Rye is also a good source of phytochemicals, including phenolic acids, lignans, benzoxazinoids, and alkylresorcinols. The number of phytochemicals detected in rye is continually increasing, and currently stands at almost two thousand chemical species, which may uncover additional therapeutic benefits.

Most of the rye grown in the United States comes from Oklahoma, North Dakota, Wisconsin, Pennsylvania, and Minnesota. The biggest rye producing countries in the world are Germany, Poland, and Russia.

Resources

Hillman, G., R. Hedges, A. Moore et al. "New evidence of Lateglacial cereal cultivation at Abu Hureyra on the Euphrates." *The Holocene* 11, 4 (2001): 383–393.

Hirst, K. Kris. "Domestication History of Rye." Thought Co website. June 3, 2019.

Iowa State University. "Rye Profile." Agricultural Marketing and Resource Center website. February 2022.

Joseph, Michael. "Rye Bread: An Exploration of Its Nutritional Values and Benefits." Nutrition Advance website. June 29, 2023.

Jonsson, Karin, Roger Andersson, Knud Erik Bach Knudsen et al. "Rye and health - Where do we stand and where do we go?" *Trends in Food Science & Technology* 79 (2018): 78–87.

Schreiber, Mona. Yixuan Gao, Natalie Koch et al. "Recombination Landscape Divergence Between Populations is Marked by Larger Low-Recombining Regions in Domesticated Rye." *Molecular Biology and Evolution* 39, no. 6 (2022): msac131.

Wheat

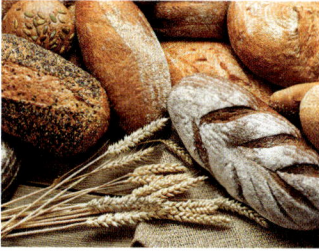

Photo by Pineapple Studio

Like barley, the origins of wheat have been traced to the Fertile Crescent, a hilly and mountainous region that extends from the foothills of the Zagros mountains in southwestern Iran, through the Tigris and Euphrates river basins in northern Iraq and southeastern Türkiye, continuing southwestward over Syria to the Mediterranean, and extending to central Israel and Jordan. Present-day wheat can trace its lineage to a clan of wild grasses called *Triticeae*, the seeds of which had a flavor that our early human ancestors enjoyed. Through over ten thousand years of human cultivation and both natural and human hybridization, literally thousands of wheat varieties have evolved.

Wheat has a long history of religious symbolism, with meanings connected to harvest and abundance, nourishment and sustenance, and resurrection and renewal. In ancient Egypt, Osiris, the god of death and rebirth, was often shown with a crown made of wheat. Grains of wheat were entombed with the pharaohs. In ancient Greece, Demeter—the goddess of agriculture, grain, and bread—sustained humankind with the earth's rich bounty. She and her daughter Persephone were the central figures of the Eleusinian Mysteries, a religious tradition that predated the Olympian pantheon. Based on a Bronze age agrarian cult, they are considered the most famous of the secret religious rites of ancient Greece.

In ancient Rome, wheat was connected to Ceres, the goddess of farming, grain, and fertility. In the First Epistle to the Corinthians,

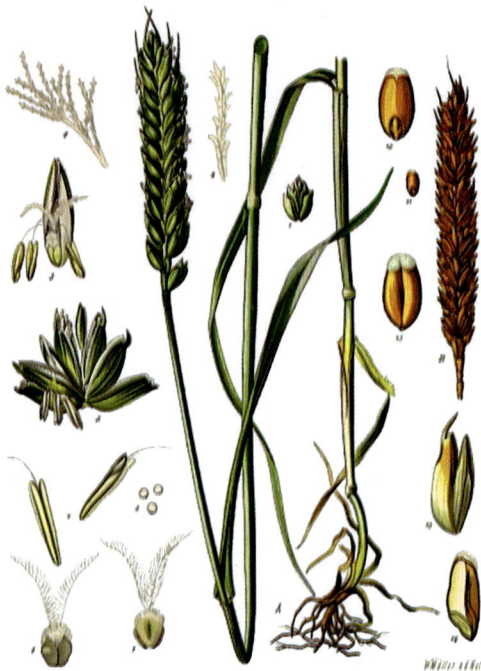

Wheat in
a drawing
by Walther
Otto Müller,
in Köhler's
*Medizinal-
Pflanzen*, 1887.

The Holy Bible describes Jesus using bread as a symbol of Christ's body during the Last Supper. When Christians partake of the Eucharist, they believe they are connecting with Jesus through the bread.

Wheat is considered an adaptable crop, as it thrives in a wide range of environments. Cultivation of wheat gradually began to spread, beginning some ten thousand years ago, from the Fertile Crescent to central Asia, southeastern Europe, and northern Africa. Wheat was said to have been introduced to the British Isles around five thousand years ago. Milling wheat for flour only became common in the twelfth century, but by the turn of the nineteenth century wheat was Great Britain's most significant crop grown for human consumption.

Wheat was first grown in the United States and Canada during the seventeenth century. It is now one of the major crops grown in the United States, with some 50 million acres (approx. 20 million hectares) devoted to wheat production. There are six major types of wheat grown in the United States for flour, and each type is best suited for a specific use or uses:

- Hard Red Winter: flat bread, rolls, croissants, Asian noodles
- Hard Red Spring: hearth breads, rolls, croissants, bagels, pizza dough
- Soft Red Winter: cakes, cookies, crackers
- Soft White: noodles, crackers, cereals, pastry
- Hard White: Asian noodles, whole wheat flour, pan breads or flat breads
- Durum: pasta

Other products made from wheat include wheat bran, spelt, khorasan wheat (kamut), couscous, farro, semolina, bulgur, farina, wheat germ, cracked wheat, matzo meal, and mir (a cross between wheat and rye). Couscous is probably the most famous; made from steamed balls of semolina flour, it forms the basis for many traditional North African dishes, especially those of Algeria, Morocco, Tunisia, and Mauritania. Although believed to have been created by Berbers, in what is now Algeria and Morocco, sometime between the eleventh and thirteenth centuries CE, couscous-based cuisine has extended beyond northern Africa to include Europe and North America. "The knowledge, know-how, and practices related to the production and consumption of couscous" was included in UNESCO's list of *Intangible Cultural Heritage* in 2020.

Over the past several years, per capita consumption of wheat in the United States and Canada has been declining because consumers want to remove refined carbohydrates (i.e., simple carbs from white flour products) from their diets. Although demand for whole wheat products is increasing, many consumers have chosen to give up wheat foods altogether. There are also concerns of gluten intolerance, a major cause of celiac disease. Gluten is found in wheat and other grains, including barley and rye. It is a protein that gives grain-based foods their soft, chewy texture, and allows bread to rise and retain moisture. Although an estimated 1–2 percent of the world's population suffer from celiac disease, many cases are undiagnosed. This has led consumers to opt for gluten-free grains like corn, oats, brown rice, quinoa, millet, and buckwheat.

Whole wheat is a nutritious food. It contains the bran (the outer layer that provides dietary fiber), the germ (the nutritious core of the kernel that contains many antioxidants), and the endosperm (the starchy middle layer of the grain). *Processed wheat*, which is made into white flour, only contains the endosperm. In addition to providing dietary fiber, whole wheat contains protein, B vitamins (especially niacin, thiamine, and folate), and a variety of minerals, including phosphorous, magnesium, and potassium.

As opposed to processed wheat, which is high in simple carbohydrates, whole grain wheat is a good source of complex carbohydrates which help regulate blood sugar. The glycemic index (GI) of whole wheat flour is forty-five, which puts it in the "low" category, while the GI of white flour is eighty-five, which is well into the "high" category. Whole grain wheat also contains many antioxidants, including phenolic acid, ferulic acid, cryptoxanthin, flavonoids, lutein, and zeaxathin—the latter two have been found to support eye health, and may lower the risk of cataracts and age-related macular degeneration.

A major article about wheat published in a recent issue of *Comprehensive Reviews in Food Science and Food Safety* highlighted whole grain (including whole wheat) products and their proven clinical benefits:

Epidemiological studies have found that consumption of whole grain products may reduce the risk of chronic diseases such as obesity, type 2 diabetes, cardiovascular diseases (CVDs), and cancer. The health-promoting effects of whole grain products, such as whole wheat products, can be attributed to their dietary fiber (DF) and phytochemical constituents. (Tian et al. 2022, 2275)

The United States is the fourth largest wheat producer in the world—after China, India, and Russia—and is also a major wheat exporter. The most important wheat-growing states are Kansas ("The Wheat State"), North Dakota, Montana, and California. Canada is the world's fifth largest wheat producer. Wheat is grown on some 50,000 Canadian farms from coast to coast, although the majority of Canadian wheat is grown in Alberta, Saskatchewan, Manitoba, and British Columbia. Most of Canada's wheat crop is exported to countries that include the United States, Indonesia, Bangladesh, Peru, Japan, and Italy.

Resources

I. W. Tian, Y. Zheng, W. Wang et al. "A comprehensive review of wheat phytochemicals: From farm to fork and beyond." *Comprehensive Reviews in Food Science and Food Safety* 21 (2022): 2275.

Brog, Shayna. "Wheat: The History of Wheat." Storymaps. March 20, 2021.

"Canada's Wheat Story." What About Wheat? website. Accessed February 13, 2024.

de Sousa, T., M. Ribeiro, C. Sabença, and G. Igrejas. "The 10,000-Year Success Story of Wheat!" *Foods*10, no.9 (2021): 2124.

Feldman, Moshe, et al. "The Origin of cultivated wheat." In *The Wheat Book*, 2001, 1–56.

"Glycemic Index of Grains." Glycemic Index Guide. Accessed February 13, 2024.

"Health Benefits of Wheat." WebMD. November 8, 2021.

Hutcherson, Aaron. "A guide to couscous: The history, different types and how to cook with it." *The Washington Post.* May 14, 2021.

Iowa State University. "Wheat," Agricultural Marketing Research Center website. February 2022.

"The Natural History of Wheat," Encyclopedia.com. Accessed February 13, 2024.

Rhys, Dani. "Powerful Symbolic Meanings of Wheat." Symbolsage.com. September 19, 2023.

Tian, W., Y. Zheng, W. Wang et al. "A comprehensive review of wheat phytochemicals: From farm to fork and beyond." *Comprehensive Reviews in Food Science and Food Safety* 21 (2022): 2274–2308.

"Wheat: An Essential Grain." WheatWorld.org. National Association of Wheat Growers. Accessed February 13, 2024.

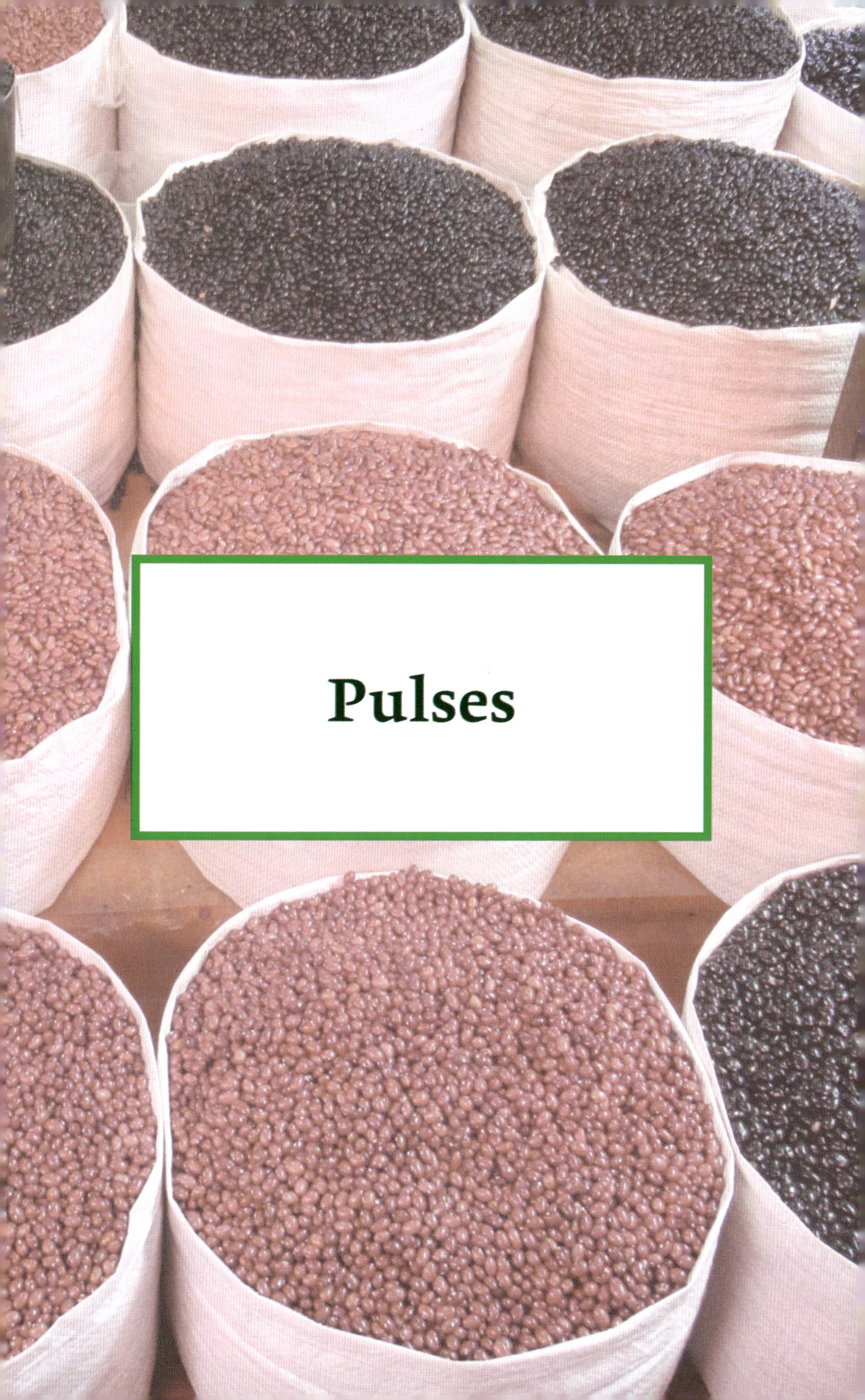

Pulses

*P*ulses are the edible seeds of plants in the legume family. The United Nations Food and Agriculture Organization (FAO) recognizes eleven types of pulses, which include dry beans, dry peas, chickpeas, cow peas, pigeon peas, and lentils. The term "pulses" is limited to crops harvested solely as dry grains, which differentiates them from other vegetable crops that are harvested while still green, like green beans and green peas, which are included in the "vegetable" section of this book.

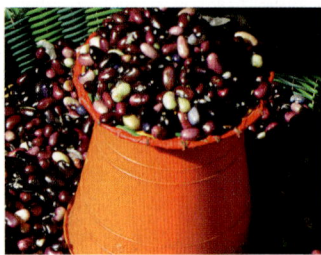

Bean

Dried beans are perhaps the most important staple food in the world. Rich in protein and essential nutrients, beans are the primary resource for people living in Latin America and Africa. In some African countries—such as western Kenya and Rwanda—per capita consumption of dried beans is over 160 kilograms (353 pounds) a year. By contrast, per capita yearly consumption in Latin America is between 12–18 kilograms, while in the United States it is just 3 kilograms (6.6 pounds) a year.

Legumes—also called *pulses*—are plants with edible seeds. Among legumes, common beans (*Phaseolus vulgaris*) are a rich world resource of biodiversity with two primary centers of domestication that flourished between 4,300 and 8,000 years ago: Central America (including Mexico) and the Peruvian Andes. The Middle American gene pool for beans has been found to extend from Mexico through Central America and into what is today Venezuela; the Andean legume gene pool is found to extend from southern Peru to northwestern Argentina.

Bean cultivation gradually moved north from Mexico through what is now the United States, often grown by Indigenous peoples along with corn and squash. After the "discovery" of the New World by European explorers, dried beans were introduced to Europe, and from there cultivation spread to Africa and Asia. The commercial cultivation of dry edible beans originated in New York State in the early 1800s, and later spread west to Michigan.

Dried beans include literally dozens of varieties: The best known are pinto, navy, black, Great Northern, red kidney, pink, lima, and black-eyed peas. Mung beans and Adzuki ("red") beans are especially popular in China and Japan, while mung beans (green gram), kidney beans, and matki (Turkish) beans are the rage in India, Pakistan, and Bangladesh. Fava beans are a popular staple in Greek and Middle Eastern cuisines. Pinto, great northern, small red, and pink beans are indigenous to Mexico, while black, navy, and small white beans originated in the tropical lowlands of Central America. Dark and light red kidney beans, white kidney beans, and cranberry beans have verified Andean ancestry.

Aside from serving as a major food source to people around the world, beans and other legumes protect the environment. They are desirable in crop rotations because they break up disease and pest cycles, provide nitrogen, improve soil microbe diversity and activity, improve soil aggregation, and conserve soil moisture.

For many Americans who grew up in the 1950s and 1960s, canned baked beans were their primary exposure to beans. Fortunately, the perception of beans as "boring" is changing fast due in part to the growing popularity of plant-based diets and Tex-Mex culture. Dried beans are among the most versatile of foods, and creative chefs use different types of beans in a dazzling variety of soups, chilis, salads, dips, and casseroles.

Beans are used in hundreds of ethnic dishes around the world: pinto beans work especially well in Mexican dishes such as refried beans and burritos; fava beans can be made into many Middle Eastern and Mediterranean dishes; kidney beans are an essential part of Indian cuisine; small red and green beans (including mung and adzuki) are popular in Asian dishes and snack foods; while black beans make excellent Latin–American-style soups, chilis, and dips. At a time when food prices have become sky-high, dried beans remain one of the most budget-friendly foods one can buy. While not as convenient to use as canned beans, dried beans can easily be soaked in water overnight and cooked the following day.

Dried beans are universally recognized as a nutrient-dense and healthy food source due to their high protein, dietary fiber, and vitamin and mineral content, which includes B-vitamins, iron, potassium, phosphorous, and folate. Beans are also a rich source of slowly digestible starch, which classifies them as a low glycemic food. Some bioactive compounds present in beans are reported to help protect us from cardiovascular diseases, hypertension, diabetes, high cholesterol, and cancer.

A peer-reviewed article appearing in the journal *Nutrients* addressed the extensive variety of phytochemicals in beans, and revealed their documented health benefits:

> [P]hytochemicals found in beans and legumes are considerably beneficial in improving blood cholesterol levels, glycemic status, providing vascular protection, and reducing markers of chronic inflammation. Furthermore, SCFAs [short-chain fatty acids] produced from the fermentation of complex dietary fiber and resistant starches in beans are important in supporting healthy gut microbial population and diversity. Increased butyrate production positively influences the gut microbiome in the reduction of body weight, body fat, and improved insulin sensitivity. (Mullins and Arjmandi 2021, 531)

In the 2023 Netflix documentary *Live to 100: Secrets of the Blue Zones*, researchers found that the top five pillars of blue zone (communities with the world's highest longevity rates) diets are whole grains, vegetables, greens, beans, and tubers such as sweet potatoes. They specifically found that eating a cup of beans a day is associated with an extra four years of life expectancy.

The largest dried-bean producing countries in the world today are Brazil, India, China, Myanmar, and Mexico. Canada is also an important leader in bean production, and exports beans to more than seventy countries. Most of Canada's beans are grown in Ontario, Manitoba, Saskatchewan, and Alberta. The major bean-producing states in the U.S. are North Dakota, Michigan, Minnesota, Nebraska, and Idaho; about 30 percent of the dried bean crop in the United States is exported.

Resources

Aubrey, Allison. "7 habits to live a healthier life, inspired by the world's longest-lived communities." *Shots: Health News from NPR*. National Public Radio website. September 9, 2023.

Hirst, K. Kris. "The Domestication of the Common Bean." ThoughtCo. com. July 3, 2019.

Iowa State University. "Dry Edible Bean Profile." Agricultural Marketing Resource Center website. February 2022.

"Love Canadian Beans." Ontario Bean Growers. Love Canadian Beans website. 2022.

Mensack, Megan M., Vanessa K. Fitzgerald, Elizabeth P. Ryan et al. "Evaluation of diversity among common beans (*Phaseolus vulgaris L.*) from two centers of domestication using 'omics' technologies." *BMC Genomics* 11, 686 (2010).

Mullins, A. P., and B. H. Arjmandi. "Health Benefits of Plant-Based Nutrition: Focus on Beans in Cardiometabolic Diseases." *Nutrients*13, 2 (2021): 519–31.

Pavek, P. L. S. "Plant fact sheet for pea (Pisum sativum L.)". *USDA - Natural Resources Conservation Service*. Pullman, WA. September 2012.

Uebersax, Mark A., et al. "Dry beans (*Phaseolus vulgaris* L.) as a vital component of sustainable agriculture and food security—A review." *Legume Science*. June 9, 2022.

Chickpea

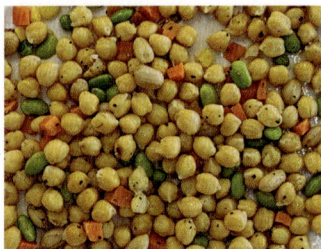

Chickpeas—also known as garbanzo beans (*Cicer arietinum*)—are a staple of Middle Eastern, African, and Indian cuisines. They are the world's second most widely grown legume, after the soybean.

The wild version of chickpeas (*Cicer reticulatum*) is only found in parts of what is today southeastern Türkiye, Syria, and the West Bank (Palestine); it is likely that chickpeas were first domesticated about 11,000 years ago. Chickpeas were part of the culture that first developed farming, called the "Pre-Pottery Neolithic" period, which existed between 10,000–8800 BCE. Chickpeas then spread to Mediterranean Europe around 6000 BCE, and to India around 3000 BCE. The ancient Greeks grew chickpeas from at least the time of Homer, during the eighth century BCE, and cultivation practices were soon followed by the Romans, Albanians, and Egyptians.

Known for their nutty, earthy flavor and slightly grainy texture, domesticated chickpeas are large, roundish, and light brown in color. They have an interesting, bumpy surface. Two main varieties of chickpeas are the larger, round, light-colored *Kabuli-type* that are common in the United States, Europe, and northern Africa. The smaller, darker-and-lighter colored, rough-coated *Desi-type* is popular in India, Iran, and Mexico.

Like other legumes, garbanzos are extremely versatile. Highly valued in Indian, Turkish, Ethiopian, Middle Eastern, Greek, Italian, and Spanish cuisines, they can be added to salads or used in soups, curries, stews, or stir-fried, pasta, or rice dishes. When prepared in a food processor or blender, and ground into a paste, chickpeas can be made into veggie burgers or meatless meatballs, called falafel, a beloved food throughout the Middle East. They can also be seasoned and roasted whole for a tasty snack. In southern Europe, chickpeas are made into flour for traditional flatbreads and fritters. When pureed and blended with tahini, garlic, olive oil, and lemon juice, chickpeas make a delicious and nutritious hummus spread; once a specialty food confined to vegetarians and adventurous eaters, hummus has become one of America's most popular plant-based foods, and is available in almost every supermarket in the United States and Canada.

Like other dry legumes, chickpeas are high in protein, dietary fiber, unsaturated and polyunsaturated fatty acids, as well as folate, iron, magnesium, manganese, phosphorus, potassium, and zinc. Chickpeas also contain several phytochemicals that, when eaten as part of a balanced, plant-rich diet, may help prevent the development of chronic health problems including diabetes, heart disease, and cancer. Because it is a high-bulk food, chickpeas provide a sensation of fullness without the calories, making it valuable in helping to control weight.

A recent article about the phytochemicals in chickpeas and their associated health benefits was published in the *World Journal of Pharmacy and Pharmaceutical Sciences*:

Chickpeas (*Phaseolus vulgaris L*) have several bioactive components associated with health benefits, such as alkaloids, anthocyanins, carbohydrates, catechins, fiber, and flavonoids phytic acid, quercetin, saponins, steroids, tannins, and terpenoids and trypsin inhibitors. Therefore, chickpeas have various biological activities, including analgesic, anti-inflammatory, antibacterial, antidiabetic, diuretic, antioxidant, hypocholesterolemic, and anti-obesity. Also, chickpeas (*Phaseolus vulgaris*) have been shown to have vigorous antidiabetic activity and may be useful in developing new antidiabetic therapies. (Para et al. 2020, 442)

The major chickpea producing countries are India, Australia, and Türkiye. Most of the chickpeas grown in the United States come from Montana, Washington, Idaho, and North Dakota.

Resources

"Chickpeas (Garbanzo Beans)." The Nutrition Source. Harvard T.H. Chan School of Public Health. Accessed February 9, 2025.

de Candolle, Alphonse. *Origin of Cultivated Plants*. New York: D. Appleton and Company, 1908, 323–24.

Hirst, K. Kris. "The Domestication History of Chickpeas." ThoughtCo. com. May 30, 2019.

Mull, Amanda. "In the Future, Everything Will Be Made of Chickpeas." *The Atlantic*. March 14, 2019.

Para, Uci, Boy Chandra, and Harrizul Rivai. "Overview of Phytochemistry and Pharmacology of Chickpeas (*Phaseolus vulgaris*)." *World Journal of Pharmacy and Pharmaceutical Sciences* 9 (2020): 442–61.

Wikipedia. "Chickpea." Accessed February 9, 2025.

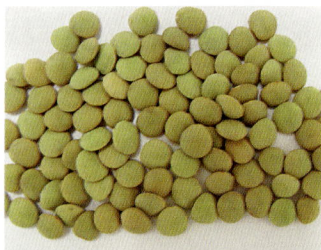

Lentil

Photo by GeorgeVandemark, USDA ARS

The lentil (*Lens culinaris*) is the world's oldest cultivated "pulse." As mentioned at the beginning of this section, pulses—also called legumes—are harvested for their dried seeds for both human and livestock food. As one of the earliest human foods, lentils remain a staple in southern Asia (especially India), the Middle East, Mediterranean Europe, and parts of northern Africa. Lentils are used in a wide range of dishes, and are highly nutritious. They also contain a variety of phytochemicals that promote good health.

The lentil was one of the first plants to be domesticated by humans in the Middle East's Fertile Crescent, together with wheat and barley. Wild lentils (*Lens orientalis*) were gathered by humans as early as 23,000 years ago, as evidenced in archeological sites in what are today Israel and Syria. Lentils were probably domesticated from stands of the wild plant somewhere between what is now southern Türkiye to the north and Jordan to the south.

When agriculture spread outside the Fertile Crescent, lentils were part of the first set of crops introduced to Greece and the rest of Europe. Lentils showed up in Greece by 6000 BCE, and were featured in wall drawings in Egyptian tombs at Thebes dating to 2400 BCE. Lentils are mentioned in some translations of the Bible in Genesis 25: 29–34, when firstborn Esau sells his birthright to Jacob for lentil stew.

By the fifth millennium BCE, the lentil was cultivated by farmers in the colder and more humid environments of central Europe. Lentils also spread to the Indian subcontinent, where it became a staple food for the Harappan civilization, which flourished in the Indus valley from 2500–1700 BCE. Lentils eventually made their way to the Americas by Spanish and Portuguese traders during the early sixteenth century, although they didn't become an important crop until 1916, when lentil cultivation began in the state of Washington. Lentils gained popularity as an affordable alternative to meat in the United States during World War II.

Lentils exist in a spectrum of colors, including yellow, orange, red, green, brown, and black. The three most common types of lentils include *brown* (European) lentils, which are sold dry in nearly every supermarket, and are popular as main dishes, or in soups, stews, pasta dishes and casseroles; *green* (French) lentils, which are firmer and used extensively in salads; and *red* lentils, which are small, sweet, and quick-cooking, and are as versatile in the kitchen as their brown cousins. Lentils can also be sprouted to enjoy by themselves or added to salad.

There are dozens of lentil varieties, and many can be found in specialty food stores and southern Asian markets. The majority were developed in India, the world's largest lentil consumer—almost half of all lentils grown in the world are eaten by Indians. Lentils are called *dal* in India, and masoor (red) dal, tuvar (pigeon pea) dal, moong (yellow) dal, and urad (black) dal are among the most popular lentils in Indian cuisine.

Lentils are good for you. In addition to providing dietary fiber and protein, key minerals include iron, potassium, magnesium, and zinc. They are a good source of B vitamins including folate, thiamine, and niacin. Lentils also contain important micronutrients like *polyphenols*, which fight cell damage and maintain nerve health. A recent article appearing in the *International Journal of Molecular Sciences* highlights the connection between eating lentils and human health:

> The evidence demonstrated that the consumption of lentils is highly associated with reductions in the incidence of degenerative diseases including diabetes, cardiovascular disease (CVD), and cancers. There has been an increase in scientific interest of the study of lentils as a functional food due to their high nutritional compositions, nutritive value, and the presence of bioactive secondary metabolites. These bioactive compounds in lentils play a vital role in the prevention of degenerative diseases in humans and a significant role in improving health. (Ganesan and Xu 2017, 2390)

Recent scientific studies have also found that lentils help reduce blood pressure, improve heart health, support the digestive system, and boost energy. As a natural cholesterol-free, gluten-free, and high-protein plant food, they can easily be incorporated into special diets for diabetic, gluten-free, vegan, vegetarian, and weight management purposes.

Canada is the world's largest producer of lentils, followed by India, Australia, Türkiye, and Nepal. The Canadian province of Saskatchewan is the largest producer of lentils in North America, followed by the states of Washington, North Dakota, and Idaho. The city of Pullman in Washington state hosts the National Lentil Festival every year, which features the world's largest bowl of lentil chili, along with a lentil cook-off, cooking demos, sporting events, and a parade.

Resources

Cleveland Clinic. "Lentils: The Big Health Benefits of Tiny Seeds." health-essentials. October 4, 2022.

Crossley, Trista. "Lentil Farming in Washington." HistoryLink.org. September 2021.

Ganesan, K., and B. Xu. "Polyphenol-Rich Lentils and Their Health Promoting Effects." *International Journal of Molecular Sciences* 18, 11 (2017): 2390–2413.

Keshavarz, Reza. Chelsea Didinger, Ann Duncan, Henry Thompson. "Pulse Crops and their Key Role as Staple Foods in Healthful Eating Patterns." Colorado State University Extension website. September 2020.

Liber, M., Isabel Duarte, and Ana Teresa Maia et al. "The History of Lentil (*Lens culinaris*) Domestication and Spread as Revealed by Genotyping-by-Sequencing of Wild and Landrace Accessions." *Frontiers in Plant Science* 12 (2021): 628439.

Sandhu, J., and S. Singh. "History and Origin." In S. S. Yadav, D. L. McNeil, and P. C. Stevenson, eds., *Lentil*. Dordrecht: Springer Verlag, 2007.

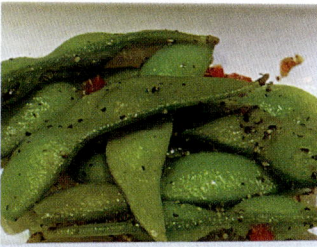

Soybean

The soybean (*Glycine max*), one of the world's most economically important crops, provides more than one quarter of the world's protein consumed by both humans and livestock. Although most of the soybeans grown in North America are fed to farm animals, the versatile plant has become an increasingly important food source for health-conscious consumers in the United States and throughout the world. It is the world's foremost provider of vegetable protein and oil, and is among the most versatile of human foods.

Recent genetic studies have found that cultivated soybeans were domesticated from their wild progenitor (*Glycine soja*) in temperate regions of China some five thousand years ago. During the Zhou Dynasty (1050–256 BCE), soybeans were designated one of the Five Sacred Grains (the others were wheat, barley, rice, and millet). The soybean was then known as *shu*, and boiled beans were eaten whole. The nutritious leaves of the plant were also eaten. Soybean cultivation later spread to what are now Korea and Japan from 300–200 BCE; they were introduced to Europe in the sixteenth century.

The soybean's timeline in North America is both fascinating and complex. In 1765, soybean seeds from China were first introduced to what was then the British colony of Georgia; five years later, Benjamin Franklin sent soybean seeds to a friend to plant in his garden. During the Civil War, soldiers used soybeans as "coffee berries" to brew "coffee" when real coffee beans were scarce. In the late 1800s, American farmers began to grow soybeans as forage for cattle.

In 1904, the renowned American agricultural scientist and inventor George Washington Carver began studying the soybean at the Tuskegee Institute in Alabama. His discoveries expanded the use of soybeans to include protein and oil for human consumption. During World War I (1914–18), Americans began using soybeans as an extender for wheat flour, and also as an alternative to meat. In 1929, American soyfoods pioneer William J. Morse left for a two-year expedition to collect soybean varieties and learn about soybean products in China, Japan, Manchuria, and Korea. He brought back more than ten thousand soybean varieties for American researchers to study. Some of these varieties were responsible for the rapid ascension of the United States becoming the world leader in soybean production.

The soybean has become one of the most versatile of human foods. Since the Zhou dynasty, Chinese cuisine has evolved to become arguably the most sophisticated in the world, and ways of preparing soybeans have evolved along with it. *Tofu*—also known as bean curd—is a cheese-like "low-tech" product made from curdling soymilk. This process dates back at least two thousand years, and now encompasses a variety of foods that include silken tofu, deep fried tofu burgers, firm and pressed tofu, smoked tofu, and frozen tofu. Tofu is considered a nutritious and low-fat alternative to meat, and is the most widely-used soy product in the world.

Soy milk is believed to have existed in China since at least 82 CE. It remains a popular breakfast drink in China and other Asian countries, and has become a popular milk substitute in many other parts of the world.

Textured soybean protein (TSP), developed in the 1960s, is "high tech" development made by texturizing concentrates, isolates, or

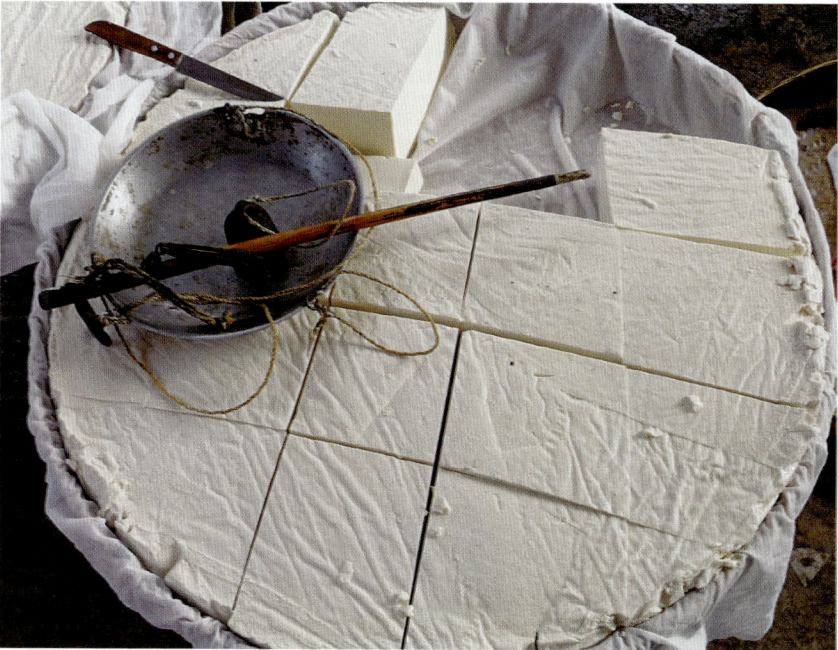

Traditionally made fermented tofu.

defatted soybean flour. It can be made into a wide variety of high-protein meat analogs that look and taste like chicken, bacon, ham, sausage, or beef. In addition to soy flour, soybean oil, and soy sauce, other popular soy-based foods include miso, tempeh, edamame, and natto (all developed in Japan), along with black bean paste (from black soybeans), margarine, soybean oil, soy-fortified breakfast cereals and pastas, soy cheese, soy creamer, and soy yogurt.

Unlike most other sources of plant-based protein, soy provides all nine essential amino acids that are needed for healthy bones and muscles. Most of the fats in soybeans are polyunsaturated and contain omega-3 and omega-6 fatty acids, which support heart health. In addition to protein and dietary fiber, soybeans are high in potassium and iron. The isoflavones found in soybeans may help strengthen the bones of women who have passed menopause. Based on studies among Asians, eating soy products may also help prevent breast cancer in woman and prostate cancer in men.

A peer-reviewed article appearing in the April 2021 issue of the *International Journal of Molecular Sciences* mentions that soybeans contain no fewer than fourteen beneficial phytochemical substances including phytic acid, triterpenes, phenolics, flavonoids, lignans, carotenoids, and coumarins, as well as protease inhibitors, oligosaccharides, and dietary fibers. The authors also stressed that these compounds are believed to help prevent cancer, delay aging, kidney failure, obesity; control healthy cholesterol levels; inhibit HIV; and prevent gallstone formation, senile dementia, and hyperlipidemia—an abnormally high concentration of fats or lipids in the blood. They also reported that soybean consumption promotes diuretic action, suppresses arteriosclerosis, provides relief from constipation, and prevents cardiovascular diseases:

> Soybean also contains substances that are involved in intestinal regulation, have antioxidative properties, prevent osteoporosis, lower blood pressure, have antithrombotic [reduce blood clots] effects,

boost immunity, and promote liver functions, and therefore, can be inferred to be closely related to the prevention of certain chronic diseases. (Kim et al. 2021, 4055)

In 2020–2021, global soybean production reached 362 million tons. The United States is the world's leading producer of soybeans, followed by Brazil, Argentina, China, and India. In the United States, the largest soybean-producing states include Illinois, Iowa, Minnesota, Indiana, and Ohio, while the three biggest soybean producers in Canada are Ontario, Québec, and Manitoba. Most of the soybeans grown in the United States and Canada are fed to livestock as soybean meal. Soybean oil can be made into biodiesel, and can also be converted to make paints, plastics, and cleaning products.

Resources

"At a Glance." Soy Canada website. Accessed October 8, 2023.

Dong, L., C. Fang, Q. Cheng et al. "Genetic basis and adaptation trajectory of soybean from its temperate origin to tropics." *Nature Communications* 12, (2021): 5445.

Frysh, Paul. "Health Benefits of Soy." WebMD. August 28, 2023.

Kim, I. S., C.H. Kim, and W.S. Yang. "Physiologically Active Molecules and Functional Properties of Soybeans in Human Health - A Current Perspective." *International Journal of Molecular Sciences* 22, 8 (2021): 4054–80.

"Major soybean-producing US States from 2018 to 2022." Statista.com. Accessed October 8, 2023.

Quinlan, Erica. "History of the soybean: Learn about soy's journey in U.S." Agrinews website. August 15, 2021.

Shurtleff, William, and Akiko Aoygaki. "History of Tofu, page 1." SoyInfoCenter.com. 2004.

"Soy Story." EatingChina.com. Accessed October 8, 2023.

"The Soybean, Its History, and Its Opportunities" *U.S. Soy: International Buyers' Guide.* June 2006.

"World Soybean Production by Country." AtlasBig.com. Accessed October 8, 2023.

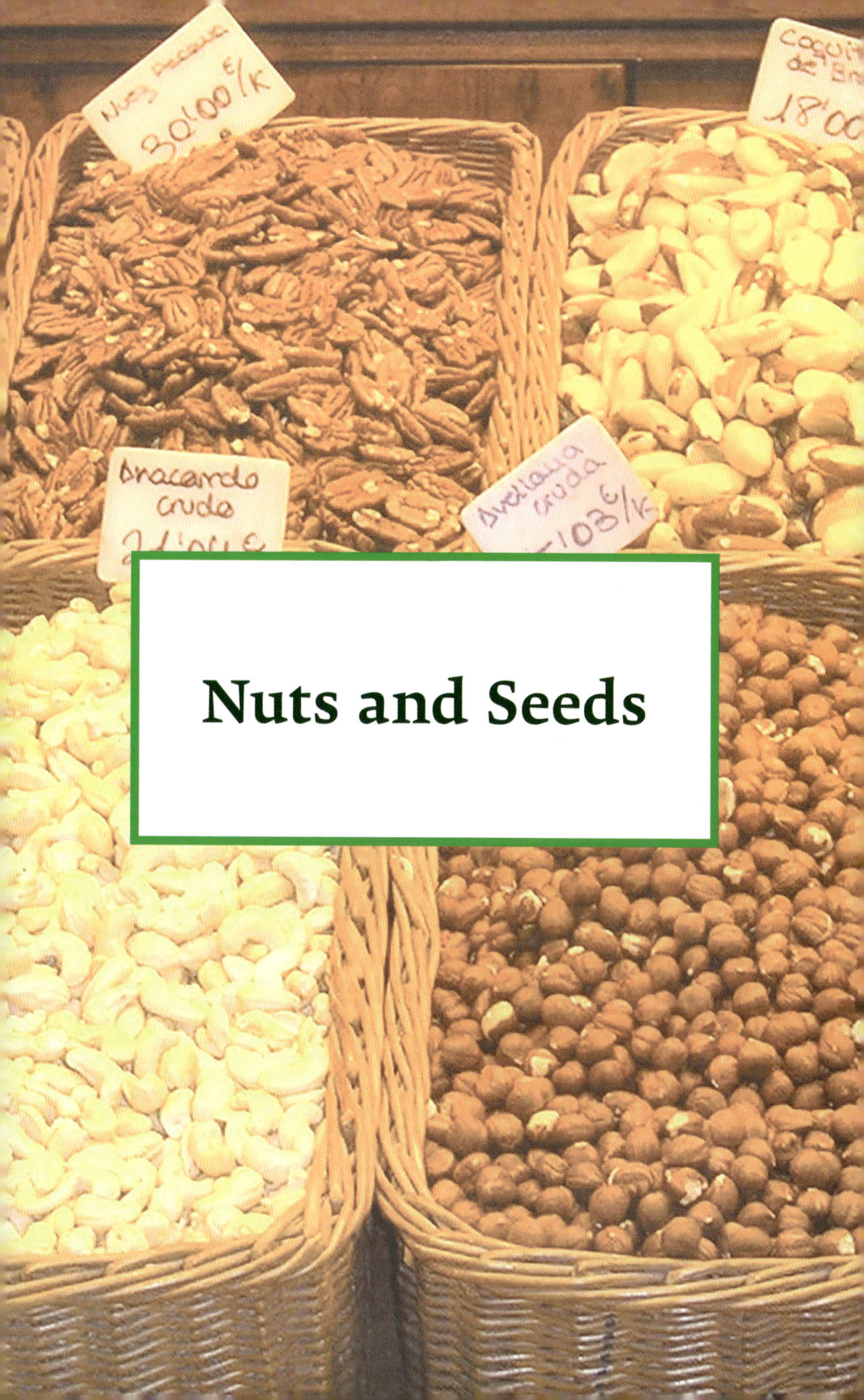

Nuts and Seeds

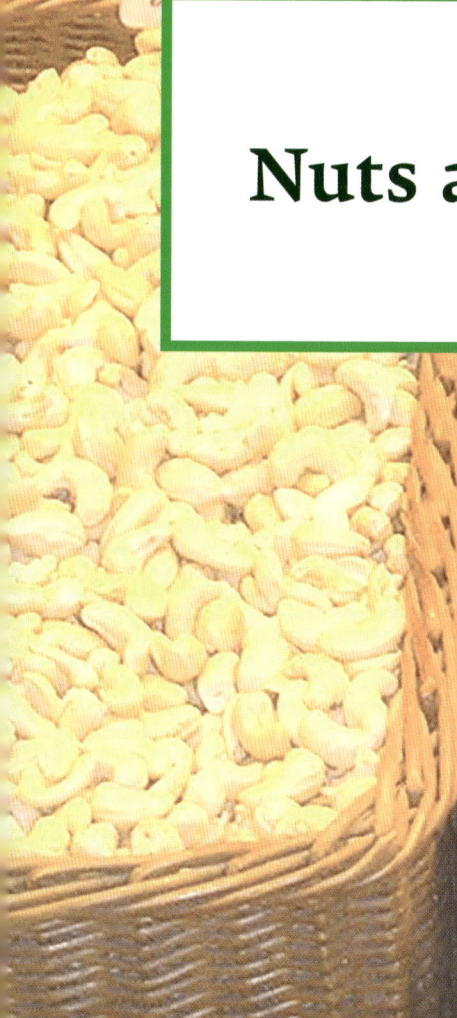

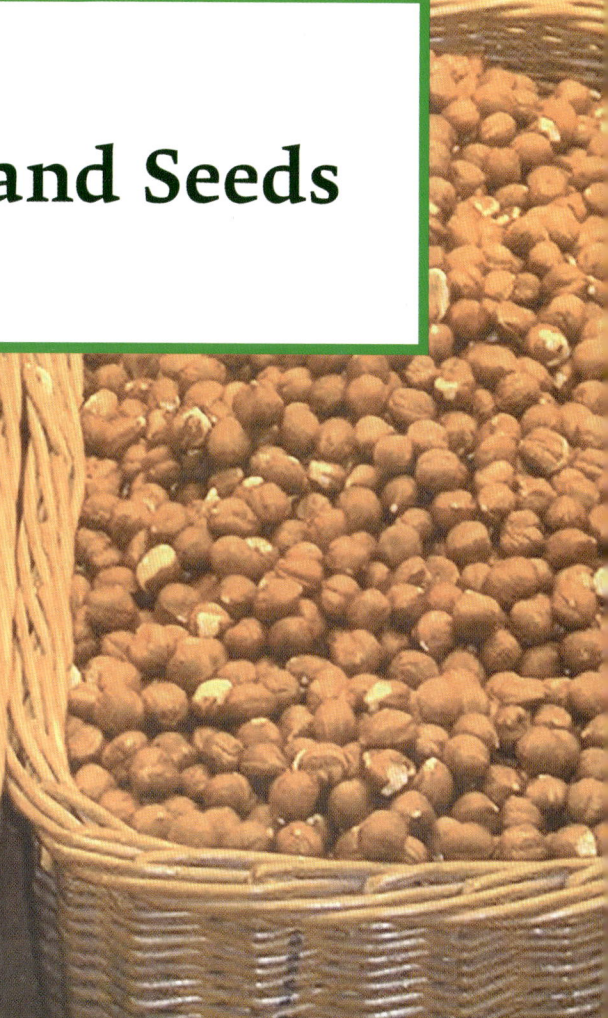

Nuts are defined as fruits that consist of a hard or tough shell that "protects a kernel which is usually edible." Although a wide variety of dry seeds have also been classified as nuts, the most accepted definition of "nut" implies that the shell does not open on its own to release the seed. In common use, a "tree nut" is any nut that comes from a tree. However, the peanut—which is actually a legume—is included in this section because it is eaten as a nut. This section will also include edible seeds such as pumpkin, sesame, and sunflower.

Although several types of nuts have been prescribed by traditional medical practitioners in both China and Persia (or Iran) to improve brain function for centuries, new research has found that nutrients and other phytochemicals found in nuts can help improve memory and overall brain function—several can even help prevent and treat Alzheimer's disease. A recent article appearing in the peer-reviewed journal *Clinical Nutrition* (Nijssen et al. 2023, 1067) focuses on the clinical effects of eating walnuts, pistachios, cashews, and hazelnuts on twenty-eight individuals with a median age of sixty-three. It reported that "Longer-term mixed nut consumption as part of a healthy diet beneficially affected brain vascular function, which may relate to the observed beneficial effects on memory in older adults. Moreover, different characteristics of the peripheral vascular tree [blood circulation] also improved."

Resources

Nijssen, K., R. Mensink, J. Plat, and P. J. Joris. "Longer-term mixed nut consumption improves brain vascular function and memory: A randomized, controlled crossover trial in older adults." *Clinical Nutrition* 42, no. 7 (2023): 1067–75.

Almonds

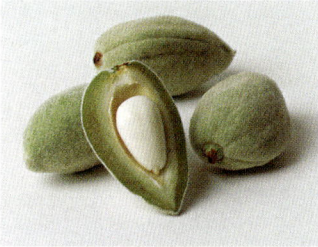

Photo via USDA ARS

Like the pecan and walnut, almonds (*Prunus amygdalus*) are commonly identified with the United States, although evidence shows that they are indigenous to the western Mediterranean region known as the Levant, which presently includes Syria, Lebanon, Israel, Palestine, Iran, and parts of Türkiye. Historically, almond trees grew wild and were later cultivated, as early as 3000 BCE. Cultivation in the Mediterranean Basin is documented by the presence of almonds among the artifacts found in historical places, such as the tomb of King Tutankhamen in Egypt and the Franchthi Cave in Greece.

Almonds were referenced in the first book of the Bible. (Genesis 43:11 indicates they were a prized food to be given as gifts:

> Then their father Israel said to them, "If it must be so, then do this: take some of the choice fruits of the land in your bags, and carry down to the man a present, a little balm and a little honey, gum, myrrh, pistachio nuts and almonds.

Wild almonds were bitter and contained a number of toxic substances, including cyanide. Yet, a recent study published in the journal *Science* found that a single genetic mutation "turned off" the ability of the plant to make the toxic compound thousands of years ago, which opened the door to the tree's domestication. Almond cultivation spread across southern Europe by the tenth century CE, but it wasn't until the

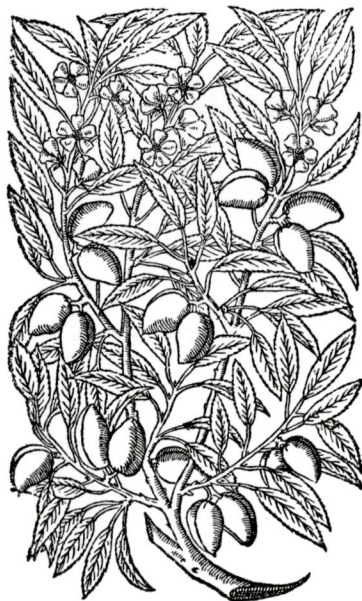

Almonds, from
John Gerarde,
The Herball, London,
1597

mid-1700s that the first almond groves were planted in California. It took another one hundred years for an almond crossbreed to be cultivated that thrived in the dry Californian climate.

Almonds are a perfect snack food by themselves, but also pair well with raisins and other dried fruits. Almonds are a major ingredient in granola cereals and energy bars. They can also be turned into almond oil; a gluten-free alternative to wheat flour; and as a high-protein, non-dairy alternative to cow's milk.

In addition to protein and dietary fiber, almonds are an important source of vitamin E—in fact, they contain more vitamin E than any other tree nut. Almonds also contain biotin, monosaturated fats, calcium, magnesium, and phosphorus. The numerous phytochemicals in almonds have been shown to possess a range of bioactivity including antioxidant, anti-inflammatory, and antiviral properties. They also fight the development of tumors and regulate cholesterol in the blood. Along with hazelnuts and walnuts, almonds have long been a part of traditional Persian medicine, used to improve brain function.

A 2017 article published in the peer-reviewed journal *Pharmacological Research* highlighted the neuroprotective properties of almonds—along with hazelnuts and walnuts—and their potential to help prevent and even treat symptoms of Alzheimer's disease:

> Beyond the molecular activities attributed to the phytochemicals, the use of these tree nuts could be more considered in scientific researches as the effective nutrients for prevention or even management of AD [Alzheimer's disease]. (Gorji et al. 2018, 115)

The United States produces about 78 percent of the world's almonds, some 2.25 million pounds a year. The vast majority of American almonds come from California. Other major producers include Spain, Australia, Iran, and Türkiye.

Resources

"Almonds." The Nutrition Source. Harvard T.H. Chan School of Public Health. Accessed October 3, 2023.

Gorji, N., R. Moeini, and Z. Memariani. "Almond, hazelnut and walnut, three nuts for neuroprotection in Alzheimer's disease: A neuropharmacological review of their bioactive constituents." *Pharmacological Research* no. 129 (2018): 115–127.

Iowa State University. "Almonds." Agricultural Marketing Resource Center website. August 2021.

Ladinsky, G. "On the Origin of Almond." *Genetic Resources and Crop Evolution* 46 (1999): 143–47.

Martínez-Gómez, P., Raquel Sánchez-Pérez, Federico Dicenta et al. "Almond." In: Kole, C. (ed.) *Fruits and Nuts. Genome Mapping and Molecular Breeding in Plants*, Vol 4. Berlin and Heidelberg: Springer Verlag, 2007.

May, H. G., and B. M. Metzger, eds. *The Holy Bible*. New York: Oxford University Press, 1973, 55.

Neilson, Susie. "How Almonds Went from Deadly to Delicious." *The Salt*. National Public Radio website. June 13, 2019.

Sánchez-Pérez, R., S. Pavan, R. Mazzeo et al. "Mutation of a bHLH transcription factor allowed almond domestication." *Science* 364, no. 6446 (2019): 1095–98.

Wikipedia. "Almonds." Accessed October 3, 2023.

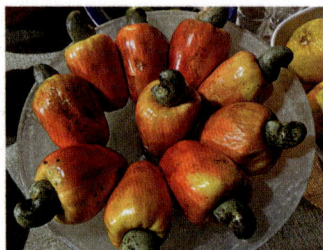

Cashew

Photo by Karen Murray

Like many other nuts, cashews are the fruit of a tree. Cashew trees produce a long, fleshy fruit called a *cashew apple*, which resembles a small pear. At the end of this fruit grows the kidney-shaped cashew nut we are familiar with. Cashew nuts are encased in a double shell containing a poison called anacardic acid, a powerful irritant. The Tupi, an Indigenous people who lived in pre-colonial Brazil, ate cashews and showed early European colonists how to remove the shell so the nut could be eaten safely. To this day, cashew nuts are normally sold shelled and roasted.

The cashew (*Anacardium occidentale*) is indigenous to northeastern Brazil. It was first introduced to the West Indies and Central America by Portuguese traders, who later brought the cashew to the Portuguese colony of Goa (now part of India) in the late sixteenth century. The nut was introduced from there to eastern Africa. In addition to tropical regions of Brazil and India, major African producers include Mozambique and Tanzania. The cashew reached the United States and Canada in the 1920s, but didn't become a popular food until the 1940s. The major producers of cashew nuts today include the Ivory Coast (Côte d'Ivoire), India, Vietnam, the Philippines, and Tanzania.

In the United States and Canada, cashew nuts are consumed mostly

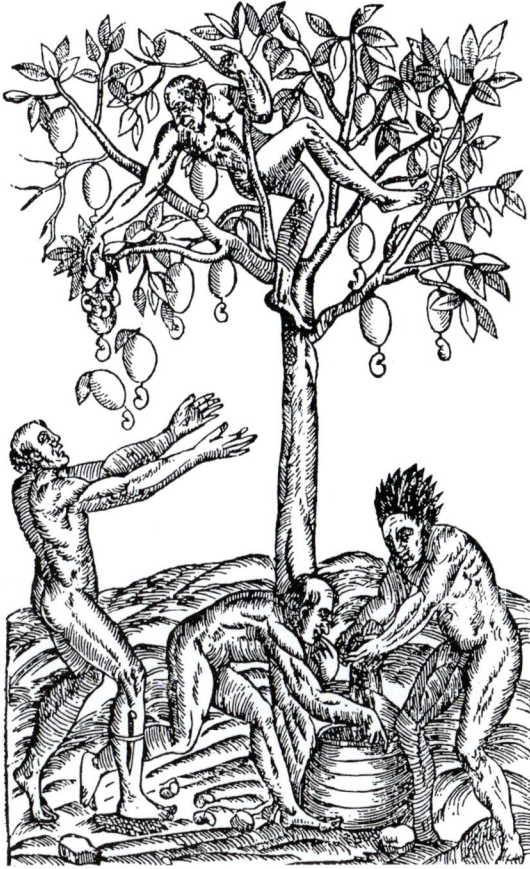

LES SINGVLARITEZ

Early drawing of a cashew tree and fruit, by the French Franciscan priest André Thevét, circa 1590.

as a snack food, either alone or as an ingredient in trail mix, fruit smoothies, or protein bars. In India, the cashew is a popular addition to chicken and vegetarian dishes, and can also be added to salads. Cashew nuts can even be made into commercial dairy-free ice cream, yogurt, cheese, and dips.

Like almonds and Brazil nuts, cashews are a good source of protein. They also have the highest magnesium content per serving of any tree nut. And, like most nuts, cashews are a good source of dietary fiber, healthy fats, B vitamins, and vitamin E.

Recent research has found that eating cashew nuts on a regular basis can decrease total blood cholesterol and especially LDL, or "bad" cholesterol. Since they are a good source of both protein and zinc, eating cashews helps strengthen the immune system, while its phosphorus and magnesium content contribute to greater bone health. The antioxidants in cashews—especially polyphenols and carotenoids—"mop up" free radicals and help reduce the risk of heart disease, cancer, type 2 diabetes, Parkinson's disease, Alzheimer's disease, and multiple sclerosis. Cashew nuts have also been linked to reducing the symptoms of colitis and painful degenerative joint disease, such as osteoarthritis.

Resources

Agrawal, Ashish. "History of Cashew Nut a World's Most Famous Nut." *Go Nuts! Blog.* October 26, 2020.

Berry, A. D., and S. A. Sargent. "Chapter 19 - Cashew apple and nut (*Anacardium occidentale* L.), in Elhadi M. Yahia, ed., Technology and Nutrition, *Postharvest Biology and Technology of Tropical and Subtropical Fruit.* Cambridge, UK: Woodhead Publishing, 2011, 414–423e.

Bolling, B. W., C. Y. Chen, D. L. McKay, and J. B. Blumberg. "Tree nut phytochemicals: composition, antioxidant capacity, bioactivity, impact factors. A systematic review of almonds, Brazils, cashews, hazelnuts, macadamias, pecans, pine nuts, pistachios and walnuts." *Nutrition Research Reviews* 24, 2 (2011): 244–75.

"Cashew plant." *Encyclopaedia Britannica.* Accessed October 7, 2023.

Fusco, Roberto, Rosalba Siracusa, A. F. Peritore et al. "The Role of Cashew (*Anacardium occidentale* L.) Nuts on an Experimental Model of Painful Degenerative Joint Disease." *Antioxidants (Basel)* 9, no. 6 (2020): 511.

Picard, Caroline. "All of the Nutritional Facts and Health Benefits of Cashews." *Good Housekeeping.* December 23, 2020.

Peterson, Elizabeth. "Where Do Cashews Come From?" Live Science website. June 30, 2014.

Shubrook, Nicola. "10 Health Benefits of Cashew Nuts." BBC Goodfood website. Accessed October 7, 2023.

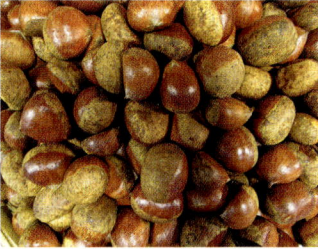

Chestnut

Chestnuts (*Castanea*) are represented by several species of trees in the beech family (Fagaceae). The chestnut tree was once among the most common trees in North America, ranging from Maine to Georgia, and west to the Mississippi River. The European settlers of North America found that the Eastern Woodlands was virtually one solid chestnut forest. Chestnut trees, called "The King of the Forest," numbered into the billions. Recent DNA studies indicate that the ancestor of the American chestnut (*Castanea dentata*) originated in China and found its way to what is now North America via Europe during the Eocene geological epoch, which lasted from about 56–34 *million* years ago. The first explicit proofs of chestnut cultivation in Europe can be dated, using palynological data (referring to the study of microorganisms and microscopic fragments of mega-organisms often found in sediments and rocks) from several regions in the Anatolian Peninsula, northeastern Greece, and southeastern Bulgaria, to 3700 BCE

The American chestnut was one of the earliest trees to be domesticated in the United States, and chestnuts were a major source of food for both livestock and people. The Ojibway, Iroquois, and Mohican tribes treasured chestnuts and used them for food and medicine. Chestnuts were roasted or ground into flour to make chestnut bread. In addition, many of the animals that Native Americans ate as food, such as deer, wild turkey, rabbits, raccoons, and squirrels, nourished themselves on chestnuts. Chestnut wood was used for kindling and woodworking.

The Chinese chestnut—known as *Castanea mollissima*—has a lineage that predates the American variety. Wild chestnuts were first mentioned in Chinese poetry over five thousand years ago, and have a planting history there that goes back at least three thousand years. Chinese chestnuts later spread throughout Asia. Another variety, known as sweet chestnut or Spanish chestnut (*Castanea sativa*), also has its genetic roots in China, and has grown wild in southern Europe and Asia Minor for millions of years. It is said that this species survived the last Ice Age over 11,000 years ago.

In *Origin of Cultivated Plants*, Alphonse de Candolle mentions that ancient chestnut forests ranged from the Caspian Sea to what is now Portugal, as well as the mountainous areas of what are now Algeria and Tunisia. Eight chestnut varieties were recognized by early Roman botanists, while the "best" chestnuts were once found near Naples and in Sardis, an ancient city (now an archeological site) in what is now western Türkiye.

The fungal pathogen "chestnut blight," which began in 1904, decimated between 90 and 99 percent of the American chestnut trees by the 1950s. It not only altered the ecology of American forests, but eliminated an important food source for billions of forest animals that relied on chestnuts for their survival. It also destroyed an important source of nourishment for humans and their livestock. Eventually, blight-resistant European and Asian chestnut trees replaced some of the originals, but domestic chestnut production in the United States and Canada remains relatively small; most chestnuts eaten in North America are imported. Korea and China are the world's biggest producers, together growing more than 40 percent of the world's chestnuts. Other major chestnut-producing countries include Italy, Türkiye, Bolivia, Japan, Spain, and Portugal.

Most chestnuts are enjoyed roasted and peeled, and are often sold shelled and precooked in snack-sized packages. Chestnuts can be made into flour for baking, and are added to soups, salads, and stir-fried dishes. According to *Good Housekeeping*, cooked chestnuts pair well with a variety of other foods including apples, cabbage, brussels sprouts, sage, thyme, and mushrooms.

Chestnuts have long been valued for their medicinal properties. In Traditional Chinese Medicine, chestnuts—eaten cooked or raw—are believed to strengthen the spleen, tonify the kidneys, strengthen the joints, and activate blood circulation to resolve swelling. Traditional Chinese doctors prescribe them for nosebleeds, scrofula, diarrhea, vomiting, sores, and weakness in the waist and knees. Native Americans healers used chestnuts to treat whooping cough, heart conditions, and chafed skin.

Chestnuts are rich in nutrients. They are a good source of dietary fiber and complex carbohydrates, which provide long-term energy. Chestnuts also contain potassium and several antioxidants (especially vitamin C and carotenoids), plus polyphenols such as gallic acid and tannins. These nutrients and plant compounds protect body cells from free-radical damage and may help protect against chronic health problems including heart disease, cancer, and diabetes. In fact, laboratory analysis shows that the antioxidant content of chestnut is higher than many other fruits, beans, and cereal products, thus making it an attractive food with added health benefits.

Resources

Chang, X., F. Liu, Z. Lin et al. "Phytochemical Profiles and Cellular Antioxidant Activities in Chestnut (*Castanea mollissima* BL.) Kernels of Five Different Cultivars." *Molecules* 25, 1 (2020):178.

de Candolle, Alphonse. *Origin of Cultivated Plants*. New York: D. Appleton and Company, 1908, 353.

Hochmuth, Robert C., Robert D. Wallace, Peter J. Van Blokland et al. "Production and Marketing of Chestnuts in the Southeastern United States." University of Florida. Institute of Food and Agricultural Sciences. October 4, 2018.

Li, Rui, Anand Kumar Sharma, Junchao Zhu et al. "Nutritional biology of chestnuts: A perspective review." *Food Chemistry* 395 (2022): 133575.

Li, Xingpeng, Hongzhe Jiang, Xuesong Jiang et al. "Identification of

Geographical Origin of Chinese Chestnuts Using Hyperspectral Imaging with ID-CNN Algorithm." *Agriculture* 11, 12 (2021):1274.

Wikipedia. "*Castanea sativa.*" Accessed October 7, 2023.

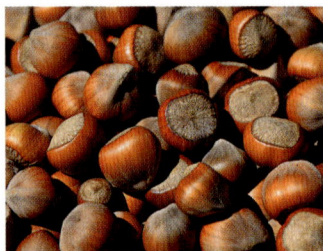

Hazelnut

Photo by Linnearodrigs

People have eaten hazelnuts (*Corylus*) since at least the Mesolithic era, which took place between 5,000 to 15,000 years ago in Europe and roughly 10,000 to 20,000 years ago in the Middle East. Today, hazelnuts—also known as filberts—are the world's third most commonly grown nut, after almonds and walnuts.

Hazelnuts are believed to be indigenous to Asia Minor, an area that includes most of modern-day Türkiye. Common opinion, based on a statement by Pliny the Elder in his work *Naturalis Historia*, is that the hazelnut originated in Pontus (on the northern coast of Türkiye) and was introduced from there to ancient Greece. Recent DNA research shows that hazelnut cultivars spread mostly from east to west, and the nuts were likely domesticated independently in what are now Türkiye, Greece, Italy, and Iran. Hazelnut cultivation was also believed to have been introduced from Italy to Spain (and the rest of the Roman Empire) by the early Romans. The European hazelnut (*Corylus Avellana*) was considered a symbol of wisdom and knowledge, as well as fecundity and fertility. The name Corylus comes from the Greek word *korylos*, which means helmet, referring to the husk covering the nut.

The American hazelnut (*Corylus americana*) is native to the eastern and central United States and the extreme southern parts of eastern and central Canada. Many Indigenous tribes, including the Cherokee, Ojibway, Dakota, and Iroquois, picked hazelnuts in the forest and used them in soup, bread, and corn pudding. They also ate hazelnuts raw, either alone or with honey, and stored them as food for the winter. Hazelnuts were also a major source of food for the animals that Native Americans hunted for food, including deer, moose, squirrels, rabbits, turkey, grouse, and pheasants. American hazelnuts are believed to have been cultivated in the United States since the 1700s.

Today, hazelnuts are used raw or cooked in many dishes. They can be shelled and enjoyed like other tree nuts, or can be ground up and used as flour for bread, biscuits, and sweets. They can also be an ingredient in stuffing or added to salads, soups, pastas, and stir-fried dishes. Filberts are widely used in the confectionary industry, especially when combined with chocolate. Nutella—a chocolate and hazelnut spread that originated in Italy—has been a worldwide favorite since the 1946.

Like other tree nuts, hazelnuts are good for health. They contain high amounts of dietary fiber, protein, B vitamins (especially thiamin), and vitamin E. They also provide iron, phosphorous, magnesium, and manganese. Recent studies have indicated that eating hazelnuts may help prevent constipation, protect the body against cell damage, reduce levels of harmful cholesterol, improve insulin sensitivity, support heart health, reduce inflammation, and even improve sperm count. As mentioned earlier, along with almonds and walnuts, hazelnuts have long been a part of traditional Persian medicine used to improve brain function. Hazelnuts in particular are valued for their ability to reverse brain atrophy. A 2017 article published in the peer-reviewed journal *Pharmacological Research* highlighted the neuroprotective properties of hazelnuts—along with almonds and walnuts—and their potential to help prevent and even treat symptoms of Alzheimer's disease.

The main hazelnut producing countries are Türkiye, Italy, Spain, the United States, and Greece. Türkiye is the top hazelnut producer and exporter, with approximately 70 percent of the world's production and 82 percent of its export, followed by Italy with nearly 20 percent of production and 15 percent of the world's export. Today, 99 percent of the hazelnuts grown in the United States come from Oregon's Willamette Valley, an area with a history of production that dates back over one hundred years.

Resources

Boccacci, P., and R. Botta. "Investigating the origin of hazelnut (*Corylus avellana* L.) cultivars using chloroplast microsatellites." *Genetix Resources and Crop Evolution* 56, (2009) pp. 851–859.

Gorji, N., R. Moeini, and Z. Memariani. "Almond, hazelnut and walnut, three nuts for neuroprotection in Alzheimer's disease: A neuropharmacological review of their bioactive constituents." *Pharmacological Research* 129 (2018): 115

Kokosal, A. Ýlhami, ed. "Hazelnut Production." *Inventory of Hazelnut Research, Germplasm and References*. Ankara: Food and Agriculture Organization, 2002.

Muehlbauer, Megan, John Capik, and Thomas J. Molnar. "Choosing Plants for a Hazelnut Orchard in New Jersey." New Jersey Agricultural Experiment Station website. Rutgers University. May 2021.

Paquin, Grace. "Hazelnut." Washington College. 2024.

"What are the Health Benefits of Hazelnuts?" Medical News Today website. November 27, 2018.

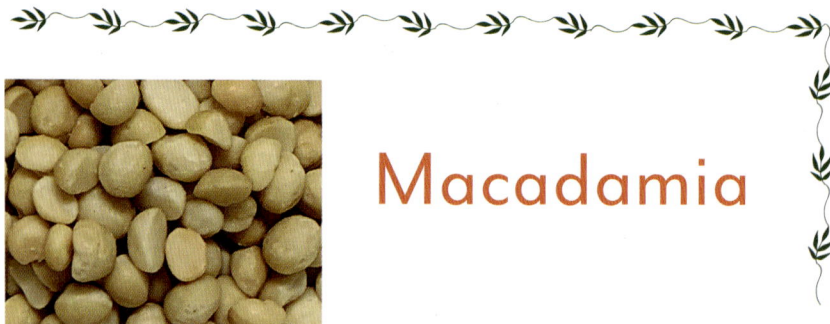

Macadamia

Although indigenous to Australia, Macadamia nuts (*Macadamia* spp.) are closely identified with Hawai'i, America's largest producer of this crunchy, creamy, and very delicious nut.

Like some other nuts, the history of the macadamia goes back thousands—if not millions—of years. The early aboriginal Budjilla people in Queensland feasted on macadamia nuts—known to them as "kindal-kindal" and "boombera"—and used its oil as a base for liniment as well as face and body paint.

In 1843, the German explorer Ludwig Leichhardt was the first recorded non-aboriginal to come across macadamias in the bush and collect them. The German-Australian botanist Baron Ferdinand von Mueller (known as "the father of Australian botany") introduced the macadamia nut to the world in the late 1850s. He named the nut to honor his friend John Macadam, an Australian chemist and physician.

Macadamia trees were first brought to Hawai'i's Big Island from a single grove in Queensland in 1881 by William Purvis, while other trees were brought to Honolulu in 1892 by R. A. Jordan, which formed the basis for macadamia nut cultivation in Hawai'i. Commercial cultivation didn't begin there until 1921. Macadamia trees are multiplied through grafting, which involves cutting off part of one tree and attaching it to another. Modern macadamia trees take between five and eight years to bear fruit.

Macadamia nuts are among the most expensive of tree nuts, and are primarily marketed as a gourmet snack food to be eaten raw or roasted. They are also used in confectionary (such as chocolate-covered macadamias), baking, ice cream, and its oil is used as an ingredient in high-end skin care formulas. While macadamia nuts don't provide as much protein as other nuts, they contain dietary fiber, manganese, thiamin, copper, and monosaturated fat, which has been found to significantly lower the risk of heart disease.

In addition, macadamia nuts are rich in phytochemicals that contribute to good health. A recent article published in *Biointerface Research in Applied Chemistry* focused on these plant compounds and their therapeutic value:

The phytochemical compounds [are] comprised of flavonoid, pro-anthocyanidin, and other polyphenols compounds. These phyto-chemical compounds can promote a wide range of pharmacological activities such as antioxidant, anti-inflammatory, anti-dyslipidemia, dietary controlled, antimicrobial, chemopreventive [cancer preventive], and NAFLD [Non-Alcoholic Fatty Liver Disease] prevention. (Insanu et al. 2021, 11480)

By 2020, the world's two largest producers of macadamias were South Africa and Australia, followed by Kenya, the United States (Hawai'i), and China.

Resources

"A Brief History of Macadamia Nuts." HawaiiOceanProject.com. July 25, 2018.

Ginis, Elizabeth. "Australian Macadamias: History in a Nutshell." *Australian Geographic*. August 9, 2017.

Insanu, M., R. Hartati, F. Bajri, and I. Fidrianny. "Macadamia Genus: An Updated Review of Phytochemical Compounds and Pharmacological Activities." *Biointerface Research in Applied Chemistry* 11, 6 (2021): 14480–89.

Iowa State University. "Macadamia Nuts." Agricultural Marketing Resource Center website. November 2021.

Katz, Brigid. "Most of the World's Macadamias May Have Originated from a Single Australian Tree." *Smithsonian Magazine*. June 4, 2019.

Moyski, Nicole. "The History of the Macadamia Nut." Accessed October 10, 2020.

Sibulali, Ayabong. *Market Intelligence Report: Macadamia Nuts Industry*. Western Cape Government (Agriculture). March 2021.

Wikipedia. "Macadamia." Accessed October 10, 2023.

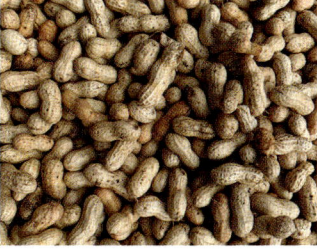

Peanut

In the United States, peanuts (*Arachis hypogeea*) are considered a flavorful and nutritious nut, and are closely identified with former President (and peanut farmer) Jimmy Carter and the American South. Yet, few people know that peanuts are actually legumes, relatives of dried beans, lentils, and chickpeas. Like tree nuts, the peanut actually begins to grow above ground, but matures *underground* (that's why they are often called *groundnuts* in England and other English-speaking countries).

Although no fossilized remains of peanuts have been found, ancient Inca graves along the coast of what is now Peru contain jars intended for holding peanuts to nourish the dead with food in the afterlife.

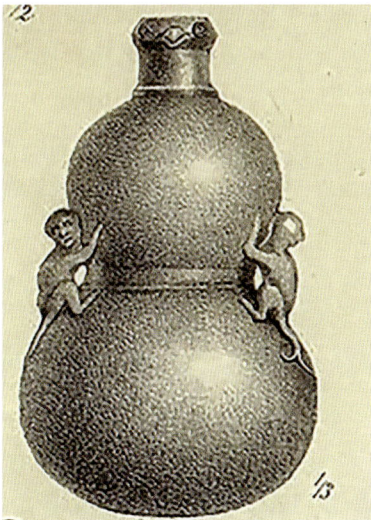

Early Inca jar shaped like a peanut.
From Alcide d'Orbigny, Voyage dans l'Amérique méridionale *(1844).*

For as long as people have been making pottery in South America (3,500 years or so), they have been making jars shaped like peanuts and decorated with peanuts. Pre-Columbian tribes in central Brazil also ground peanuts with maize to ferment into an intoxicating beverage for celebrations.

Spanish explorers found peanuts growing in what is now Mexico, and brought peanut plants back to Spain. Traders eventually introduced peanuts to Africa and Asia. When Africans were brought to North America as slaves during the seventeenth to nineteenth centuries, peanuts came with them. Records show that peanuts were grown commercially in South Carolina from around 1800, and used for oil, human food, and animal food.

By the early 1900s, the celebrated American botanist George Washington Carver and others developed new varieties of peanuts, and improvements were made in cultivation and harvesting practices. Roasted and salted peanuts later became a popular snack food in America, and peanut butter became a favorite childhood treat. Peanut butter, believed to have been introduced by food pioneer John Harvey Kellogg (of Kellogg's cereal fame) in 1895, became a staple food for American troops serving in Europe during World War I.

Peanuts are mostly enjoyed as peanut butter, which is spread on bread or crackers, and pairs well with bananas. Peanuts are also eaten directly from the shell, either raw or roasted, or roasted without their shell (either dry or in oil), with or without salt. They are a popular ingredient in trail mix, energy bars, and many types of candy. Peanuts can also be used in stir-fried or noodle dishes, or added to salads. In Thailand, peanuts are made into dipping sauce for spring rolls and other finger foods.

Although peanuts cause severe allergies in some individuals, they are generally considered a superfood, packed with nutrition. In addition to protein, peanuts contain monounsaturated and polyunsaturated fats that help decrease "bad" LDL cholesterol and increase "good" HDL cholesterol. In addition to vitamins and minerals (including vitamins B_3, B_6, E, and folic acid and minerals iron, magnesium, and zinc), peanuts contain bioactive compounds (including polyphenols, phytosterols, and antioxidants) that help protect against heart disease, inflammation, and cancer. A peer-reviewed article in the journal *Future Foods* highlights the phytochemicals in peanuts and their contribution to good health:

> Peanut and peanut products positively affect human health with their nutrients (lipid profiles) and bioactive compounds such as phytosterols, phenolic compounds, stilbenes, lignans, and isoflavonoids. These bioactive compounds protect against cardiovascular disease, type 2 diabetes mellites, and cancer. (Çiftçi and Suna 2022, 100140-1)

The authors added that peanut consumption is recommended to include the skin of the nut because it contains higher concentrations of some of the bioactive ingredients mentioned above.

Eating peanuts may also increase longevity. A large-scale study found that people who regularly ate any kind of nuts (including peanuts) were less likely to die of any cause than were people who rarely ate nuts. The fact that peanut farmer and former President Jimmy Carter celebrated his one-hundredth birthday in October 2024—shortly before he passed away the following January—is one example of this possibility.

The United States is the fifth largest producer and a major exporter of peanuts, which contributes over four billion dollars to the U.S. economy every year. Four basic varieties, including the Runner, Virginia, Spanish, and Valencia, are commercially grown. The largest peanut producers in the world are China, India, Nigeria, and Sudan.

Resources

Çiftçi, S., G. Suna. "Functional components of peanuts (Arachis Hypogaea L.) and health benefits: A review." *Future Foods* 5 (2022): 100140.

"Health Benefits of Peanuts." WebMD. November 22, 2022.

"The History of Peanuts." *Virginia Carolinas Peanuts*. AboutPeanuts.com. Accessed February 9, 2025.

Iowa State University. "Peanuts." Agricultural Marketing Resource Center website. August 2022.

Kershner, Ellen. "The Truly Bizarre Origins of Peanut Butter." DailyMeal. com. May 15, 2023.

"Peanuts Rise to Superfood Status." The Peanut Institute website. September 17, 2018.

"World Peanut Production by Country." AtlasBig.com. Accessed October 10, 2023.

Wright, D. L., B. L. Tillman, I. M. Small et al. "Management and Cultural Practices for Peanuts." *University of Florida Extension*. 2020.

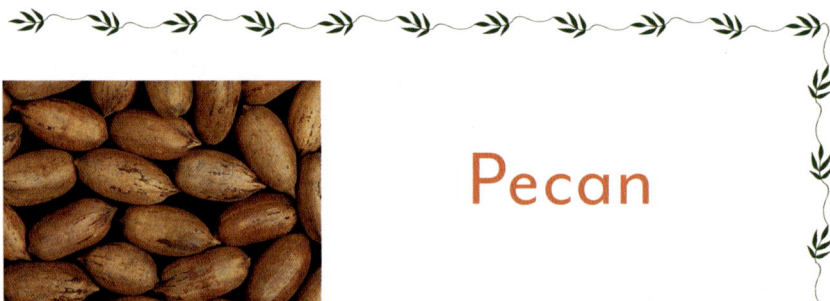

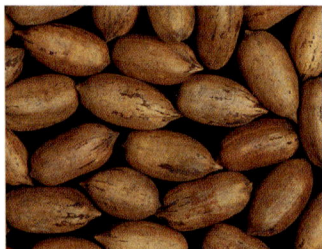

Pecan

Photo by Scott Bauer, USDA ARS

Like its distant cousin the walnut, the pecan can trace its lineage back millions of years, to when the Juglandaceae family of plants divided into walnuts and hickory nuts, of which the pecan is a descendent. Unlike the modern-day walnut (*Junglans regia*), the pecan is considered indigenous to the temperate regions of North America, as indicated by its Latin botanical name *Carya illinoinensis*. The name pecan is said to come from the Algonquian word meaning "nut." The Cree referred to it as *pakan* (hard-shelled nut), the Ojibwa *bagaan*, and the Abenaki as *pagan*.

Native Americans consumed wild pecans for centuries before they were "discovered" by Spanish explorers during the sixteenth century in what are now Texas, Louisiana, and Mexico. The Spanish are also credited with introducing the pecan to Europe, Asia, and Africa. European settlers quickly adopted the tasty and nutritious pecan into their diets. Thomas Jefferson is said to have cultivated pecans at his plantation in Monticello, and gave seedlings to George Washington, who grew them at Mount Vernon.

Wider cultivation of pecans began in the American southeast in the early nineteenth century, when European settlers thinned wild pecan stands and used the surrounding grass for animal grazing. Botanists experimented with grafting techniques, although they weren't widely adopted until the late 1800s. The arrival of the railroads facilitated commercial sales and distribution to major cities. The pecan is grown mainly in Georgia, Texas, Oklahoma, and New Mexico. It is also an important nut crop in Mexico, where it is known as the *pacana* or *nuez lisa* (smooth nut). The Texas legislature named the pecan the official state tree in 1919. Alabama named the pecan its official state nut in 1982, followed by California (as one if its four official state nuts) in 2017.

Pecans are generally enjoyed shelled and raw, and are also a popular ingredient in desserts (i.e., pecan pie and ice cream), energy bars, candy, smoothies, and breakfast cereals.

Like other tree nuts, the pecan is rich in dietary fiber and is a good source of protein, which promotes growth and enhances immunity. Pecans also contain monosaturated fat, which can reduce the risk of heart disease and cancer. They are an excellent source of B vitamins (especially thiamin, pantothenic acid, and pyridoxine) as well as magnesium, phosphorous, zinc, manganese, and copper. Manganese and copper have been found to boost overall metabolic health, may contain anti-inflammatory properties, and may potentially help reduce the risk of high blood pressure and heart disease. Finally, pecans have more flavonoids—a type of antioxidant found mostly in fruits and vegetables—than any other tree nut. People who eat diets high in flavonoids have been found to be less likely to develop chronic health problems, such as heart disease, diabetes, some types of cancer, and cognitive decline due to aging.

An article appearing in the December 2022 issue of the *Journal of Agriculture and Food Research* described the phytochemicals found in pecans and their health benefits:

> Similar to walnuts in chemical composition, pecans represent a rich source of healthy fats and polyphenolic compounds and have been shown to reduce or prevent diseases such as coronary heart disease, gallstones, obesity, metabolic syndrome, cancer, inflammation, hypertension, and diabetes. (Tong et al. 2022, 100387)

The authors of this article observed that while global demand for pecans has increased over the years, sales in the United States have not, with most pecan consumers being educated, older adults. They suggested that, given the health benefits pecans can provide, educational strategies to promote them—especially digital media—would be a valuable asset in improving public health, especially among younger consumers.

Resources

Harper, Douglas. "Pecan (n.)." Online Etymology Dictionary. Accessed September 13, 2023.

"History of Pecans." Texas A&M University Extension. Accessed September 13, 2023.

London, Jaclyn. "9 Health Benefits of Pecans That'll Make You Go Nuts." *Good Housekeeping.* December 6, 2017.

"Pecan." *Encyclopaedia Britannica.* July 14, 2023.

Reedy, Victor R. and Ronald Ross Watson, eds. *Nuts and Seeds in Health and Disease Prevention.* Cambridge, MA: Academic Press, 2011, 881–89.

Tong, Xiao, Amy Szacilo, Hsiangting Chen et al. "Using rich media to promote knowledge on nutrition and health benefits of pecans among young consumers." *Journal of Agriculture and Food Research* 10 (2022): 100387.

Wikipedia. "Pecan." Accessed February 9, 2025.

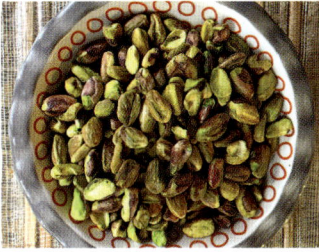

Pistachio

The pistachio (*Pistacia vera*) is indigenous to western Asia and Asia Minor, with a range that extended from present-day Syria to the Caucasus and Afghanistan. Archaeological evidence in Türkiye indicates that humans were eating pistachios as early as 7000 BCE. Along with almonds, they were mentioned in Genesis 43:11:

> Then their father Israel said to them, "If it must be so, then do this: take some of the choice fruits of the land in your bags, and carry down to the man a present, a little balm and a little honey, gum, myrrh, pistachio nuts and almonds."

In Persia, the pistachio was considered a luxury food. Legend has it that pistachios were a favorite of the Queen of Sheba, who ruled during the tenth century BCE. Alexander the Great (334–323 BCE) is said to have introduced pistachios to Greece. Later, under the rule of the Roman Emperor Tiberius (first century CE), the nut was introduced to Italy and Spain, and soon spread to other Mediterranean regions. Its modern name comes originally from the Middle Persian word *pistakē* and the Italian *pistacchio*.

The first pistachio tree was brought to California in 1854 by Charles Mason, who sold seeds for experimental plantings. He also introduced pistachios to Texas and several other southern states. This was followed by the arrival of several small trees from France in 1875, which were planted in Sonoma, California. The United States Department of

Agriculture grew a variety of pistachio species at its Plant Production Station in Chico beginning in the early 1900s. In 1929, the American botanist William E. Whitehouse traveled to Persia, returning to California the following year with some twenty pounds (ten kilograms) of individually selected pistachio nuts. The first test plots were soon planted; trees take seven to ten years to mature. Only one tree bore fruit, which Whitehouse named the "Kerman" after a Persian carpet-making town. After Whitehouse's death, scientists propagated and strengthened the Kerman by budding it to heartier rootstock varieties.

After many years of experimenting, plantings began to emerge in California during the 1960s, and commercial production began in the late 1970s. Over the past four decades, the cultivation of pistachio trees (primarily in California's San Joaquin Valley) have grown substantially. California now produces some 99 percent of all pistachios grown in the United States, with the rest produced in Arizona and New Mexico. Major pistachio producers worldwide include Iran, Türkiye, Syria, and China.

Unsalted pistachio nuts are the ultimate healthy snack food, whether eaten alone or added to salads, ice cream, yogurt desserts, nut bars, trail mix, casseroles, or stir-fried dishes. A major "problem" with pistachios is that once one begins eating them, it is often difficult to stop. Nutritionists suggest that by buying them in the shell, consumption will be slower and one will feel the satisfaction of feeling full without eating too many. Like other tree nuts, pistachios are not a low-calorie food, and eating a small handful a day is considered adequate for most people.

In addition to offering a "complete" protein, like animal-based foods, pistachios are rich in dietary fiber, vitamin B_6, and essential minerals like potassium. Pistachios are also rich in monounsaturated and polyunsaturated fats, which have been found to reduce LDL ("bad") cholesterol. They are also a major source of antioxidants, including vitamin E, polyphenols, and the carotenoids lutein and zeaxanthin. Two of these antioxidants are not found in other nuts. In addition to helping reduce free-radical damage in general, pistachios have been linked to a decreased risk of developing macular degeneration.

A landmark article detailing the phytochemical properties of pistachios and their health benefits was published in the July 2022 issue of the peer-reviewed journal *Nutrients*. The authors—three of the four are affiliated with the Department of Food Science at Cornell University (Yuan et al. 2022, 3002)—described pistachios as "[. . .] a nutrient-dense food containing a unique profile of good-quality protein, fats, minerals, vitamins, and antioxidants, such as carotenoids and polyphenols, with cellular antioxidant activity." In addition to the health benefits of eating pistachios, as described earlier, their research focused on the possible anticancer properties of pistachios.

They found that pistachio phytochemical extracts showed potent activities against human breast, liver, and colon cancer cells *in vitro*, with exceptionally high activity seen against human breast cancer cells. Pistachio phytochemical extracts were also shown to inhibit growth in all three varieties of cancer cells (breast, liver, and colon). These findings point to the potential of using pistachios as part of both cancer prevention and treatment.

Resources

Cleveland Clinic. "3 Reasons Why Pistachios Can Boost Your Health." healthessentials. February 4, 2020.

"Pistachio Origin." Iran Dried Fruit blog. June 28, 2024.

"History: Pistachio Origins." American Pistachio Growers website. 2017.

"History of the Pistachio." HeartoftheDesert.com. October 19, 2020.

Laguaite, Madeline. "Health Benefits of Pistachios." WebMD. August 28, 2022.

May, H. G., and B. M. Metzger, eds., *The Holy Bible* (New York: Oxford University Press, 1973), 55.

Yuan, W., B. Zheng, T. Li, and R. H. Liu. "Quantification of Phytochemicals, Cellular Antioxidant Activities and Antiproliferative Activities of Raw and Roasted American Pistachios (*Pistacia vera* L.). *Nutrients*14, 15 (2022): 3002.

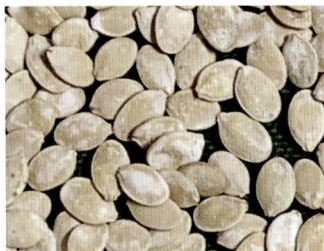

Pumpkin Seed

As mentioned earlier, pumpkins are a member of the squash family, which contains several dozen major species. Although pumpkin was originally an important food crop among Native Americans living in what are now Mexico and the United States, most of the "sugar pumpkin" variety of squash (*Cucurbita maxima*) grown in the United States today (primarily in Illinois and Indiana), and the Connecticut field pumpkin (*Cucurbita pepo*) is used to provide jack-o'-lanterns for Hallowe'en.

The nutritious flesh of the pumpkin is sometimes used to make pumpkin pie, muffins, or soup. However, both pumpkin flesh and especially pumpkin seeds are usually considered waste products and discarded. Fortunately, both pumpkins in general and pumpkin seeds in particular are finally becoming recognized for their flavor, nutritional value, and numerous health-giving properties.

Pumpkin seeds have enjoyed a long history in traditional medicine: traditional Chinese doctors and Ayurvedic medical practitioners in India have utilized pumpkin seeds for treating kidney disorders, prostate diseases, intestinal parasites, and skin infections for centuries. The nutritional and therapeutic value of pumpkin seeds has only recently begun to be examined by modern nutritionists and medical researchers.

Pumpkin seeds (*Cucurbita* spp.) are not limited to the jack-o'-lantern type of pumpkin Americans are most familiar with, but are found in varieties popular in Mexico, India, and China, including *Cucurbita pepo*, *Cucurbita maxima*, and *Cucurbita moschata*. Pumpkin seeds are especially becoming a popular food source in Africa, due in part to their availability as well as their nutritional and medicinal benefits. All varieties of pumpkin seeds are enjoyed by people around the world for their appealing flavor and texture.

Pumpkin seeds have been praised by nutritionists for their high protein content and useful amounts of the essential fatty acid linoleic acid. Pumpkin seeds contain remarkably high proportions of essential amino acids. They are also good sources of zinc, phosphorous, magnesium, potassium, and selenium, leading one group of researchers to call pumpkin seeds a "nutritional powerhouse."

A recent peer-reviewed article published in *Scientific African* highlighted the many health-giving properties of pumpkin seeds:

> Some of these bioactives and minerals act simultaneously at different or identical target sites with the potential to impart physiological benefits, promote well-being, and reduce the risk of non-communicable disorders such as tumors, microbial infections, hyperglycemia and diabetes, oxidative stress associated complications, prostate disorders, and urinary bladder complications. (Dotto and Chacha 2020, e00575)

The authors also addressed therapeutic activities of pumpkin seed extract (PSE), which include liver protective, wound healing, hair-growth stimulating, anthelmintic [kills parasitic worms], antioxidant, and chemoprotective properties which help protect the body against harmful effects of chemotherapy.

The authors added that "the low sodium and high potassium contents in the pumpkin seeds translate to a significant clinical implication for improving cardiovascular health." Ongoing research is investigating the value of pumpkin seeds in the prevention and treatment of diabetes, internal parasites, cancer, and anemia. In addition, researchers are exploring the positive effects of pumpkin seeds on the central nervous system, especially with regard to social phobias and insomnia.

Pumpkin seeds have experienced a growth in popularity in recent years, and are usually consumed either toasted (and sometimes salted) by themselves or enjoyed in trail mix, smoothies, or as an ice cream topping. They can be cooked along with rice, are a good addition to hot cereals, and can be added to tossed salads. Pumpkin seeds are also used in the baking industry, primarily as flour in biscuits and bread.

Pumpkin seeds are often found in natural foods stores or in the "snack food" section of supermarkets and convenience stores. Although pumpkin seeds are a healthy food, some preparations are fried in oil and contain large amounts of salt, making them a high-sodium food.

Here is an easy way to roast raw seeds straight from the pumpkin.

> **Roasted Pumpkin Seeds**
>
> Preheat oven to 300 degrees Fahrenheit (150 degrees C).
>
> After cleaning the seeds and allowing them to dry, spread them in a thin layer on an oiled or parchment paper lined baking tray.
>
> Bake for about thirty minutes, or until you hear the seeds begin to pop.
>
> After removing them from the oven, the seeds can be lightly tossed in a small amount of olive oil and your choice of seasoning (salt, paprika, oregano, cumin, chili powder, etc.) if desired.
>
> Spread the seeds again on the baking sheet and bake for another twenty minutes.

Resources

Afifa, Aziz, Sana Noreen, Waseem Khalid et al. "Pumpkin and Pumpkin Byproducts: Phytochemical Constitutes, Food Application and Health Benefits." *ACS Omega* 8, 26 (2023): 23346–23357.

Batool, M., M. M. A. N. Ranjha, U. Roobab et al. "Nutritional Value, Phytochemical Potential, and Therapeutic Benefits of Pumpkin (*Cucurbita* sp.)." *Plants (Basel)* 11, 11 (2022):1394.

Dotto, Joachim M., and James S. Chacha. "The potential of pumpkin seeds as a functional food ingredient: A review." *Scientific African* 10 (2020): e00575.

KC. "Pumpkin & Pumpkin Seeds Benefits, Properties in Traditional Chinese Medicine (TCM)." *Nature Health.* August 7, 2023.

Monica, Sarah Jane, J. R. Sheila, C. Madhanagopal et al. "Chemical composition of pumpkin (Cucurbita maxima) seeds and its supplemental effect on Indian women with metabolic syndrome." *Arabian Journal of Chemistry* 15, no. 8 (2022): 103985.

"Pumpkin." Drugs.com. November 30, 2022.

Yadav, M., S. Jain, R. Tomar et al. "Medicinal and biological potential of pumpkin: an updated review." *Nutrition Research Reviews* 23, 2 (2010):184–190.

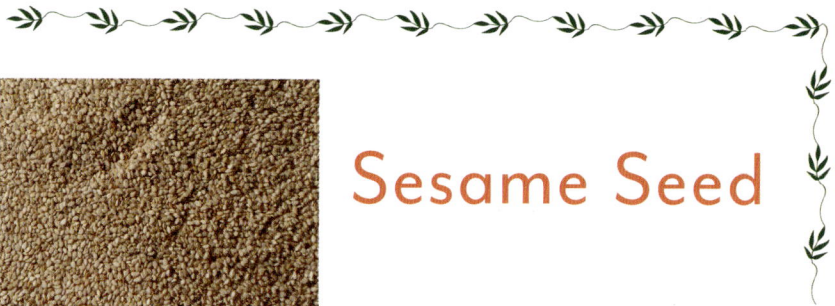

Sesame Seed

Sesame (*Sesamum indicum*) is one of the world's oldest cultivated crops. It is believed to have originated in what is today Pakistan, at the archeological site of Harappa, located in the Indus Valley, more than five thousand years ago. The plant was brought to Mesopotamia around 2500 BCE, where it was highly prized for its oil (the oil content in sesame seeds ranges from 45 to 60 percent).

The oldest source of oilseed known to humanity, a primary feature of this ancient plant is pods that open when ripe, revealing hundreds of tiny white seeds (they also grow in a variety of colors including shades of black, brown, gray, and gold). Hardy and drought-resistant, cultivated sesame plants eventually spread throughout Asia, Africa, and the area around the Indian Ocean by humans traveling by both land and sea.

This vast area ranges from India to Greece, and includes countries in northern Africa such as Egypt, Sudan, and Morocco. Various sources have claimed that sesame seeds were first used in China five thousand years ago, although recent archeological evidence shows a history of sesame cultivation in China for only seven hundred years.

Sesame has long been a subject of literature and legend. It was mentioned in ancient Mesopotamian cuneiform texts dating from 2400 BCE and was described in both the *Tebtunis Papyri*, dating from the second millennium BCE, and the *Medical Papyrus* from Thebes in 1552 BCE. Sesame seeds found buried in the tomb of King Tutankhamen date from around 1350 BCE. Xenophon, the Athenian philosopher and historian, documented sesame cultivation in Armenia by the fifth century BCE. In addition to using sesame oil ancient Egyptians ground sesame seeds for flour and early Romans ground the seeds with cumin to make a special paste to spread on bread. The famous Arabic expression "open sesame," from the medieval *One Thousand and One Nights* tale of "Ali Baba and the Forty Thieves," refers to the sesame pod's ability to suddenly split open, revealing a veritable treasure of seeds, a suggestion of abundance, money, and magic.

Sesame seeds have a distinctive nutty flavor and are utilized extensively in the cuisines of the Middle East and Asia. Tahini (ground sesame seeds) is widely used to make hummus and baba ghanoush, two popular Middle Eastern delicacies. Tahini also makes a tasty addition to sauces and salad dressings, can be drizzled on burgers or falafel dishes, and can be enjoyed as a "butter" to spread on bread. Whole sesame seeds are used to flavor and garnish various foods, especially breads and other baked goods. Halvah—made with crushed and sweetened sesame seeds—is a favorite Middle Eastern confection. Sesame seeds are often added to *daifuku*, a Japanese treat made with glutinous rice and bean paste. I have often enjoyed black sesame candy, a popular treat from Taiwan, Japan, and China that can be found in Asian supermarkets in Europe and North America.

Sesame also has a long history as a medicinal plant. Medieval Arabs applied sesame oil to the skin to treat burns and itching. They also used roasted sesame seeds combined with poppy or linseeds as a medicine to increase sperm production and sexual stamina. In addition to prescribing sesame oil to treat burns, twelfth-century Armenians used sesame as an anointing oil in Christian ceremonies.

Black sesame seeds have been part of Traditional Chinese Medicine since the 1600s, and are used in herbal preparations that treat liver and kidney problems. Sesame has been a part of India's Ayurvedic medical tradition, which dates back more than two thousand years, to treat diabetes, high cholesterol, skin problems, and arthritis.

Sesame seeds are rich in protein and contain a wide variety of nutrients including high amounts of copper, manganese, and calcium. They also contain vitamin B_1 (thiamin), magnesium, and zinc. When taken with traditional diabetes medications, sesame oil has been found to enhance effectiveness in regulating blood sugar. In addition to several antioxidants, sesame seeds and oil contain *sesamol*, a phytochemical with anti-inflammatory, antioxidant, antidepressant, and neuroprotective properties. It is believed to stop cell mutation, prevent liver damage, inhibit the aging process (especially regarding the formation of wrinkles due to prolonged and repeated UV exposure), and support the immune system in general. Other bioactive components present in sesame seeds have been found to exhibit therapeutic benefits including antioxidant activity, anticancer impacts, constipation protection, and anti-diabetes properties.

Since sesame seeds are not grown in North America, they are imported. The biggest global producer of sesame seeds is Sudan, followed by Myanmar, Tanzania, India, and Nigeria.

Resources

Bedigian, D. "History and Lore of Sesame in Southwest Asia." *Economic Botany* 58, 3) (2004): 329–353.

Gupta, Diksha, and Deepak Soni. "Sesame Seeds." Tata Img website. Updated August 29, 2022.

"Health Benefits of Sesame Seeds." WebMD. November 30, 2022.

"Hei Zhi Ma." Me&Qi.com. Accessed February 9, 2025.

Li, M., J. Luo, M. A. Nawaz et al. "Phytochemistry, Bioaccessibility, and Bioactivities of Sesame Seeds: An Overview." *Food Reviews International* 40, 1 (2024): 309–335.

Qiu, Z., Y. Zhang, D. Bedigian et al. "Sesame Utilization in China: New Archaeobotanical Evidence from Xinjiang." *Economic Botany* 66 (2012): 255–263.

"Sesame." *Encyclopaedia Brittanica.* Updated January 7, 2025.

Wikipedia. "Sesame." Accessed February 9, 2025.

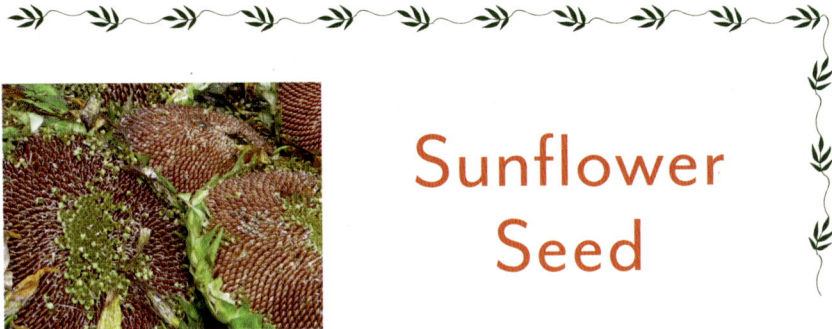

Sunflower Seed

The sunflower (*Helianthus annuus*), believed to be indigenous to the Western Plains of North America, has grown wild in many areas of the United States, Canada, and Mexico for millennia. They are believed to have been domesticated by Native Americans over five thousand years ago, with sunflower seeds being used as a foodstuff even before the cultivation of corn.

Sunflowers were also used as a medicinal crop and a source of dye, and sunflower oil was used for ceremonial body painting and applied to pottery (as greenware) help make it more water repellent. Among the Zuni people of what is now New Mexico, the fresh or dried root of the sunflower plant was chewed by traditional healers before sucking venom from a snakebite and applying a poultice of the chewed root to the wound. (This compound poultice of the root was applied with much ceremony in the case of rattlesnake bites.) Among other folk healers, various parts of the sunflower have been found efficient in traditional medicines to treat dysentery, cough, skin rashes, and diarrhea.

It is said that when wild sunflowers were tall and in bloom, they were a popular food for bison, which in turn improved the quality of their meat. Many other native peoples of the Americas considered the sunflower a sacred plant; the sunflower was a symbol of the solar deity of the Aztecs and the Otomi of what is now Mexico, as well as for the Incas of Peru and Bolivia.

Spanish explorers are believed to be the first Europeans to collect the sunflower in North America; by 1580, it had become a common garden flower in Spain. Early English and French explorers also brought sunflowers to their respective countries, and they were soon spread along established trade routes to Italy, Egypt, Afghanistan, Russia, India, and China.

Sunflowers became an important oilseed crop in Russia, which is now the world's largest producer of sunflowers (Ukraine ranks second). Sunflower cultivation is widespread throughout other parts of Europe and Asia, including Romania, Türkiye, and China. The United States ranks as the sixth-largest producer of sunflowers in the world, with Argentina being the largest producer in Latin America.

Before 1966, sunflower acreage in the United States was devoted primarily to non-oilseed varieties. The center of sunflower cultivation is believed to have originated in the American Southwest, or in the Mississippi or Missouri River valleys. European settlers began to cultivate sunflowers in the early 1800s as an easy-to-grow supplementary food. Later, sunflowers were planted as garden ornamentals. They were also grown to feed to farm animals in the late 1800s and early 1900s. Expanded world production of the sunflower resulted primarily from the development of high-oil varieties by plant scientists, and more recently by the development of hybrids.

Sunflower seeds are sold as a snack food both raw or roasted, with or without salt and/or seasonings added. Sunflower seeds can be processed into sunflower butter, a good alternative to peanut and other nut butters. They are also a popular ingredient in protein bars and trail mixes. Sunflower oil is commonly used as a healthy oil for cooking and salad dressings; sunflower seeds are sold as food for birds.

Sunflower seeds have a strong nutritional profile. They are high in protein, which supports immunity, and dietary fiber, which enhances the growth of friendly gut bacteria and promotes regularity. They are also a good source of vitamins E, B$_1$, and B$_6$, as well as minerals including iron, copper, selenium, manganese, zinc, magnesium, and potassium. In addition to supporting healthy bones and joints, and improving brain function, magnesium has been found to lower blood pressure. It also may have a positive effect on mood, and can reduce anxiety and depression. The chlorogenic acid found in sunflower seeds can help reduce blood sugar levels.

Sunflower seeds are rich in "healthy fats" that provide a number of health benefits including lowering the risk of developing diseases like high blood pressure and heart disease. Sunflower seeds contain phytosterols, which are closely related to heart health and have been shown to reduce levels of LDL ("bad") cholesterol; sunflower seeds have more phytosterols than any other seed. Sunflower seeds also have a high monounsaturated fat and omega-6 content, which are known for their inflammation fighting benefits. The vitamin E and selenium found in sunflower seeds have been linked to helping prevent colon cancer.

A recent article published in the journal *Food Science & Nutrition* focused on the nutritional and health properties of sunflowers:

> The health benefits of sunflower oil, meal, and other products are limitless, as they possess anticancer, antioxidant, antihypertensive, anti-inflammatory, hypocholesterolemic, skin-protective, analgesic, and antibacterial activities. Their effects on the muscles, blood vessels, and nerves are also known. Sunflower oil is also efficient in the treatment of colds, coughs, dysentery, constipation, and diseases like urinary, bronchial, pulmonary, and laryngeal infections. (Adeleke and Babalola 2020, 4675)

The main concern with eating sunflower seeds is that they are high in calories—especially when roasted in oil. Many people find them delicious and even somewhat addictive, which can lead to weight gain. This is why nutritionists recommend that consumption of sunflower seeds should not exceed one quarter cup (60 ml) a day. Added salt is a health concern as well, which can counter the seeds' natural blood pressure-reducing benefits. Nutritionists also recommend that sunflower seeds be eaten only without the shell in order to prevent possible bowel blockage when consumed in large amounts.

Resources

Adeleke, B. S., and O. O. Babalola. "Oilseed crop sunflower (*Helianthus annuus*) as a source of food: Nutritional and health benefits." *Food Science & Nutrition*8, 9 (2020): 4666-4684.

"Health Benefits of Sunflower Seeds." Nourish by WebMD. Reviewed October 15, 2024.

Netshiomvani, Takalani. "The 14 Amazing Health Benefits of Sunflower Seeds-Nutrition and How to Eat Them." *For Care Education and Research* (2022).

"Sunflower Production." North Dakota State University. NDSU Extension Service. 2007.

Wikipedia. "Common Sunflower." Accessed February 9, 2025.

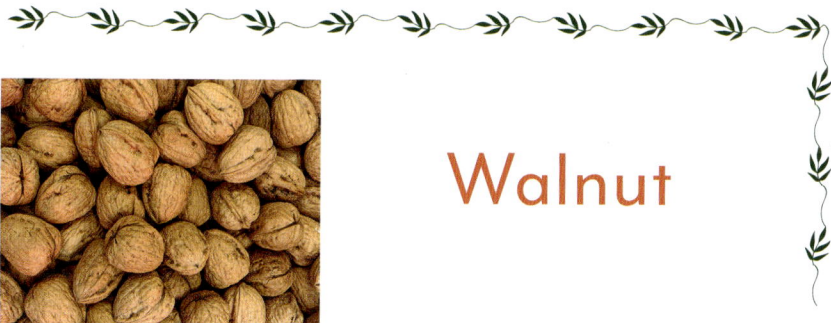

Walnut

Walnuts (Juglandaceae) are among the world's most popular tree nuts. Fossilized remains of the modern walnut's predecessors found in Central Europe date back over five million years. It is believed that birds, squirrels, and other small animals spread nuts to other parts of Europe.

Over millennia, the Juglandaceae family divided into walnuts and hickory nuts, of which the modern-day pecan is a descendent. As in Europe, birds, squirrels, and other rodents are credited with spreading these nuts to both North America and Asia. Later, human migration also facilitated the spread of nuts.

There are presently more than forty different species of walnuts, although the most cultivated—"English," "Persian," or "Common" walnut (*Juglands regia*)—is believed to have originated in Persia more than nine thousand years ago. Recent research has shown that the Persian walnut is the result of hybridization between two long-extinct species that occurred around 3.45 million years ago, making it one of humanity's most ancient foods. Fossilized remains of the ancestors of *Juglands regia* found in northeastern China date back 2.79 million years, to the late Pleistocene to Pliocene eras.

Persian walnuts were traded on the Silk Road that connected the Middle East to Asia, and also by British merchants in western Europe (hence the name "English" walnut). Commercial walnut cultivation in the United States began in 1867 near Santa Barbara, California, and eventually spread north to California's Central Valley, where most of America's walnuts are grown today.

Walnuts are usually eaten on their own as a healthy snack, but can also be added to salads, pasta dishes, breakfast cereals, soups, and baked goods. They are also used to make walnut oil, which is used in salad dressings and is usually expensive.

In addition to protein and dietary fiber, walnuts are a good source of omega-3 fatty acids and vitamin E. They are rich in antioxidants which help reduce "bad" LDL cholesterol levels. The monounsaturated and polyunsaturated fats in walnuts have been found to also lower LDL cholesterol levels, while their omega-3 fatty acids may reduce the risk of heart attack and stroke. Like other tree nuts, walnuts contain dietary fiber, which helps lower cholesterol and promotes the growth of healthy gut bacteria. Fiber also makes us feel full, so we eat less. Walnuts are a source of L-arginine, an amino acid that has been shown to lower blood pressure, improve cholesterol, and support blood vessel health.

Researchers at the Marshall University School of Medicine in West Virginia have identified several biochemicals—including n–3 (omega-3) fatty acids, tocopherols, beta-sitosterol, and pedunculagin—found in walnuts that have cancer preventative properties. Their research showed promise in slowing the proliferation of breast, prostate, kidney, and colon cancers. Other emerging research shows that walnuts may contribute to cancer prevention through several compounds working together—ellagitannins, melatonin, and gamma-tocopherol may each work through different paths to reduce oxidative stress, inflammation, and gene expression which, especially in combination, may lead to cancer. Because walnuts are usually eaten raw, nutritionists advise that they have greater antioxidant abilities than nuts which are eaten roasted.

Walnuts—known as *hu tao ren* in Traditional Chinese Medicine—are believed to strengthen the kidneys, lungs, and large intestines. Since the meat of the walnut resembles the two lobes of the human brain, traditional Chinese doctors consider walnuts an excellent "brain food." As mentioned earlier, walnuts, almonds, and hazelnuts have long been a part of traditional Persian medicine, and have been prescribed to improve brain function.

A 2017 article published in the peer-reviewed journal *Pharmacological Research* highlighted the neuroprotective properties of walnuts—along with almonds and hazelnuts—and their potential to help prevent and even treat symptoms of Alzheimer's disease (AD) by providing macronutrients, micronutrients, and phytochemicals which affect several pathways in AD pathogenesis (the process by which the disease develops). The authors conclude, "Beyond the molecular activities attributed to the phytochemicals, the use of these tree nuts could be more considered in scientific researches as the effective nutrients for prevention or even management of AD. (Gorji et al. 2018, 115)"

After studying dozens of research papers, the authors of an article published in *Current Pharmaceutical Design* singled out walnuts as the best potential nut to be used in an alternative therapy to help treat memory loss:

> A number of scientific studies have demonstrated their [referring to nuts] actions against inflammation, oxidative damage, the aging process, as well as dementia or memory loss. However, only walnuts, followed by almonds, hazelnuts, and pistachios, have shown promising results in empirical studies for memory improvements. (Arslan et al. 2020, 4712)

The United States is the world's second largest producer of walnuts after China, followed by Chile, Ukraine, and France. In addition to domestic consumption in the United States, walnuts are a major agricultural export, primarily to Germany, Turkey, China Japan, and Spain.

Resources.

Arslan, J., A.U. Gilani, H. Jamshed et al. "Edible Nuts for Memory." *Current Pharmaceutical Design* 26, 37 (2020): 4712–4720.

"California Walnuts: Today, Tomorrow and Years to Come." California Walnut Board. January 23, 2018.

Feng, Xiaojia, H. Zhou, S. Zulfiqar et al. "The Phytogeographic History of Common Walnut in China." *Frontiers in Plant Science* 9 (2018): 1399.

Frei, Jonas. "A Brief History of Juglandaceae." *Arnoldia* 78, no. 3. (2021).

Gorji, N., R. Moeini, and Z. Memariani. "Almond, hazelnut and walnut, three nuts for neuroprotection in Alzheimer's disease: A neuropharmacological review of their bioactive constituents." *Pharmacological Research* 129 (2018): 115.

Hardman, W. E. "Walnuts have potential for cancer prevention and treatment in mice." *The Journal of Nutrition* 144, 4 (2014): 555S–560S.

Kitzerow, Rebecca M. H. "Walnuts and Your Brain—A Chinese Medicine Superfood." *Always Well.* December 19, 2018.

"Nuts and your heart: Eating nuts for heart health," Mayo Clinic. Accessed August 8, 2023. "Walnuts: Support a Cancer-Preventive Diet." American Institute for Cancer Research website. Accessed July 15, 2023.

Zhang, Bo-Wen, Lin-Lin Xu, Nan Li et al. "Phylogenomics reveals an ancient hybrid origin of the Persian walnut." *Molecular Biology and Evolution* 36, no. 11 (2019): 2451–61.

Other Foods

This section includes plant foods that do not easily fit into the previous food categories in this book, based on the ways they are normally consumed. For example: although coffee comes from a tree and its beans can be botanically classified as "seeds," roasted coffee beans are used primarily as a beverage and not something you would add to trail mix, like sunflower or pumpkin seeds.

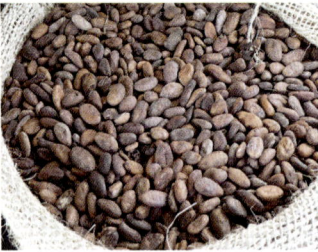

Chocolate

Chocolate has been called "the best-known food that nobody knows anything about." When most of us think of chocolate, a tasty candy bar pops into mind, likely from Hershey in Pennsylvania, or from producers in Switzerland or Belgium. Yet, like many other foods, the history of chocolate has deep roots that go back thousands of years, to one of the world's most ancient civilizations.

Chocolate is made from the fruit of the cacao tree (*Theobroma cacao*), which is indigenous to Mexico and Central America. The fruits are called *pods*, and each pod contains around forty cacao beans. The beans are then dried and roasted before processing.

The origin of chocolate has been traced to the Olmecs, who lived in what are now the Mexican states of Tabasco and Veracruz. Archeologists believe the Olmecs used cacao beans ground into a bitter tasting ceremonial drink beginning in about 1500 BCE. The use of cacao as a sacred drink used for rituals of birth, marriage, and death eventually spread to the Maya and Aztecs, who believed the cacao bean had magical properties. In Aztec culture, cacao beans were considered more valuable than gold, and were reserved for royalty. Emperor Moctezuma II drank the beverage regularly, which was often flavored with chili peppers and spices. The word "chocolate" is derived from the Aztec Nahuatl word *xocolatl*.

Chocolate is believed to have been introduced to Europe by either Christopher Columbus or Hernán Cortés, whose army overthrew the Aztec Empire in 1521. Chocolate soon became a popular drink in Spain, France, and Italy, with the bitter flavor offset with sugar, cinnamon, and other seasonings. The Spanish introduced chocolate to Florida in 1641, and the first chocolate house in America opened in Boston by 1683. By the time of the Boston Tea Party, in 1773, cacao beans had become a major import. According to botanist Alphonse de Candolle, the Spanish also brought cacao beans from Acapulco to the Philippines in both 1674 and 1680, "where it succeeded wonderfully."

Powdered cocoa was invented by the Dutch chemist Conrad van Houton in 1828, which later evolved into what is now called "Dutch cocoa." To make cocoa powder—which is used to make chocolate— cacao beans are fermented, dried, roasted, crushed and ground. When compared to unsweetened cocoa powder, unsweetened cacao nibs are higher in calories, fat and protein, but lower in carbohydrates, fiber and iron. Generally speaking, cacao products are good sources of selenium, magnesium, chromium and manganese. Plus, the darker the chocolate, the higher the cacao content, and the higher the mineral content.

In 1847 the first chocolate bar was developed in England by molding a paste made of sugar, chocolate liquor, and cocoa butter. Milk chocolate was created by mixing powdered cacao with powdered milk and sugar, by Daniel Peter in Switzerland in 1876. But milk chocolate didn't become popular until Peter and his friend Henri Nestlé started the Nestlé Company, which brought milk chocolate to the mass market several years later. In 1879, Swiss chocolatier Rudolf Lindt invented a machine to aerate chocolate, giving it a smooth, easy-to-eat consistency.

While chocolate ranks as one of humanity's most decadent treats, dark chocolate has been praised by nutritionists for its health benefits due to its high concentration of cacao solids, made from cacao beans that are rich in antioxidants including flavonols and polyphenols. Because dark chocolate contains less sugar and fat than milk chocolate or white chocolate, it provides higher amounts of cacao solids: dark chocolate has between 50 and 90 percent cacao solids, while milk chocolate contains 10 to 50 percent. Flavonols in chocolate have been found to improve blood circulation and lower blood pressure, and are also considered beneficial in fighting cell damage due to aging. They may even offer protection from the sun's ultraviolet rays. Polyphenols have been found to reduce cortisol levels, a stress hormone. They also have mood-enhancing properties. On top of these benefits, dark chocolate is also a good source of essential minerals including iron, magnesium, phosphorous, copper, and zinc.

Chocolate is an extremely popular food, mostly enjoyed as candy bars and other chocolate treats. It is also used as a flavoring for smoothies and other blended drinks, as well as ice cream and pastry. Cocoa remains a popular drink whether served hot or cold.

Yet, as the demand for chocolate increases, the expansion of cacao plantations has destroyed rainforests, especially in western Africa. Both chocolate companies and consumers are searching out fair-traded cacao that not only provides farmworkers with adequate wages but helps protect the environment as well. Fair trade ensures that producers have the tools to cope with changes in the environment—including climate, severe weather, and pestsand evolve more sustainable production models.

Cacao beans are cultivated in fifty-six countries around the world. The major cacao producing countries are the Ivory Coast, Ghana, Indonesia, Nigeria, Cameroon, Brazil, and Ecuador. The United States is a major importer of both cacao beans and processed chocolate: Americans eat 2.8 billion pounds of chocolate each year. However, per capita chocolate consumption in the United States pales in comparison to that of some European countries. The Swiss consume some 8.8 kilograms (twenty-two pounds) of chocolate per person a year, while the Austrians place second, with some 8.1 kg (twenty pounds) each year. In the United States, per capita yearly consumption is only 4.5 kilograms (ten pounds) a year. The Chinese rank among the world's lowest chocolate consumers, with per capita annual consumption of only 0.10 kg, less than a single four-ounce chocolate bar a year.

Resources

Cleveland Clinic. "Dark Chocolate Health Benefits." healthessentials. March 10, 2022.

"Cocoa Producing Countries 2023." World Population Review website. 2023.

de Candolle, Alphonse. *Origin of Cultivated Plants*. New York: D. Appleton and Company, 1908, 314.

Fiegl, Amanda. "The History of Chocolate." *Smithsonian Magazine*. March 1, 2008.

"History of Chocolate." History.com. August 10, 2022.

"Which country eats the most chocolate in 2024?" World Population Review website. 2024.

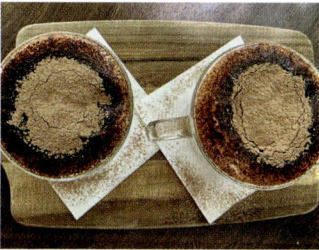

Coffee

I drank my first cup of coffee as a sixteen-year-old exchange student in Bogotá, Colombia. At home, my parents called it a drink "for adults" and hadn't allowed my brother and me to have more than an occasional sip. I was surprised that my Colombian host family served coffee to their teenage children at every meal. Drinking my first small cup of steaming *tinto* (rich, black coffee) was a rite of passage that I will always remember.

Darkly colored, bitter, and slightly acidic, coffee is a stimulant primarily due to its caffeine content (1,3,7-trimethylxanthine is the chemical name for caffeine). Available in more than two thousand varieties and served in myriad ways, coffee has become the most popular hot beverage in the world. It has even become the number one hot beverage in Taiwan and Japan, both known for their ancient tea drinking traditions. Coffee is also very popular in China, especially in the large cities. The Shanghai International Coffee Culture Festival recorded 9,553 coffee shops in Shanghai at the end of 2023, the highest number of coffee shops in any city in the world.

There are two major coffee varieties: Arabica and Robusta. Arabica coffee beans are richer in aromatic substances, along with hints of various types of fruit. Robusta coffee has a more "earthy" flavor that can be very bitter. Robusta beans are generally cheaper than Arabica beans, and are mainly grown in the lowlands of Brazil and Vietnam, while Arabica beans are grown primarily in the highlands of Colombia, Central

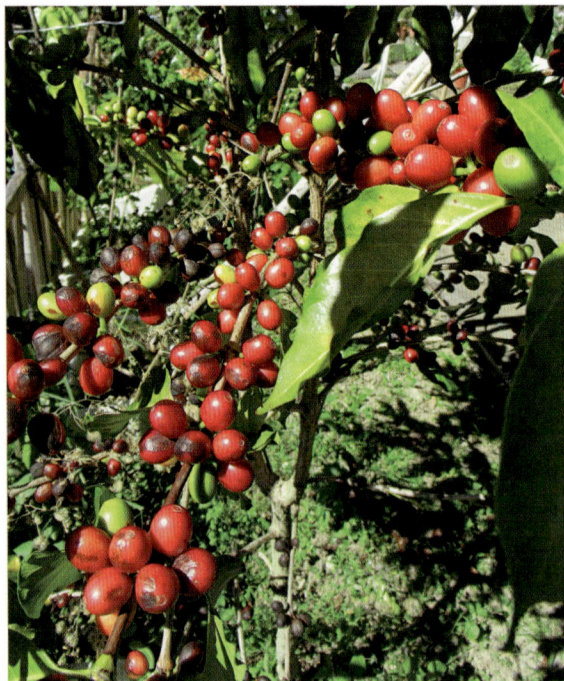

Berries on a coffee plant.

America, Africa, and Indonesia. Like wine, the quality and flavor of coffee depends on the terroir in which the coffee plants are grown, such as soil, climate, rainfall, sun exposure, and temperature. Quality also depends on how the beans are harvested, stored, and roasted.

Like most people, I believed that coffee originated in either Colombia or Brazil—two of the world's largest exporters of coffee beans. But recent studies have found that the coffee plant originated in the highlands of Ethiopia, where some of the world's finest coffees are grown today, including the Sidamo, Harrar, and Yirgacheffe varieties. According to legend, the coffee plant was discovered by a goat herder named Kaldi around 850 CE, who observed increased physical activity in his goats after they consumed raw coffee beans from the tree.

It appears that coffee plants were taken across the Red Sea to what is now Yemen during the fourteenth century, and cultivated there. Sufi monks were among the first to brew coffee as a stimulating beverage to help them to pray through the night.

Although first prohibited by Muslim clerics due to its properties as a stimulant, coffee eventually became a favorite drink among Arabs, primarily men. The Ottoman Empire introduced coffee throughout the European continent during the 1500s. It is said that Pope Clement VIII (1536–1605) forbade consumption of what his advisors called "Satan's drink" until he tried it himself. He is reported to have said, "Why, this Satan's drink is so delicious that it would be a pity to let the infidels have exclusive use of it." By the end of the seventeenth century, coffee consumption was flourishing throughout much of Europe.

Coffee has a long history as a beverage to share with friends. The first coffeehouses appeared in Mecca during the 1600s, and in Constantinople (now Istanbul) in the 1700s. These coffeehouses became popular gathering places for men to enjoy social activities that included conversation with friends, smoking, listening to music, and playing board games. Coffeehouses soon began to thrive in European cities like Budapest, Vienna, Rome, Berlin, London, and Paris, and coffeehouse culture later spread throughout the world. Although coffeehouses have existed in the United States since the 1800s, the most recent trend began in 1966, when Alfred Peet, known as the "godfather of gourmet coffee" opened Peet's Coffee and Tea near the University of California campus in Berkeley. Originally a source of packaged coffee and tea, his store grew into a chain of gourmet coffeehouses. Starbucks soon followed, and world "coffee culture" changed forever.

Although they grew coffee in limited amounts, Yemen was the world's main producer of coffee throughout the seventeenth century, until cultivation spread to the Dutch East Indies, now known as Indonesia, in 1690. In 1714, the mayor of Amsterdam presented a gift of a coffee seedling to King Louis XV of France, who had it planted in the *Jardin royal des plantes médicinales* (the Royal Garden of Medicinal Plants) in Paris.

In 1723, a young naval officer named Gabriel de Clieu obtained a seedling from the King's plant and transported it to the French island of Martinique in the Caribbean. The coffee seedling soon multiplied, and is credited with the spread of over 18 million coffee plants on Martinique over the next fifty years. This seedling is believed to be the ancestor of all the coffee trees that have been planted throughout the Caribbean and Central and South America—mostly in Brazil and Colombia—beginning in the eighteenth century. Coffee cultivation was established in the Kingdom of Hawai'i in 1825, and its premium-grade Kona coffee is still grown there today.

Today coffee is cultivated throughout the moist subtropics and high-altitude regions of the world, including Africa, Asia, and Latin America. During the late nineteenth and early twentieth centuries, machines were invented to grind and roast coffee beans on a commercial scale, and methods to remove the caffeine from green beans were introduced.

As a hot drink, coffee is brewed from the roasted and ground seeds (or beans) of the plant. Coffee can be prepared in a variety of ways, including espresso, French press, pour over or drip, or by using a filter or coffee bag. Many coffee drinkers prefer their brew black (with or without sweetener), or coffee can be enjoyed with milk, cream, or non-dairy creamer, and made into drinks such as caffè latte, cappuccino, or Frappuccino (a trademarked beverage available at Starbucks). Many cold prepared coffee drinks are high in fat, sugar, and calories, and often include whipped cream and flavorings like caramel and mocha. Canned coffee—both hot and cold—is sold in vending machines throughout Japan, and canned or bottled varieties are becoming popular in North America as well. Coffee is also used to flavor candies, liquors, and pastries.

Although many believe that coffee is unhealthy, recent medical and nutritional research has found that coffee is actually a healthy drink when consumed in moderation. Nutritionists at the Johns Hopkins University School of Medicine point out that, in addition to caffeine, coffee contains a variety of antioxidants and other phytochemicals that can reduce the possibility of premature death from heart disease, stroke, type 2 diabetes, and kidney disease, especially among women. Studies have also found that drinking coffee on a regular basis can strengthen the body's DNA and support liver function while decreasing the risk of developing Alzheimer's disease, colorectal cancer, heart failure, stroke, and Parkinson's disease.

However, nutritionists suggest that consuming coffee with sugar, cream, or chemical flavorings like caramel and mocha substantially add unwanted calories from sugar and fat, and reduce the health benefits of coffee. They recommend drinking coffee black or with low-fat creamer and little or no sweetening.

Finally, coffee contains caffeine. The positive aspects of caffeine include better mental focus and alertness, while negatives can include nervousness, anxiety, and insomnia. For this reason, nutritionists generally suggest drinking caffeinated drinks like coffee in moderation.

Resources

de Candolle, Alphonse. *Origin of Cultivated Plants*. New York: D. Appleton and Company, 1908, 416-17.

Francis, John K. "Coffea arabica L. Rubiaceae." Factsheet of U.S. Department of Agriculture, Forest Service. August 2007.

"History of coffee." *Wikipedia*. Accessed February 9, 2025.

McDonnell, Stephen. "City of cafes: Shanghai's love affair with coffee." BBC. July 30, 2024.

Myhrvold, Nathan. "History of Coffee." *Encyclopaedia Britannica*. September 22, 2023.

"9 Reasons Why (the Proper Amount) of Coffee Is Good for You." Johns Hopkins Medicine website.

"The History of Coffee." National Coffee Association website. Accessed September 28, 2023.

Travisan, Andrea. "What are the factors that affect coffee quality?" *Eureka Blog*. Accessed September 28, 2023.

Wikipedia. "Pope Clement VIII." Accessed September 28, 2023.

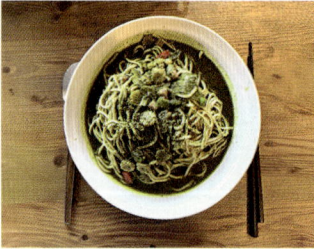

Pasta

Pasta's earliest roots have been traced to ancient China during the Shang Dynasty (1600–1045 BCE), where pasta was made from either wheat or rice flour. A popular myth states that Italian merchant explorer Marco Polo discovered pasta during his travels to China in the thirteenth century, although pasta appeared in ancient Greece during the first millennium BCE. It also appears that Africa had its own form of pasta at that time, made with *kamut*, also known as Khorasan wheat.

The works of the Greek physician Galen during the second century CE mention *itrion*, a homogeneous compound of flour and water used to create a type of boiled dough. The *Jerusalem Talmud* records that *itrium* was a popular food in Palestine from the third to fifth centuries CE. In what is now Italy, the existence of pasta can be traced to the Etruscan civilization, which flourished in the regions we now call Lazio, Umbria, and Tuscany in the fourth century BCE. During the first century CE, the Roman poet Horace mentioned a food called *lagana*, which consisted of fine sheets of dough—believed to be an ancestor of modern-day lasagna.

The Italian people have long been celebrated for their creativity and innovation, and, like much of Italian culture, pasta was a culinary art form that flourished during the Renaissance. By the fourteenth century, pasta had become a staple food in Rome and Florence. In later centuries, many different types of pasta became available in dried forms, which made it more accessible to the general public. Before the introduction of tomatoes to what is now Italy in the sixteenth century, pasta was accompanied by traditional ingredients still popular today: oil and garlic, ricotta cheese, or a paste made of fresh herbs (pesto). Yet, thanks in part to the arrival of tomatoes, pasta—along with many varieties of tomato sauce—has become synonymous with Italian cuisine today.

Historians have credited Thomas Jefferson with popularizing pasta in the United States. During an extended stay in Paris from 1784–1789, Jefferson ate what he called "macaroni" and liked it so much be brought back several cases of the pasta to Virginia. He reportedly asked a friend to bring back more pasta from Naples when his supply ran out.

During the late nineteenth and early twentieth centuries, more than four million Italian immigrants—mostly from central and southern Italy—settled in the United States. Their culinary traditions arrived with them, and pasta soon became a popular food enjoyed by people of many ethnicities. Italian-style pasta is available in many different forms, including spaghetti, fusilli, lasagna, ravioli, rigatoni, orzo, farfalle, and capellini. Traditional Italian pasta is made with two simple ingredients: wheat flour and water. As culinary customs have become more sophisticated, Italian-style pasta can now be made from other dried ingredients, including whole wheat, lentils, spinach, tomatoes, buckwheat, corn, or rice.

Noodles (made primarily with wheat or rice) have remained one of the most beloved foods in China, and are enjoyed in Chinese homes and restaurants throughout the world. Chinese cuisines offer dozens of types of noodles that vary according to their region of origin. Visitors to China, Hong Kong, Taiwan, and Singapore can often see chefs making fresh noodles by hand in restaurant windows and at traditional markets. In Japan, the most famous noodles include soba, ramen, and udon, which have also found their way into a variety of other Asian cuisines.

Instant noodles—mostly in the form of ramen from Japan, China, and Korea—are among the world's most popular fast foods. Adapted from traditional Chinese Yi noodle soup, instant ramen was developed by Taiwan-born Momofuku Andō, of Japan's Nissin Foods, in 1971. Instant noodles have since become one of the most ubiquitous fast foods on the planet, with over one hundred billion servings consumed annually. According to 2023 data provided by the World Instant Noodles Association (yes, there actually is such a group), people living in China and Hong Kong consume over forty-five billion servings a year, followed by Indonesia (14.26 billion), and Vietnam (8.48 billion servings). The United States ranked sixth, with Americans consuming just over 5.15 billion servings of instant noodles a year.

Many different types of pasta (whether instant or otherwise) are enjoyed all over the world. In fact, a global survey by the charity Oxfam has named pasta as the world's most popular dish ahead of meat, rice, and pizza.

Resources

Avery, Tory. "Uncover the History of Pasta." The History Kitchen. Public Broadcasting System website. July 26, 2012.

Buckley, Julia. "How this fruit became the star of Italian cooking." CNN Travel. March 20, 2021. Accessed April 14, 2025.

"Global Demand of Instant Noodles, Top 15." Instantnoodles.org. World Instant Noodles Association. Accessed September 5, 2023.

"History of Pasta: Wheat + Water + Patience." DeLallo.com. Accessed September 5, 2023.

"How Pasta Became the World's Favourite Food." BBC.com. June 11, 2011.

Santonastaso, Timothy. "A Brief History of Pasta." *Italics Magazine*. May 29, 2020.

Wikipedia. "Instant Noodles," Accessed September 5, 2023.

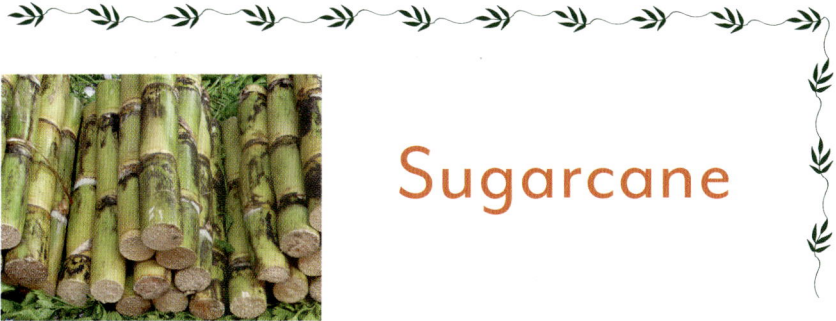

Sugarcane

Sugar is humanity's oldest known sweetener (aside from honey), and has been eaten alone or as an ingredient in a wide variety of beverages and other foods for thousands of years. Sugar traditionally comes from sugarcane (*Saccharum officinarum*), a high-yielding tropical grass whose cultivation dates back to India some three to four thousand years. The origin of the word "sugar" is from the Sanskrit term शर्करा (*śarkarā*), meaning ground or candied sugar.

From India, sugarcane cultivation spread west through the Khyber Pass in Afghanistan, and soldiers of Alexander the Great's army are known to have carried it with them to Europe from India after military campaigns in 325 BCE. Sugarcane also spread east to Southeast Asia, the Indonesian Archipelago, and New Guinea. As with many other plants, the gradual spread of sugarcane over the millennia led to several new species, especially in India and China.

Our ancestors initially chewed pieces of sugarcane stalk to extract its sweet juice. Many people who live in tropical countries continue this practice today, as it is an easy, packaged form of energy food that is available at little or no cost (sugarcane often grows wild by the roadside, and is also easily available in traditional markets throughout the tropics).

By 400 BCE, rudimentary methods for manufacturing granular sugar from sugarcane were developed in India, and Nestorian Christian monks living near the Euphrates River are believed to have refined raw sugarcane into a form of "white" sugar around 450 CE. The sugar industry in the Mediterranean region of Europe began at the time of the Arabian conquest of Egypt in 640 CE, and Arab traders introduced sugar across North Africa and into Spain by 750 CE. Christopher Columbus is believed to have brought sugarcane to the Caribbean and other parts of the Americas in the 1490s, while the Portuguese introduced sugarcane to western Africa and Brazil.

The demand for sugar was especially high in Europe. It was first used to sweeten tea, but soon became an important ingredient in chocolate and other sweets. In addition to its cultivation in Southeast Asia (especially southern China and Taiwan), sugarcane became an important crop in Brazil, Cuba, and what is now the southern United States, where the slave trade provided cheap labor, and sugarcane became a major source of income for plantation owners. Although sugarcane is no longer an important crop in the United States, it is still grown commercially in Louisiana, Florida, and Texas. The last sugar mill in Hawai'i closed in 2016. Brazil remains the biggest producer of sugarcane in the world, followed by India, China, and Thailand.

Although sugar from sugarcane remains popular today, sugars from other sources are often added to our food. In addition to sugar from certain varieties of beets, other sources of sugar include honey, molasses, maple syrup, and fruit juice concentrates. But the cheapest and most widely used sugar in American diets comes from high-fructose corn syrup, which is added to nearly every processed food imaginable: baby food, breakfast cereals, canned vegetables and sauces, breads and pastries, and candy and other sweets. The American Heart Association (AHA) notes that 47 percent of the added sugar in American diets are found in soft drinks, fruit drinks and juices, sports and energy drinks, and in commercially prepared coffee and tea. Snacks and candy provide an additional 31 percent of the added sugar that Americans consume every year. Per capita annual consumption of refined sugar in the United States is a stunning sixty-nine pounds.

Consuming large amounts of sugar can raise blood glucose levels, which can lead to a wide variety of health problems including obesity, diabetes, heart disease, colon cancer, high blood pressure, high cholesterol, kidney disease, liver disease, and even an increased risk of dementia.

Sugar provides carbohydrates—the fuel that provides the body with energy. The body breaks down foods containing carbohydrates into glucose, which can then enter the bloodstream. While it is true that a certain amount of glucose is necessary for the brain, central nervous system, and red blood cells to function properly, the AHA suggests that these needs can be met without adding sugar to our foods. Naturally occurring sugars are found in fruits, vegetables, legumes, nuts, and seeds, which also supply dietary fiber, vitamins, minerals, and healthy phytochemicals (unlike sugar).

Resources

Brumbly, Stevens M. et al. "Sugarcane." *Compendium of Transgenic Crop Plants* (2008).

Iowa State University. "Sugarcane Profile." Agricultural Marketing Resource Center website. April 2022.

Sissons, Beth. "Does the Body Need Sugar? How Much to Consume." Medical News Today website. March 30, 2021.

Wikipedia. "History of Sugar." Accessed December 1, 2023.

Wikipedia. "Sugar." Accessed December 1, 2023.

"World Sugarcane Production by Country." AtlasBig.com. Accessed December 1, 2023.

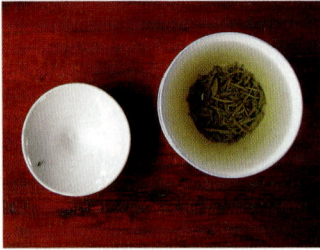

Tea

Tea (*Camellia sinensis*) is believed to be the most popular drink in the world after water and coffee. According to a Chinese legend dating from 2737 BCE, the emperor Shen Nung was sitting near a bush while his servant was boiling his drinking water, and some leaves from the bush fell into the water. The Emperor, who was also an herbalist, decided to try the infusion that his servant had accidentally created. The hot drink that resulted is now known as tea. Whether the story is true or not, the practice of using the leaves from *Camellia sinensis* to make a medicinal drink has ancient origins, and the plant began to be cultivated in China during the third century CE.

Containers for tea have been found in tombs dating from the Han dynasty (206 BCE–220 CE), and the first published account of tea cultivation, processing, and drinking appeared in 350 CE. During the Tang dynasty (618–906 CE), tea became firmly established in China, and the first book entirely devoted to tea, the *Ch'a Ching*, or "Tea Classic," was written by Lu Yu during the eighth century CE.

The first seeds for tea-producing plants were brought to Japan during the ninth century CE by Japanese Buddhist monks who had gone to China to study. As in China, tea drinking soon became an important part of Japanese culture, and cultivation spread through much of Japan by the 1200s. The well-known Japanese tea ceremony is said to have had its roots in the rituals first described in the *Ch'a Ching*.

The Dutch are believed to have brought the first consignment of Chinese tea to Europe in 1610. They also likely introduced tea to

Formosa (now Taiwan) in the early 1600s, but cultivation wasn't successful until Chinese settlers from Fujian brought tea plants to northern Formosa in 1810. Tea cultivation on the Indonesian island of Java was begun by the Dutch, who brought seeds and growing implements from Japan between 1826 and 1833. At around the same time, tea plants were found growing near the border between today's Myanmar and what is now the Indian state of Assam. The British are credited with having introduced both tea cultivation and tea culture to what is now India in 1836 and to Ceylon (Sri Lanka) in 1867.

By the early nineteenth century, tea drinking became popular in Europe—especially in Great Britain, where the British popularized the concept of afternoon tea, a daily practice in which tea is served along with sandwiches and pastry. Until the 1850s, most of the tea imported to Britain came from China, although cheaper tea from Ceylon became available during that time. As tea became more

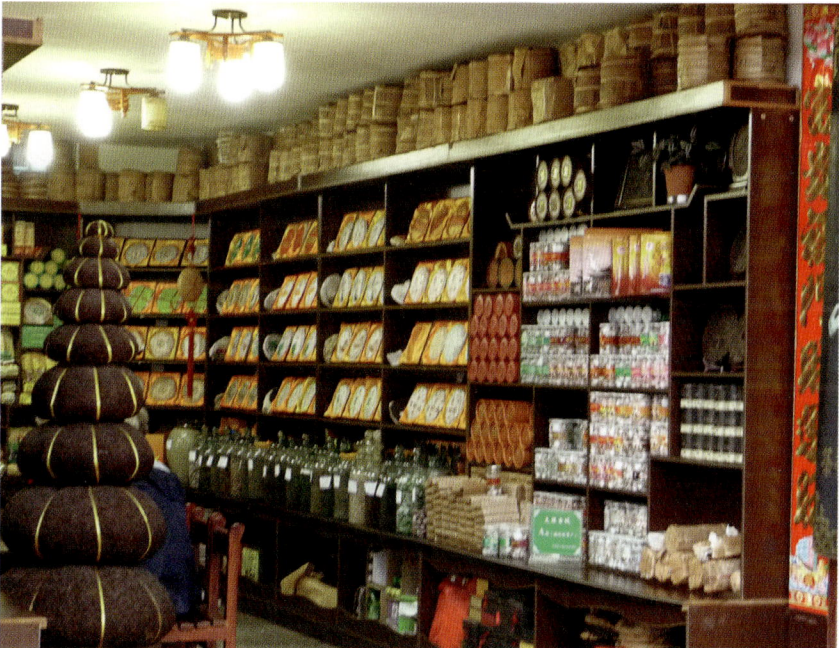

A tea shop showing numerous varieties of tea.

affordable, tea consumption increased markedly. Tea remains extremely popular in the United Kingdom, where more than 88 million cups of tea are consumed daily.

Tea drinking was as popular in the American colonies as in England, and all tea was required by the British government to be imported through Britain. The Boston Tea Party, a protest against the 1773 Tea Tax (three pence per pound) imposed by the British government on tea exports to America, sparked the Revolutionary War. The United States is the largest tea importer in the world today.

While hundreds of varieties of tea are currently enjoyed both hot and iced, the main types include *green tea*, whose leaves and buds have not undergone the withering and oxidation process used to produce black teas and oolong teas; *black tea*, a strong-tasting fermented tea popular in the West; *white tea*, which can be one of several styles that generally feature young or minimally processed leaves; and *oolong tea*. The degree of oxidation of oolong tea lies between green tea (not oxidized) and black tea (fully oxidized). The oxidation process gives oolong tea more flavor than green tea but milder than black tea, which is usually consumed with milk and sugar. Bottled iced tea has become widely available in supermarkets and convenience stores, although many tea drinkers save money by brewing tea at home to serve chilled, adding sweetener and flavorings if desired.

Bubble tea is a popular drink that has swept the world. Developed in Taiwan during the 1980s, it can be of the green, black, or oolong varieties. It almost always contains tapioca, a type of starch extracted from the cassava root, which is indigenous to South America. The tapioca in bubble tea is in the form of pearls, or "bubbles," which give this tasty cold drink its name. Bubble tea is often made with added sugar, syrups, and milk. Although a popular treat, it is not anywhere near as healthy as plain, brewed green, black, or oolong teas.

The flavor of tea varies by where the tea leaves are harvested and how they are grown and processed. Black tea is the most popular tea worldwide, followed by green, oolong, and white tea, respectively. The world's major producers of tea include China, India, Sri Lanka, and Kenya.

Tea is considered a healthy drink. Both green and black tea contains a variety of antioxidants including polyphenols, which inhibit free-radical damage to body cells. Black tea contains theaflavins and thearubigins, which are antioxidant polyphenols that help alleviate high cholesterol; they also have been found to lower the risk of high blood sugar. Drinking two to three cups of green or black tea daily has been associated with a reduced risk of premature death in general and a lower risk of heart disease, stroke, type 2 diabetes, and cancer in particular.

A peer-reviewed article appearing in a recent issue of *Food Chemistry* summarizes the phytochemicals in tea and their health-giving properties:

> The promising health recompenses of tea have been linked to its different phenolic components, which have diverse biological characteristics. Tea also contains several flavonoids, alkaloids, phenolic, theanine, etc., which are associated with antioxidant characteristics and a variety of health benefits. It can also lower the pervasiveness of neurological disorders as well as prevent different types of cancer, metabolic syndromes, cardiovascular diseases, urinary stones, obesity, and type 2 diabetes. (Bag et al. 2022, 131098)

The authors added that, because tea helps to improve health and prevents many diseases, its consumption has been regarded by medical researchers as a "health-promoting habit" that is both clinically and scientifically based.

Green, black, white, and oolong teas contain caffeine. As mentioned earlier, positive aspects of caffeine include better mental focus and alertness, while negatives can include nervousness, anxiety, and insomnia. For this reason, nutritionists generally suggest drinking caffeinated drinks like tea in moderation, and no later than four to six hours before bedtime. While decaffeinated teas won't keep you awake at night, they do not contain the antioxidant levels that caffeinated teas provide.

Resources

Altman, Nathaniel. *Taiwan: Fifty Things You Didn't Know.* Brooklyn: Gaupo Publishing, 2024, 139-40, 146.

"Are There Health Benefits to Drinking Tea?" WebMD. November 10, 2022.

Bag, S., A. Mondal, A. Majumder, A. Banik. "Tea and its phytochemicals: Hidden health benefits & modulation of signaling cascade by phyto-chemicals." *Food Chemistry* 371, no. 1 (2022):131098.

"History of Tea." UK Tea & Infusions Association website. Accessed March 28, 2024.

Peluso, I., and M. Serafini. "Antioxidants from black and green tea: from dietary modulation of oxidative stress to pharmacological mecha-nisms." *British Journal of Pharmacology* 174, 11 (2017): 1195–1208.

Sivasubramaniam, Sinnathurai. "tea." *Encyclopaedia Britannica.* September 19, 2023.

"Tea." The Nutrition Source. Harvard T.H. Chan School of Public Health. April 2023.

Index